Instrumental Methods of Drug Analysis

Instrumental Methods of Drug Analysis

Prof. Dr. G. Vidya Sagar

Principal, Veerayatan Institute of Pharmacy,
Jakhania, Mandvi-Kutch, Gujarat

and

Dean, Faculty of Pharmaceutical Sciences,
KSKV Kachchh University,
Bhuj-Kutch, Gujarat

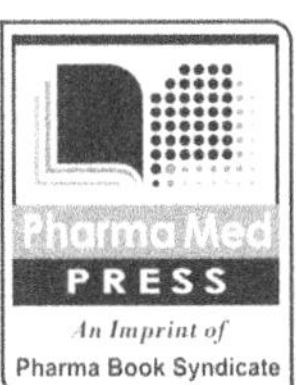

PharmaMed Press

An imprint of Pharma Book Syndicate

A unit of BSP Books Pvt. Ltd.

4-4-309/316, Giriraj Lane,
Sultan Bazar, Hyderabad - 500 095.

Published by :

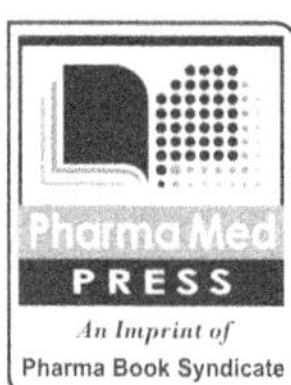

PharmaMed Press
An imprint of Pharma Book Syndicate

A unit of BSP Books Pvt. Ltd.

4-4-309/316, Giriraj Lane, Sultan Bazar, Hyderabad - 500 095.
Phone: 040-23445605, 23445688; Fax: 91+40-23445611
E-mail: info@pharmamedpress.com

ISBN : 978-93-52300-60-0 (HB)

Dedicated to My Parents

Late Shri G. C. Naidu and Smt. G. Lalitha
and all my teachers
who brought me to this stage.

"I never did anything worth doing by accident nor did any of my inventions came by accidents, they came by hard work".

- Thomas Alva Edison

Gujarat Technological University
Ahmedabad, Gujarat

Shri Manish Bharadwaj, I A S
Vice-Chancellor

Foreword

Pharmaceutical Analysis is an important branch of Pharmaceutical Sciences which deals with the various traditional, Physico-Chemical and modern analytical methods, utilizing qualitative and quantitative estimation of drugs and Pharmaceuticals, are performed. The Pharmaceutical technologist should know at every stage of the production process that both the qualitative and the quantitative composition of the Pharmaceutical materials undergoing conversion. In a Pharmaceutical Industry, no material is taken into production or released without analytical data, which characterizes its quality and stability for various purposes. These results not only form the basis of all the processing calculations but they also determine the costs of the materials which form the basis of financial estimates.

The textbook 'Instrumental Methods of Drug Analysis' by Prof. Dr. G. Vidya Sagar has been written to suit the needs of undergraduates of Pharmacy and Analytical Sciences. The book gives a lucid exposition of various modern analytical techniques like Infrared Spectroscopy, Flourimetry, Chromatographic techniques like HPLC, HPTLC and Gas Chromatography. Some of the difficult topics like NMR and Mass Spectroscopy are explained in a simple terminology. This textbook covers the syllabus of Pharmaceutical Analysis of many Indian Universities offering B.Pharm.

The textual presentation is explicit and the language simple. I am sure that this book will meet the didactic needs of the students in the subject and will find better acceptance by the teachers of Pharmaceutical Analysis and in addition to those who have special interest in the subject.

Finally, I compliment Dr. G. Vidya Sagar for his painstaking efforts in bringing out this textbook and I earnestly believe that his efforts will be suitably rewarded by wider readership among the fellow Pharmacists.

January, 2009,
Ahmedabad.

Manish Bharadwaj
Vice-Chancellor

Preface

Analysis of Drugs and Pharmaceuticals forms the backbone of research and development in Pharmaceutical Industry and Academia. This book is primarily focused towards fulfilling the requirements of B.Pharm. in Pharmaceutical Analysis, as recommended by the All India Council for Technical Education (AICTE) and adopted by major Universities in the country. The fundamental concepts have been dealt in detail in "*Basics of Drug Analysis*" and this book focuses on various Physico-Chemical and instrumental techniques and their wider application for large number of drugs.

The book is conveniently divided into several chapters, each chapter dealing with a method of instrumental analysis. The book gives a review of several conventional methods like UV, Visible and Flourimetric Spectroscopy and also deals at length, the newer techniques like HPLC, quality evaluation of Herbals etc. All the topics have been written in easy to understand and simple language with special emphasis on Pharmaceutical applications. The book will be useful to analysts, and Quality control staff of Pharmaceutical Industry.

I record my sincere thanks to faculty members of Veerayatan Institute of Pharmacy, Mandvi for their constant encouragement.

Any suggestion for the improvement of this book from the readers will be highly appreciated.

-Author

Acknowledgements

To write a book of this magnitude, one requires a lot of patience and perseverance. My teaching the subject over the last 20 years helped me to get the experience and skills to write this book. I gratefully acknowledge the unstinted support by the following friends and academicians. They helped me in going through the manuscript and offering their valuable comments.

1. Dr. N. J. Gaekwad, Chairperson, Department of Pharmaceutical Sciences, Rashtrasant Tukadoji Maharaj Nagpur University, Nagpur.
2. Prof. Pankaj Sharma, Principal, Vidyasthali Institute of Pharmacy, Jaipur
3. Prof. Dr. J. S. Dangi, Dean, Department of Pharmaceutical Sciences, Guru Ghasidas University, Bilaspur, Chattisgarh.
4. Prof. Dr. Kishor Pramod Bhusari, Principal, Shri Sharad Pawar College of Pharmacy, Wanadongri, Hingna Road, Nagpur.
5. Prof. Dr. B. Jaykar, Principal, Shri Vinayaka Mission's College of Pharmacy, Kondappanaickenpatti, Salem.
6. Prof. Milind Umerkar, Principal, Smt. Kishoribai Pharmacy College, Kamptee, Nagpur.
7. Prof. Komal Sharma, B.N. College of Pharmacy, Udaipur.
8. Prof. S. J. Deherwal, Department of Pharmaceutical Sciences, Pandit Ravishankar Shukla University, Raipur, Chattisgarh.

I gratefully acknowledge the sustained support of the management, staff and students of Veerayatan Institute of Pharmacy in writing this textbook. The successful compilation of this book was possible with the cooperation and help of my wife, Mrs. Swapna Sagar and my daughter Hasitha.

Finally I would like to place on record the services of Shri Anil Shah, Pharma Book Syndicate in bringing out the book in a most beautiful way.

-Author

Contents

CHAPTER 1

CHROMATOGRAPHY

Introduction

In 1903, Russian Botanist "Tswett" found the chromatographic technique.

Once he was doing a simple extraction and accidently he found this technique.

[The name of the scientist is actually M. Tswett]

Chromatography

Chromatography is a combination of greek words:

Chroma : Colour

Graphos : Writing

M. Tswett was successful in doing the separation of chlorophyll, xanthophyll and several other coloured substances by percolating vegetable extracts through a column of calcium carbonate.

(i) to percolate, (of liquid) to ooze ;

(ii) Percolation; percolator :

The calcium carbonate column acted as an adsorbent and the different substances got adsorbed to different extent and this gives rise to coloured bands at different positions, on the column. Tswett termed this system of coloured bands as the chromatogram and the method as chromatography.

However in majority of chromatographic procedures no coloured products are formed and the term is a misnomer.

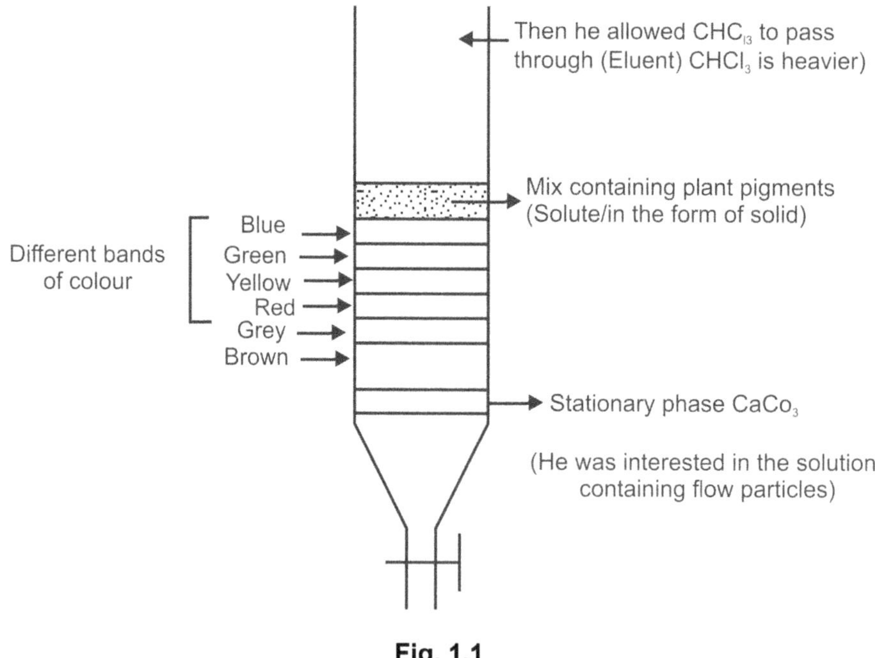

Fig. 1.1

Thus, Tswett developed a new separation technique that involved passage of mixture to be separated through a column of a finely divided powdered adsorbent.

A portion of the mixture was applied to the top of such a column and it was washed thoroughly with an organic solvent.

As the washing step proceeded, the several components in the mixture were washed down by the column at different rates, finally they separated completely in different bands.

Tswett gave the name "chromatography" because chroma means colour and graphy means zones of separation.

Mixture of colourless compounds can also be separated.

Now-a-days, chromatography is an essential method of separation.

Introduction

If we have complex mixture, extraction is very difficult as number of compounds having similar properties are present and there is also interference of other substances.

Generally separation is carried out in following order :

(i) *Single extraction:* not 100% extraction.

(ii) *Multiple extraction:* close to 100% extraction.

(iii) *Continuous extraction:* It involves use of heat, so it is not used for thermolabile material.

(iv) *Counter current distribution (CCD):* It does not involve use of heat. But multiple extraction is carried out at room temperature.

(v) *Chromatography:* Chromatography is basically an advanced continuous technique of separation involving minimum two phases.

Here the thousand times extraction at room temperature.

No heating is involved in this method, so thermolabile compounds can also be separated or extracted. So this is called as "cold separation technique".

The main two phases can be described by :

(i) Stationary Phase: It must be steady, remains at one place, bind with different solute to different extent, like

Strongly bound; Loosely bound

(ii) Mobile Phase: Continuously move in one direction.

Most loosely bound solute move fast with mobile phase whereas most strongly closely bound solute move slowly with mobile phase. So generally closely bound solute is obtained on the upper part of the column whereas loosely bound solute is obtained at the lower part of the column.

Stationary and Mobile Phase

(i) *Stationary Phase*: It must be stable and must bind with different solutes to different extent.

And to fulfil the condition of stability, it must be in the form of solid particles but we can have liquid also as a stationary phase in the form of liquid coated solid particles.

Two types of liquids can be used as stationary phase:

(a) Physically bound liquid: Here, the liquid is coated on the solid surface.

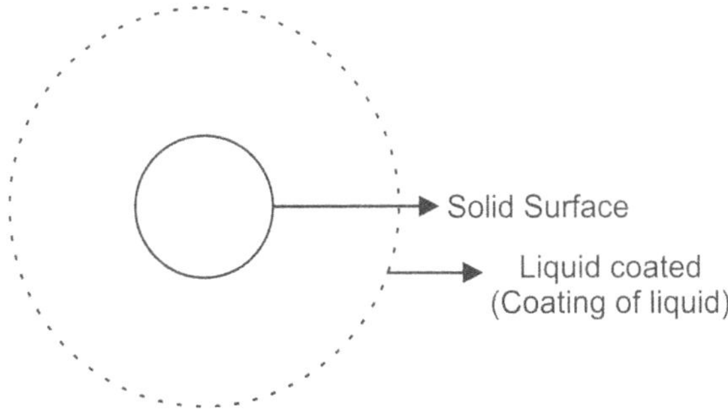

Fig. 1.2

(b) Chemically bound liquid

(ii) ***Mobile Phase*****:** It must be mobile, it must possess the flow property.

Mobile phase continuously moves in one direction.

Liquid/gas can be used as mobile phase.

S.C.F: super critical fluid is also used.

So, chromatography is a separation technique involving two phases.

Driving Forces which Make Mobile Phase to Move

(i) Gravitational force

(ii) *Pressure*: in built in cylinder or external as in HPLC.

(iii) *Electrostatic attraction*: Here electrophoretic chromatography. We arrange electrode, so liquid gets attracted

(iv) *Capillary Action*: Water/liquid rises against gravity due to capillary action in paper/cloth.

Scientific Definition of Chromatography as per USP – 2000

Chromatography is defined as a procedure by which solutes are separated by *dynamic differential migration process* in a system consisting of two or more phases, one of which moves continuously in a given direction and in which the individual substance exhibit different mobilities by reasons of differences in adsorption, partition, solubility, vapour pressure, molecular size or ionic charge density. The individual substance thus separated can be identified or determined by suitable analytical method.

Different Terms used in Definition

(a) *Dynamic Differential Migration Process:* It is a procedure or technique of separation; migration refers to movement.

There is an equilibrium between two phases, stationary and mobile phases of solute which is constantly changed and is dynamic.

[dynamic : forces which produce motion]

Explanation

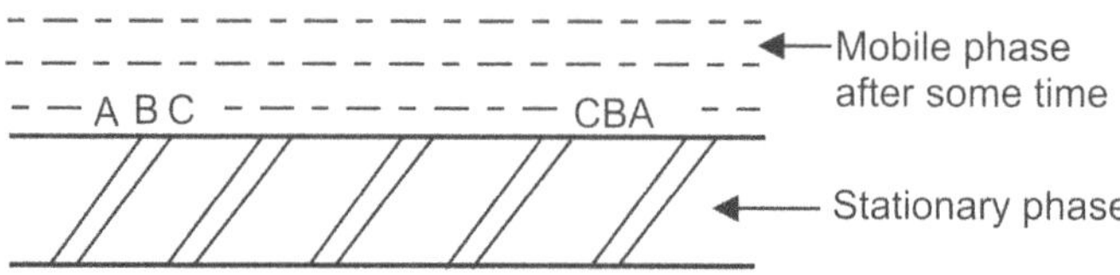

Fig. 1.3

Suppose A, B, C are three different components in the mixture.

Dynamic means forces which produce movement. So here dynamic means movements of A, B, C from stationary to mobile phase.

Differential means all the components of the mixture, here A, B, C are not having same equilibrium in mobile phase.

It is possible that A is highly soluble in mobile phase so A is moving faster and so we can say that A is less absorbed in stationary phases and so it is more soluble in mobile phase. And suppose C is less soluble in mobile phase and more soluble in stationary phase then it will move slower. So, in the (fig.1.3), initially mixture containing compounds A, B, C is then separated on the stationary phase after some time and as A moves faster in mobile phase and it will get adsorbed last on the stationary phase and C which is more soluble in stationary phase will get adsorbed first so the sequence becomes C, B, A after (some time) due to dynamic differential migration process.

Q. Why this dynamic differential migration exists?

OR

Which factors are responsible for separation of different components?

OR

Because of which factors this dynamic differential migration is possible?

Ans.

(i) Adsorption

For this stationary phase must be solid.

If one component is more absorbed from mixture, it will move slower with mobile phase as compared to the component which is less adsorbed on the stationary phase.

(ii) Partition

For this mechanism stationary phase must be liquid and immiscible with mobile phase.

If all components of mixture have different partition co-efficient between stationary phase and mobile phase then only separation can be possible.

(iii) Solubility

If component is more soluble in stationary phase then it will move slower with mobile phase.

(iv) Vapour pressure

If the solute is in gaseous phase, then we can use gaseous mobile phase.

Then here the component, which has higher vapour pressure will remain more in gaseous state and so it will move more easily in gaseous mobile phase.

(v) Molecular size or Volume

If stationary phase has more attraction towards smaller molecules, then bigger molecules will be moving faster.

(vi) Ionic Charge

Applicable for ionic molecules because intensity of positive and negative charge varies.

If we have stationary phase, which has negatively charged molecules, then one which has higher positive charge will get retained on stationary phase and others having less intense positive charge will move faster in mobile phase.

In short, originally chromatography is a separation technique but now-a-days additional instruments are attached for other analytical methods like pH meter, potentiometer etc., by which we can be able to define amount of the substance and we can also identify the substance.

So, both qualitative as well as quantitative analysis can be performed while performing chromatographic technique of separation.

With the passage of time, the routine use of chromatography as a separation technique became universal and has been extended to several areas of study, especially chemistry, biology and medicine. Apart from its use in analysis it is becoming a potential technique as a method for the preparation of very pure compounds such as in pharmaceutical industry or in the manufacture of pure chemicals.

Chromatography is probably the most important single analytical technique used today and will probably continue to be so far the foreseeable future. It is a corner stone of molecular analytical chemistry in particular. Recently its coupling with atomic absorption spectroscopy has extended its application to elemental analysis.

The information obtained by gas chromatography is particularly useful to the research organic chemist or biochemist who wants to know what material he has synthesized in the laboratory or separated from living tissue. In addition to its application to pure research, it is valuable to the industrial scientist who wants to know the composition of his competitor's product, as well as to many other people involved in the characterization of matter. It can also be used as a method of preparing very pure compounds or in manufacture of pure chemicals.

Advantages of Chromatography

- Decomposition of substances do not occur. This is important especially for thermolabile substances and substance from biological origin.
- Separation can be carried out on micro/semi micro scale, i.e., small quantity of mixtures is required for analysis.

- Chromatographic techniques are simple, rapid and require simple apparatus.
- Complex mixtures can be handled with comparative ease.

Classification of Chromatography

(I) Based upon nature of Stationary and Mobile Phase

There are different types of chromatography based on the type of stationary and mobile phases used. They are:

(i) Gas-solid chromatography.

(ii) Gas-liquid chromatography.

(iii) Solid-liquid chromatography.

[column chromatography, thin layer chromatography, HPLC (High performance liquid chromatography)]

(iv) Liquid –liquid chromatography.

[paper partition chromatography, column partition chromatography]

(II) Classification based on Instruments

(i) Column chromatography :

(a) *Adsorption column chromatography*: stationary phase is solid based on absorption principle.

(b) *Partition column chromatography*: Stationary phase is liquid.

(ii) Paper chromatography

Here stationary phase is paper.

The mode (mechanism) by which the paper is inserted, we further classify them as:

(a) *Ascending paper chromatography*: Mobile phase rises on paper due to capillary action against gravity.

(b) *Descending paper chromatography*: Paper is hung. Mobile phase moves downwards.

(c) *Circular paper chromatography*: paper is placed horizontally. Mobile phase moves from centre to periphery.

(d) *Two dimensional paper chromatography:*

Normal Phase: Mobile phase is less polar than stationary phase.

Reversal: Mobile phase is more polar than stationary phase.

[mobile phase moves from centre to periphery two times]

(iii) Thin Layer Chromatography

(i) Normal TLC

(ii) Two dimensional TLC.

(iii) Continuous development TLC

(iv) High performance/pressure TLC (HPTLC). Here, in all four techniques solid absorbent is in the form of very thin layer of stationary phase.

(iv) Gas Chromatography

Here gas is used as mobile phase with some pressure, it is constantly moving.

(a) Gas-liquid chromatography (GLC) liquid is stationary phase; partition principle.

(b) Gas-solid chromatography (GSC) solid is stationary phase; absorption principle.

(c) Capillary gas chromatography: Stationary phase is in very narrow tube having length of 100 meter.

(v) High Pressure / Performance Liquid Chromatography (HPLC)

Most popular method of chromatography in pharmacopoeia.

More than 60% analysis in pharmacopoeia are given by this method. Liquid is mobile phase.

It is allowed to flow with 300 atm (atmospheric) pressure.

(i) Normal phase HPLC (NPHPLC)

(ii) Reversal phase HPLC (RPHPLC)

(iii) Gradient flow [amount of slope:]

(iv) Isocratic [Iso : same]

(vi) Super-Critical Fluid Chromatography (SFC)

Mobile phase is neither liquid nor gas but is in between phase. [a phase between liquid and gas is used here as a mobile phase]

(vii) Ultra high Pressure Chromatography

Pressure is further increased about 3000 to 5000 atm

(viii) Electrophoretic Chromatography

Different charges at different ends and solute will move according to the charge.

III Based on the Principle of Separation

OR

Based on working principle

The main principles of separation can be either adsorption or partition. Hence they can be called as adsorption chromatography or partition chromatography.

(i) ***Adsorption Chromatography*:** When a mixture of compounds (adsorbate) dissolved in the mobile phase (eluent) moves through a column of stationary phase (adsorbent), they travel according to the relative affinities towards stationary phase. The compound which has more affinity towards stationary phase travels slower and compound which has lesser affinity towards stationary phase travels faster. Hence the compounds are separated. No two compounds have the same affinity for a combination of stationary phase, mobile phase and other conditions.

Examples where adsorption is the principle of separation: Gas-solid chromatography, column chromatography and HPLC (High performance liquid chromatography).

(ii) ***Partition Chromatography*:** When two immiscible liquids are present, a mixture of solutes will be distributed according to their partition co-efficients. When a mixture of compounds are dissolved in the mobile phase and passed through a column of liquid stationary phase, the component which is more soluble in the stationary phase travels slower. The component which is more soluble in mobile phase travels faster. Thus the components are separated because of the differences in their partition co-efficients. No two components have the same partition co-efficient for a particular combination of stationary phase, mobile phase and other conditions.

The stationary phase as such cannot be a liquid. Hence a solid support is used over which a thin film or coating of liquid is made which acts as a stationary phase.

Counter current extraction: It works on similar principle. In this two immiscible solvents flow in opposite direction. The solute mixture is distributed between these solvents, depending upon their partition co-efficient. The advantage is that fresh solvent comes in contact, therefore extraction is effective and thus solute mixture is separated into individual components.

Examples where partition is the principle of separation: Gas liquid chromatography, paper partition chromatography, column partition chromatography etc.

(iii) ***Ion-exchange Chromatography*:** In this type, an ion exchange resin is used. Reversible exchange of ions takes place between similar charged ions and that of ion exchange resin. A cation exchange resin is used for the separation of cations and anion exchange resin is used to separate a mixture of anions.

(iv) ***Gel Permeation Chromatography (Gel filtration, size exclusion chromatography)*:** A gel is used to separate the components of a mixture according to their molecular sizes. Different gels are used for different molecular weight ranges. The solvent used can be of aqueous or non-aqueous type. The stationery phase is a porous matrix. The matrix is made up of wide variety of compounds like cross-linked polystyrene, polyvinyl acetate gels, cross linked dextrans (sephadex), polyacrylamide gels, Agarose gels. The mobile phases used may be organic solvents or aqueous buffers. The most commonly used detector is differential refractiometric detector. For some class of compounds, uv-visible detector, electrochemical detectors, etc., are used.

The mechanisms involved in the separation process is because of steric and diffusion effects in pores of different gels. This technique is used in the separation of proteins, polysaccharides, enzymes and synthetic polymers.

(v) ***Chiral Chromatography*:** In this type of chromatography, optical isomers (levo and dextro form) can be separated by using chrial stationary phases.

Modification in Simple Chromatography

Wide variety of solvents are used

Mobile phase of solvent which can be water/alcohol/mix of different solvents in different proportion are used.

As per our requirement, we can apply gravity force and we can also charge rate of flow by changing pressure by pumps.

In stationary phase, we can use wide variety of compounds. (solid with smaller particle size has greater surface area).

Sometimes liquid can be used as stationary phase.

Q. How Separation is Achieved?

OR

What is the Mechanism of Separation?

OR

General Mechanism of Separation

Suppose we have a mixture of different solute A + B + C

(i) Sample mixture is introduced in a very narrow band.

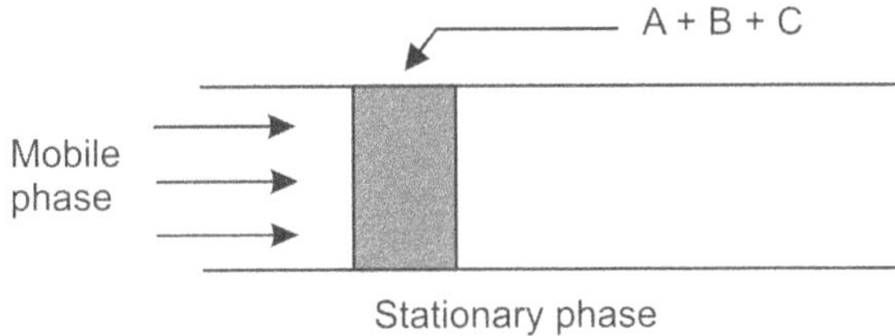

(ii) Mobile phase continuously moves in one direction.

(iii) Stationary phase binds different solute to different extent.

Suppose, compound C → Poorly bounded

B → Intermediate

A → Strongly bounded

(iv) The solutes which are not bound to stationary phase are carried foreword with mobile phase.

(v) The solute which is least retained will be moving little faster. Thus different solutes are moving with different speed.

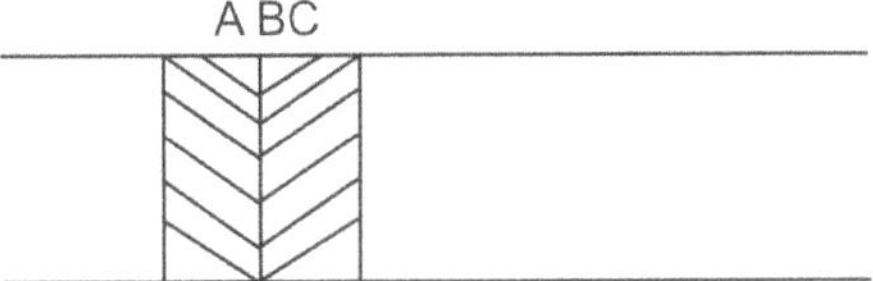

(vi) Same thing continues but as the solute moves foreword, there is spreading of concentration. This is called as "zone broadening" or "band broadening".

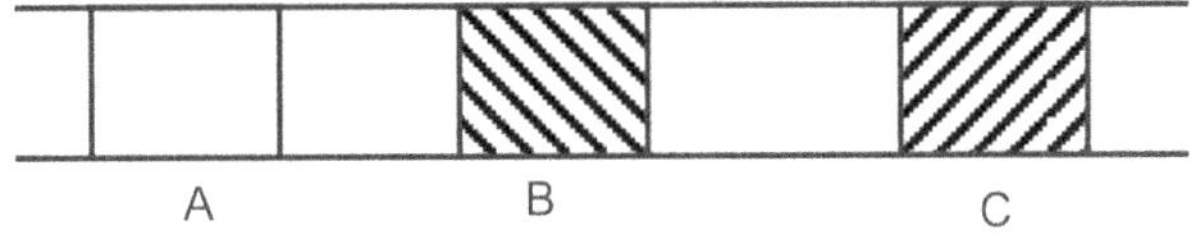

As the distance travelled by the solute is more, band broadening becomes higher and so spreading also increases.

Spreading is inversely related with separation efficiency.

More spreading of solute

⇓

inefficient separation.

Less spreading of solute

⇓

efficient separation.

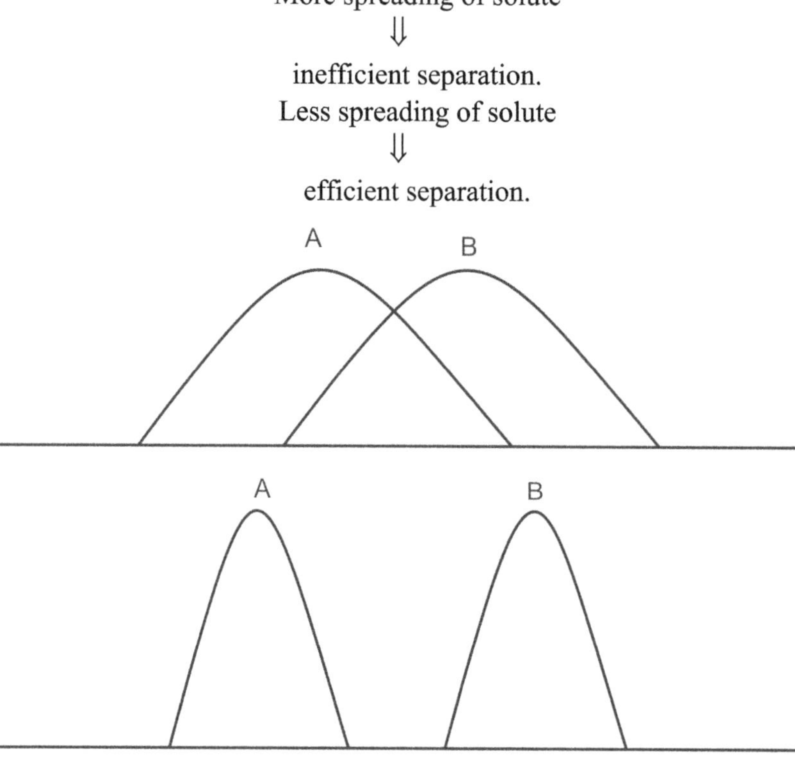

Fig. 1.4

If we have complex mixture i.e., ABC having very closely similarity in their properties, then the separation efficiency is very low.

In this case, we increase the length of tube/ stationary phase so that the distance travelled in the stationary phase increases, so separation also increases. Thus, "As the length of the stationary phase increases, the separation efficiency increases". But this is helpful only in case where the solutes to be separated have very similar properties.

"As the length of the stationary phase increases, the spreading of solute concentration also increases and due to spreading separation efficiency decreases.

So if the system is continued, then lower, less binding solute comes out of system, then intermediate, i.e., least binding and then the strongly bound compound comes out, one after another.

So, overall mechanism of separation can be explained as "separation of different compounds depends on their own intensity of tendency to bind to the stationary phase".

Chromatogram: It is the graphical expression of separated compound in chromatography.

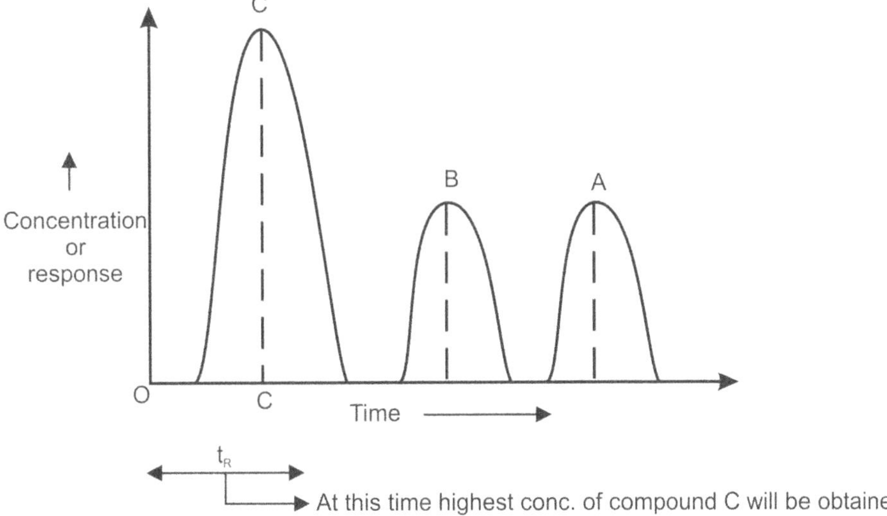

Fig. 1.5

Now, time taken by component C to get separated is

t_R : Retention time

Definition of Retention Time (t_R) : The time required from the time of introduction of sample to the system to the time to take out 50% of the solute.

At retention time, 50-50% of solute concentration on the either side means 50% solute is in the system and 50% solute is out of the system.

If the graph is like this

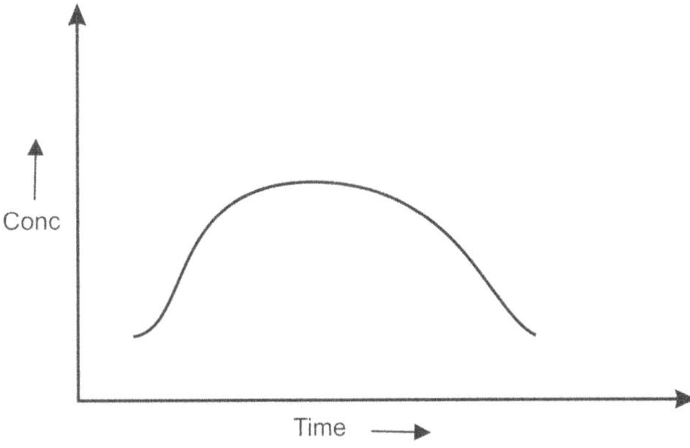

Fig. 1.6

t_R is not clear here. Such condition is not seen in ideal chromatography.

Retention volume V_R: Volume of mobile phase required to take out exactly 50% of the solute from the system and 50% will be in the system.

$$V_R = t_R \times F$$

where

t_R = Retention time

V_R = Retention volume

F = Flow rate of mobile phase (means at what rate, mobile phase is passing through)

e.g., suppose 10 ml of mobile phase comes out per minute, if t_R = 10 min. Then,

$$V_R = t_R \times F$$
$$= 10 \times 10$$
$$= 100 \text{ ml}$$

t_R is for identification/qualitative purpose, so if t_R is fixed for any compound, then we can predict which compound will come out first.

In chromatogram, height of peak/area under peak will give the concentration of the compound and it will give quantitative information also.

t_R is the characteristic of a solute. Response is expressed in concentration

Response = area under curve height/inch

One criteria is that efficiency of separation is important. Efficiency of separation means very closely related substances should be separated without overlapping.

Principle of Column Chromatographic Separation

Basically, all chromatographic systems consist of two phases. One is the stationary phase which may be solid, gel, liquid or solid/liquid mixture which is immobilised. The second is mobile phase which may be liquid or gas and flows over or through the stationary phase. The choice of stationary or mobile phase is made so that the compounds to be separated have different distribution co-efficients. This may be achieved by setting up:

(i) an adsorption equilibrium between a stationary solid and a mobile liquid phase (adsorption chromatography);

(ii) a partition equilibrium between a stationary liquid (or semi-liquid) and a mobile liquid phase (counter current chromatography and partition chromatography);

(iii) a partition equilibrium between a stationary liquid and a mobile gaseous phase (gas-liquid chromatography).

(iv) an ion-exchange equilibrium between an ion-exchange resin stationary phase and a mobile electrolyte phase (ion-exchange chromatography).

(v) an equilibrium between a liquid phase inside and outside a porous structure or molecular sieve (exclusion chromatography).

(vi) an equilibrium between a macromolecule and a small molecule for which it has a high biological specificity and hence affinity (affinity chromatography).

The principle of separation may be depicted by considering a column packed with a solid granular stationary phase to a height of 5 cm surrounded by the mobile liquid phase of which there is 1 cm^3 per cm of column means 1 cm column 1cm^3 solvent average mobile phase.

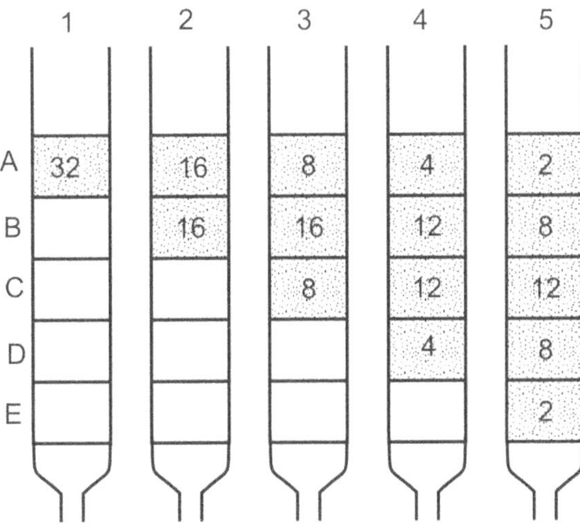

Fig. 1.7

If 32 μg of a compound is added to the column in 1 cm^3 of solvent then as this 1 cm^3 (solvent) move on the column to occupy position A, 1cm^3 of solvent will leave the base of the column. If the compound added has an effective distribution co-efficient of 1, it will distribute itself equally between the solid and liquid phases. If distribution co-efficient more or less than 1 then we need to add more? If a further 1cm^3 of solvent is introduced on to the column, the solvent in section A will move down to B taking 16 μg of the compound with it, leaving 16 μg at A. At both A and B a redistribution of the compound will occur so that there is 8 μg in the solvent and 8 μg in the solid phase. The addition of further 1 cm^3 of solvent to the column displaces the solvent in A to B and then B to C giving the distribution of the compound as shown in stage 3. Addition of a further 1 cm^3 of solvent leads to the distribution shown at stage 4, and further 1 cm^3 aliquot (such part of a number that will divide it without remainder) to the situation at stage 5.

It is apparent that after five equilibriums the compound is distributed throughout the whole column, but is maximally concentrated at the centre of the column. If a compound had an effective distribution co-efficient of less than 1, more than 50% of the compound would be left on the solid phase after each equilibrium. Although after five equilibriums some of the compound would be present throughout the column, the column. Alternatively, for a compound with an effective distribution of greater than 1, the concentration peak after five equilibriums would be below the centre of the column.

The greater the number of equilibrations that occur on a column, the greater becomes the concentration of the compound on a certain part of the column. There are, therefore, two important factors which influence the pattern of separation (resolution) of a mixture of compounds. The rate of progress of a compound through the column depends on its effective distribution co-efficient and the sharpness of the compound band on the column depends on the number of equilibrations that have taken place.

In a real situation, equilibrium occurs continuously on a column since the solution is being continuously added and, in normal working columns, thousands of equilibrations take place. Chromatography column is considered to consist of a number of adjacent zones in each of which there is sufficient space for the solute to achieve complete equilibrium between the mobile and stationary phase. Each zone is called as a theoretical plate and its length in the column is called the plate height (H) which has dimensions of length. The more efficient the column, the greater the number of theoretical plates that are involved. The way in which the number of theoretical plates (N) affects the distribution of a solute with an effective distribution co-efficient of 1 is shown in the figure given below.

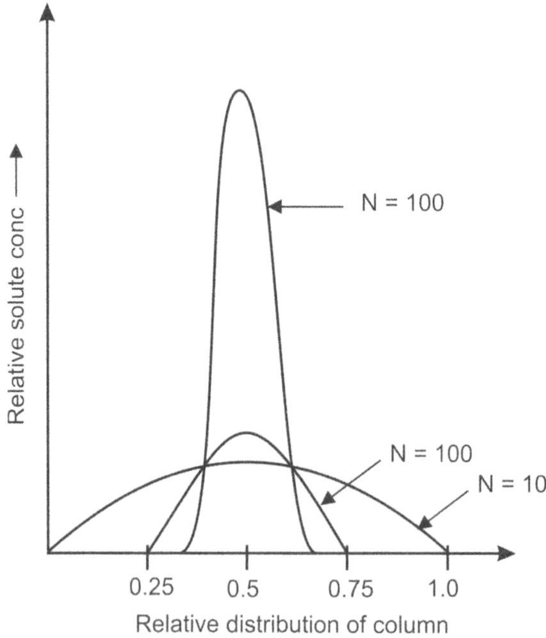

Fig. 1.8

Diagrammatic effect of the number of theoretically plates (N) on the shape of the solute band

Number of theoretical plates α Separation efficiency of column

Theories of Chromatography

(i) Plate theory

(developed/given) by Martin and Synge

(ii) Rate theory by van Deemter

(iii) Random walk or non-equilibrium theory by Gidding.

I Plate Theory

According to plate theory, a chromatographic column consists of a series of separated discrete yet continuous horizontal layers which are termed as the theoretical plates. An equilibrium of the solute between the stationary and mobile phases takes place at each of these plates. Migration of solute is then assumed to occur by a series of stepwise transfers between one plate to the other immediately below.

So, it is based on consideration that "the entire system is divided into several zones (plates) (or into small fragments/segments) with imaginary distance called height of plate" within which solute is in equilibrium between stationary and mobile phases. This imaginary distance is refered to as height/length equivalent to one theoretical plate, i.e., HETP $\Rightarrow$ symbol H or h.

The efficiency of separation in a chromatographic column gets increased as the number of theoretical plates increases. This is because the number of equilibrations will also correspondingly increase. The number of theoretical plates N refers to a measure of column efficiency.

Eg. As in case of rectification as the number of plates are increased, efficiency of rectification also increases.

Here the distillation column containing a mixture of solvents is shown in the figure.

Aim is to separate all the solvents.

Simply, the column containing 20 plates is more efficient than a column containing 7 plates

So, efficiency is calculated in terms of HETP.

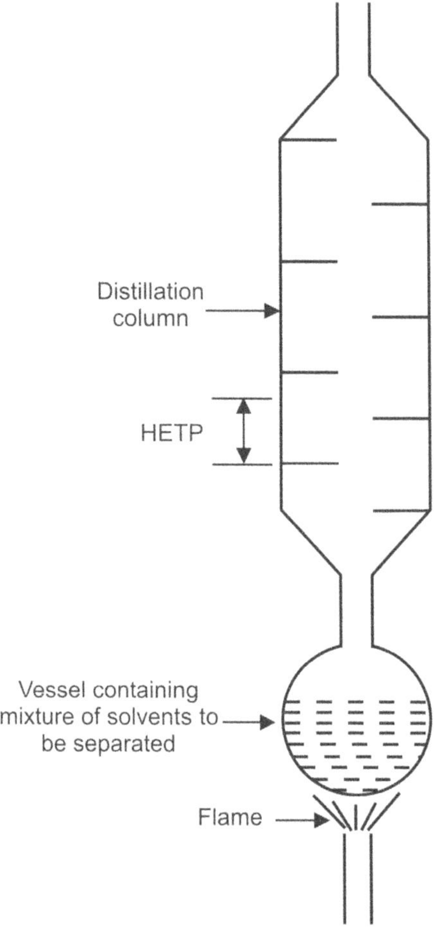

Fig. 1.9

HETP

It is the height of a layer of the column, such that the solution leaving the layer is in equilibrium with the average concentration of the solute in the stationary phase throught the layer.

OR

HETP

It is the length or height of stationary phase within which there is a perfect equilibrium of solute concentration between stationary and mobile phase.

HETP

Height equivalent to theoretical plate

OR

Height equivalent of one (a) theoretical plate.

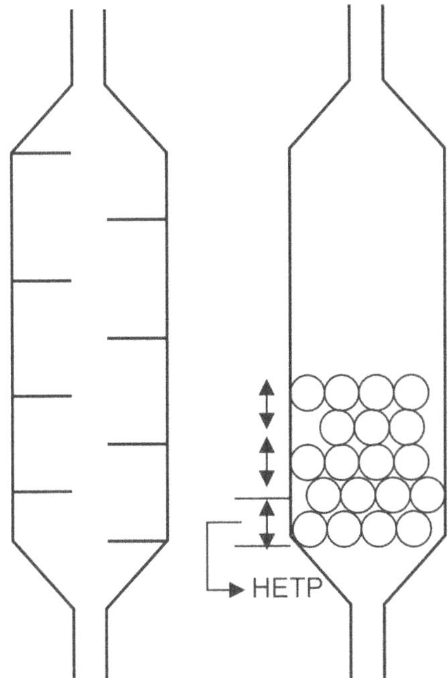

Fig. 1.10

HETP is symbolised as H or h.

$$\therefore \quad H = h = HETP$$

If column contains other packed material rather than plates then efficiency is calculated in terms of HETP

Less/lower the value of HETP $\Rightarrow$ Greater the number of plates per unit length $\Rightarrow$ higher the efficiency in column & vice versa

HETP $\uparrow$ *increases the* HETP $\Rightarrow \downarrow$ decrease in no. of HETP $\Rightarrow \downarrow$ decrease in efficiency

HETP is measured generally in the unit mm where as number of HETP is unit less.

Now,

$$n = \frac{L}{H}$$

where,

n = number of theoretical plates

L = Total length of the stationary phase

H = HETP; Height equivalent to theoretical plate.

and $H = \frac{L}{n}$; here unit must be considered.

Now, separation is directly related to number of plates.

Other relationship among no. of plates and t_R & w.

$$n = 16\left(\frac{t_R}{w}\right)^2$$

where,

t_R = retention time

w = width of peak

Separation Efficiency

It is the capacity of system to separate very closely related compounds having very similar properties with a little difference.

If it can separate enantiomer, then we can say that the efficiency of the system is high.

If confirmation isomers which have similar optical properties can be separated. Then the system is called to be having highest separation efficiency.

Now in chromatography, there will be equilibrium distribution in both phases means solute remains partially in mobile phase and partially in stationary phase

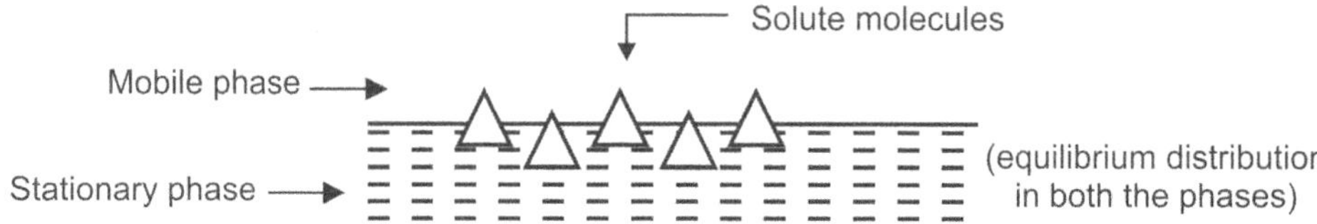

Fig. 1.11

$$S_m \rightleftharpoons S_s$$

S_m : solute concentration in mobile phase

S_s : Solute concentration in stationary phase.

So, overall

Separation efficiency α no. of plates (n)

$n \uparrow increases \Rightarrow H \downarrow decreases$

Separation efficiency α $\frac{1}{\text{HETP}}$

Derivation of Fundamental Equation of Chromatography

Chromatograph: The instrument used for separation in chromatography.

Chromatogram: The graphical expression of separated compound in chromatography.

It is outcome of separation technique.

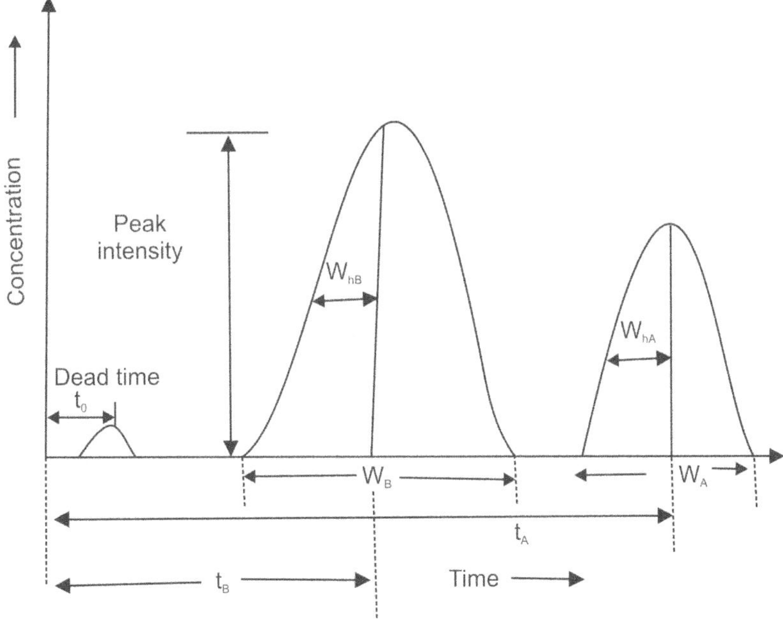

Fig. 1.12

Let us take an example of a mixture containing A & B components.

Component B is nor retained by stationary phase. So, moves faster with mobile phase while component A is retained by stationary phase. So, it moves slowly with mobile phase.

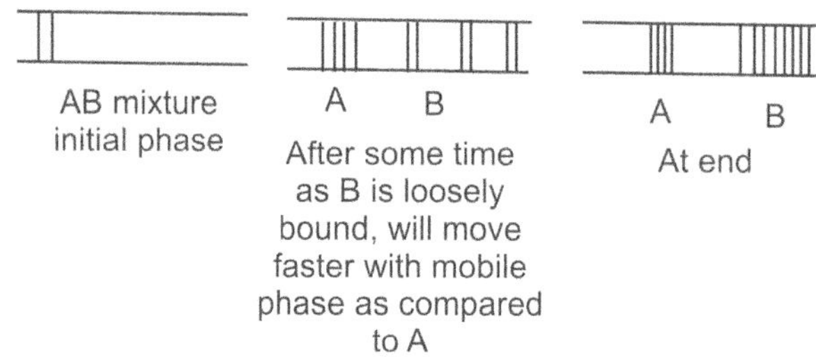

Fig. 1.13

As component B moves faster and gets separated first, so in chromatogram we will obtain the peak first for component B and then for component A.

0 (zero) time is the time when we introduce mixture.

Here in chromatogram/graph

t_B : retention time for component B.

t_A : retention time for component A.

w_B : width of peak for component B.

w_{hB} : width at 50% concentration for component B.

W_A : width of peak for component A.

W_{ha} : width at 50% concentration for component A.

Note: here width is expressed in(min) because X_{axis} is in time (min).

Definition of Retention Time (t_R)

It is the time required from time of introduction of sample to chromatographic system to the time when 50% solute comes out of the system and 50% solute remains within the system.

Retention time for different components are different. So, retention time, being characteristic of a component, is used for identification or qualitative analysis purpose.

Width of Peak

At zero height (or in graph at zero concentration) whatever width is there is called as width of peak.

Retention Volume

It is the volume of mobile phase required to take out 50% solute from chromatographic system.

It is represented by V_R.

$$V_R = F \times t_R$$

Where

F = Rate of flow of mobile phase through the system.

t_R = Retention time

V_R = Retention volume

At retention time/volume amount of analyte in column is equivalent to amount of analyte that comes out.

∴ Amount of anlyte comes out ≡ Amount of analyte in column

$$\Rightarrow V_R C_M = C_M V_M + V_s C_s$$

where

V_R = Retention volume

C_M = Concentration of solute in mobile phase

C_s = Concentration of solute in stationary phase

V_s = Volume of total stationary phase

V_M = Volume of total mobile phase

$$\therefore V_R C_M = C_M V_M + V_S C_S$$

$$= \frac{V_R C_M}{C_M} = \frac{C_M V_M}{C_M} + \frac{V_S C_s}{C_M}$$

$$= V_R = V_M + V_S \left(\frac{C_s}{C_M} \right)$$

$$\text{Now } \frac{C_S}{C_M} = K$$

$$\Rightarrow V_R = V_M = KV_S$$

This is the fundamental equation of chromatography.

$$V_M = V_O = \text{Dead volume}$$

Total volume of mobile phase that we have introduced into the system.

$$\therefore V_R = V_O + KV_S$$

It is applied in all types of chromatography.

Retention volume is different for each component

Dead Volume

It is the volume required by totally unretained solute.

If solute is totally non-reactive in both phases $\Rightarrow K = 0$

$$\Rightarrow V_R = V_M$$

This equation is applied in retention mechanism also.

This equation describes exact characteristic of solute.

In the mixture of two components A & B, if component A has higher K value the V_R will increase.

Some Important Matters

(i) If C_s is higher concentration of solute in stationary phase the value of K also increases and that's why V_R increases.

[here $K = \frac{C_S}{C_M}$ so $\uparrow$ increases in the k $\Rightarrow$ higher the binding of solute with stationary phase $\Rightarrow$ which requires more amount of mobile phase to drag 50% of concentration of solute with it out of the system].

(ii) n can also be calculated by formula

$$n = 16\left(\frac{t_e}{w}\right)^2$$

where

t_R = retetion time; w = width at base line

and $$n = 5.54\left(\frac{t_e}{w_h}\right)^2$$

where

w_h = width of half height (or at 50% concentration) of solute in both the phases.

It is expressed by α

$$\therefore \alpha = \frac{t_B - t_O}{t_A - t_O}$$

Where, t_o = dead time

Dead time

It is the minimum time required to take out any solute.

$$\therefore \alpha = \frac{t_B^1}{t_A^1}$$

Where

t_B^1 & t_A^1 adjust retention time adjust retention time = Retention time – Dead time.

Example 1

In a chromatographic separation, the retention time of a newly found ant malarial drug is 3.3 minutes and width at base line is 20 seconds. If the total length of system is 1.3 meters, calculate the number of theoretical plates/meter and HETP.

Here

t_R = 3.3 minutes

$\Rightarrow$ t_R = 198 seconds [3.3 $\times$ 60 sec]

W = 20 seconds

L = 1.3 meters

n = (?)

HETP = (?)

$$n = 16\left(\frac{t_R}{w}\right)^2$$

$$= 16\left(\frac{198}{20}\right)^2$$

$$= 16\,(9.9)^2$$

$\Rightarrow$ n = 1568.16 plates per metre

Now,

$$H = \frac{L}{n}$$

$$\therefore H = \frac{1.3}{1568.16}$$

$$\therefore H = 8.28\ \text{gg} \times 10^{-4}\ \text{metre}$$

Resolution

Separation efficiency of chromatographic method is mathematically known as resolution.

Universally, it is defined as separation of closely related compounds.

It is expressed as R or R_S.

$$R_s = \frac{2(t_B - t_A)}{W_B + W_A}$$

where

W_A or W_B = width at base line

t_B or t_A = retention time

From the above equation, if width increases then resolution decreases.

So, width of chromatographic peak should be as narrow as possible.

And time t_A & t_B should be different sufficiently i.e., difference between t_A and t_B should be more for i.e., resolution.

Separation Efficiency α Resolution (R_S)

If width of the peak increases ⇒ resolution decrease

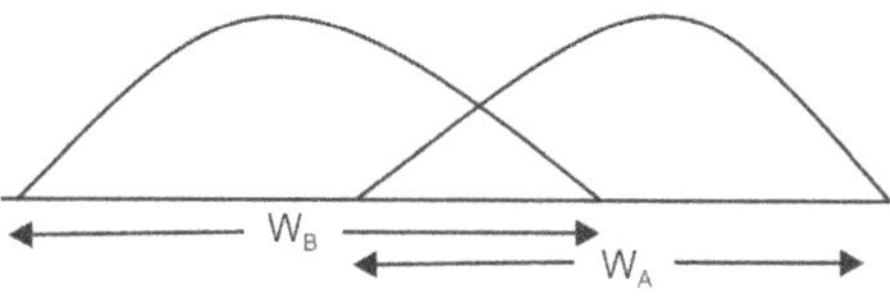

Fig. 1.14

Practically, it is observed that when R = 1, there is about 98% separation and 2% mixing

when R = 1.5 ⇒ 100% separation

when R > 1.5, we achieve the highest efficiency, means separation is more and more better as R moves above the value 1.5

when R = 1,

R = 1.5

R > 1.5

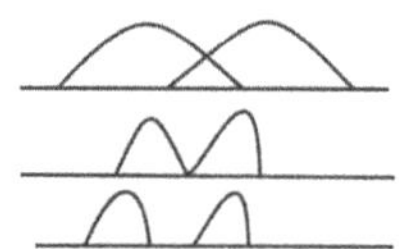

Fig. 1.15

98% separation

100% separation

Most efficient separation

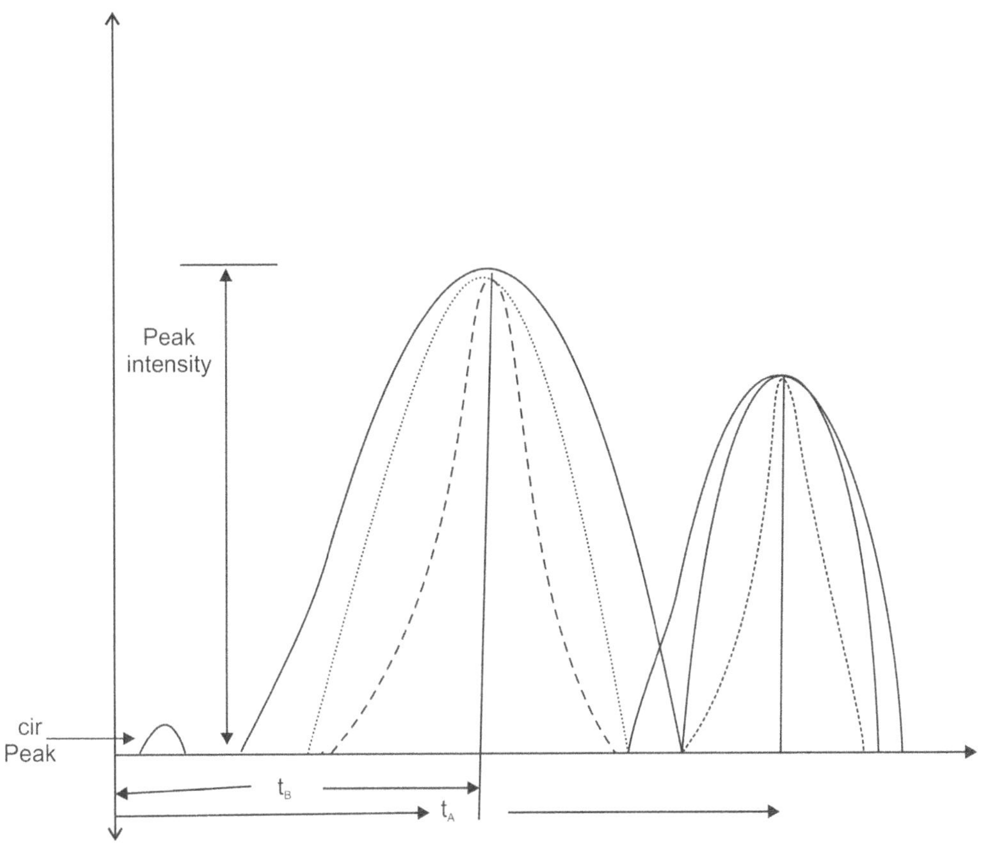

Fig. 1.16

Here retention time remains same but width is changed, so R_S varies for different width.

So, if width is minimum $\Rightarrow$ R_s would be high

Now, another formula for R_S is,

$$R_S = 1.18\,\frac{(t_B - t_A)}{W_{hB} + W_{hA}}$$

$$N = 16\left(\frac{t_R}{W}\right)^2$$

Example 2

Mixture of 2 drugs separated by chromatography having retention time of 5.2 min and 36 minutes respectively and their width at base-line are 12 seconds and 8 seconds respectively. Calculate resolution and number of plates and comment on efficiency.

Now, here for two drugs A & B;

t_A = 5.2 mintues t_B = 3.6 mintues

= 312 seconds = 216 seconds

W_A = 12 seconds W_B = 8 seconds

R_S = (?)

n = (?)

now,

$$R_S = \frac{2(t_A - t_B)}{W_A + W_B}$$

$$= \frac{2(312 - 216)}{12 + 18}$$

$$R_S = \frac{2(96)}{20}$$

$$R_S = 6.4$$

Here, R_s is greater than 1.5 so, highest separation efficiency the system is having

Difference between separation and resolution

Separation

Maxima of two solutes is measured and width is not considered.

Resolution

Width is considered here

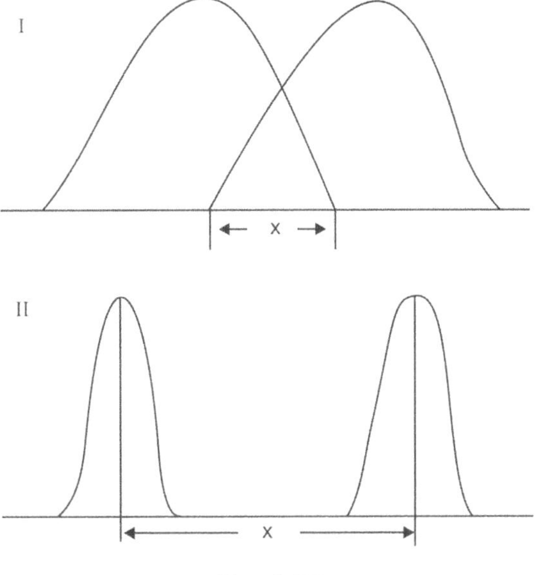

Fig. 1.17

Here, the difference ($t_B - t_n$) i.e., x is same in both, but the width of chromatographic peaks of both are different so in II resolution occurs whereas in I there is separation.

Tailing Factor

Generally, we require symmetrical peak and it is ideal.

But in some cases we get asymmetrical peak. For this, pharmacopoeia has defined tailing factor or peak symmetry factor.

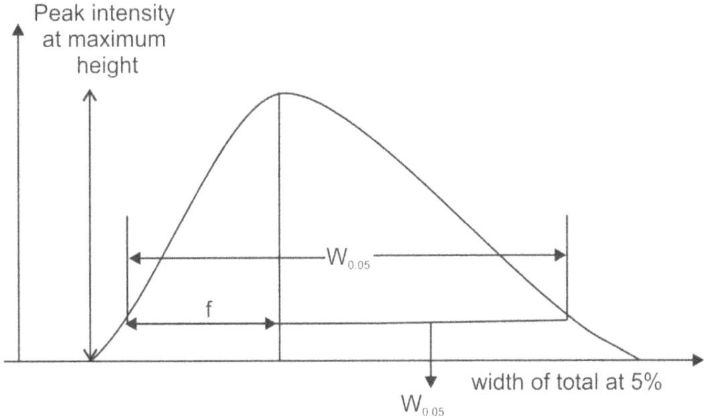

Fig. 1.18

Width at 5% of total height means $\frac{5}{100} = 0.05$, total height 100% from that we measure tailing factor of 5% of the total height.

Now tailing factor is represented by T.

$$T = \frac{W_{0.05}}{2f}$$

Where f =

If peak is perfectly symmetrical then T = 1

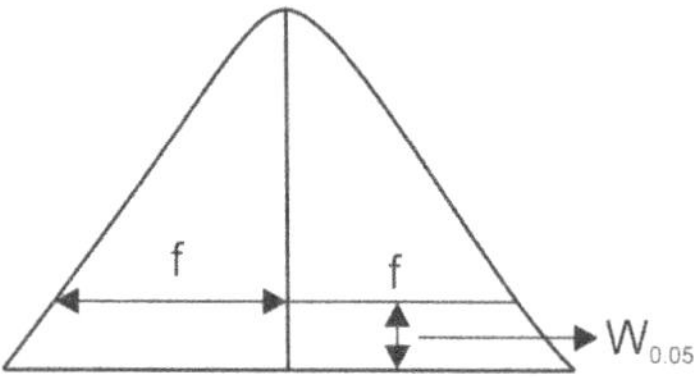

Fig. 1.19

So, if T > 1 OR T < 1 ⇒ peak is asymmetrical

Tailing value is permitted upto 1.1.

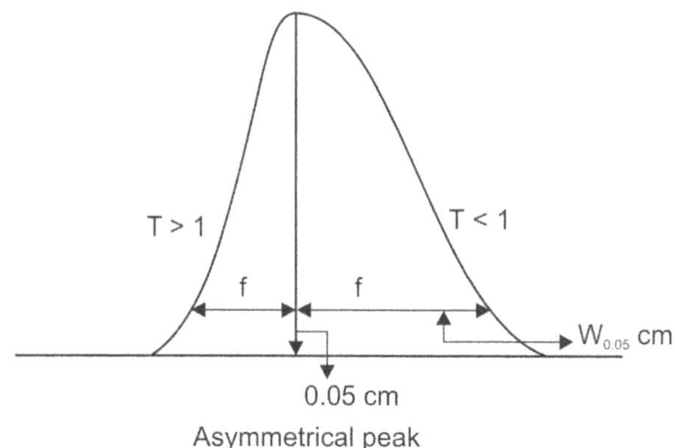

Fig. 1.20

[suppose $W_{0.05} = 6$

and f (at left side is)2

$$T = \frac{W_{0.05}}{2f} \Rightarrow \frac{6}{4} = 1.5 > 1$$

and if f (at left side is) 4

$$\Rightarrow \frac{6}{8} = 0.75 < 1]$$

II Rate Theory

OR

Van Deemter Theory

OR

Van Deemter Equation

OR

Zone Broadening Factor

OR

Factors Affecting Zone Broadning

The rate theory is able to explain the effect of variables such as mobile phase velocity and adsorbabilities which determine the width of an elution band [Elution: the separation of material by washing]. It also relates the effects of these variables on the time taken by a solute to make its appearance at the end of the column. Migration of solute particles in a column occurs in a state of confusion, each solute molecule progressing in a stop and go sequence independent of any other molecule. If a molecule is attached to the stationary phase, its migration down the column is temporarily stopped, but the zone passes on. That is to say, one molecule may get immobilised temporarily on the column while other molecules migrate. In this manner, a molecule alternates rapidly between adsorbed and desorbed states. The time a molecule spends in either phase is highly irregular and it depends upon an accidental energy gain by a molecule from its environment so as to effect a reverse transfer. A particle can migrate only if it is present in the mobile phase and as a result the migration down the column is also highly irregular. Consequently, some solute molecules may migrate rapidly whereas other may lag behind. The net result of all these random individual processes is a symmetric distribution of velocities around the mean value, which represents the behaviour of the most common or average particle. The width of zone gets increased as it migrates down the column, because more time is needed for migration to take place. Hence, the zone width is directly related to the residence or retention time on the column and inversely proportional to the mobile phase velocity. If the best use of a chromatographic column is to be made, a study of the factors that determine the time of retention of a molecule by either phase and the factors that decide zone spreading must be made.

Now if we increase velocity of the mobile phase, then the efficiency may increase or decrease $(\downarrow_{se})$ depending on the components.

This theory explains the effect of rate of flow of mobile phase on zone broadening.

Now HETP = h = measure of separation efficiency.

The concept here is same as plate theory so if value of HETP is less, then greater will be the separation efficiency.

Van Deemter observed that with increase in h, zone broadening or spreading of solute concentration increases.

Zone broadening is simply width increasing factor.

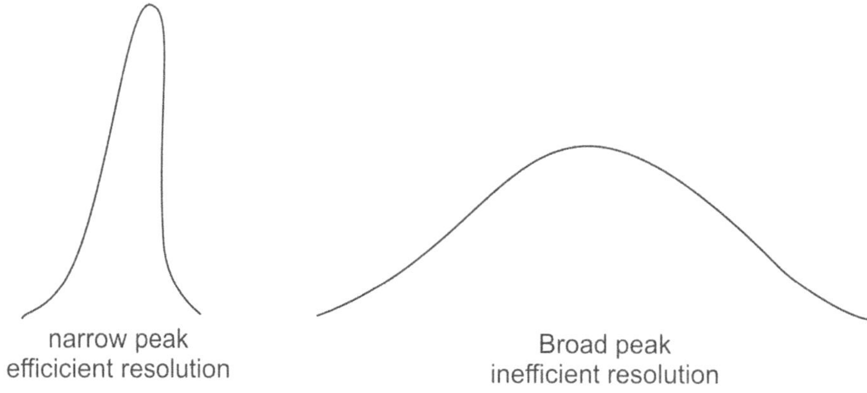

Fig. 1.21

Zone broadening is represented by H (or h), as width of peak increases broad zone also increases.

So, h should be as low as possible, because h has inverse relationship with separation efficiency.

$$\text{Separation efficiency } \alpha \ \frac{1}{\text{zone broadening}}$$

$$\text{and Separation efficiency } \alpha \ \frac{1}{H}$$

$\Rightarrow$ H α zone broadening and as width of peak (W) increases, broad zone also increases.

$$\left.\begin{array}{l} H \ \alpha \text{ zone broadening} \\ \therefore h \ \alpha \ w \end{array}\right\} \text{Zone broadening } \alpha \text{ width}$$

Now,

$$h = \frac{L}{n}$$

$$\Rightarrow \qquad h \,\alpha\, \frac{1}{n} \text{ and } h \,\alpha\, W$$

$$\Rightarrow \qquad h \,\alpha\, \frac{w}{n}$$

and

$$w \,\alpha\, \frac{1}{n}$$

$$n = 16\left(\frac{t}{w}\right)^2$$

if $h \rightarrow \uparrow$ *increases*

$w \rightarrow \uparrow$ *increases*

$n \rightarrow \uparrow$ *increases*

S.E $\rightarrow \uparrow$ *increases*

So, the theory depends on the value of h, hence it is also named as "zone broadening phenomena" or "zone broadening factor". And h is mainly concern with the speed of mobile phase that affects the separation efficiency and also with stationary phase.

Van-Deemter Equation

OR

Sources of zone broadening

Mathematical representation of this theory is known as Van-Deemter equation.

$$H = A + \frac{B}{\mu} + C\mu$$

Chromatographic peaks are generally broadened by three kinetically controlled process

(i) Eddy diffusion factor

(ii) Longitudinal diffusion factor

(iii) Non-equilibrium mass transfer factor

The magnitude of these effects are determined by such controllable variables as flow rate, particle size of packing, diffusion rates and thickness of the stationary phase.

The Van-Deemter equation was derived for gas-liquid chromatography; it provides an approximate relationship between the flow rate n of the mobile phase and the plate height H. A, B, C are constants which depends upon the properties of stationary and mobile phase. Here, the quantity A is associated with eddy diffusion, B with longitudinal diffusion and C with non-equilibrium mass transfer.

If A, B, C or μ are more or less, we have corresponding effect on H.

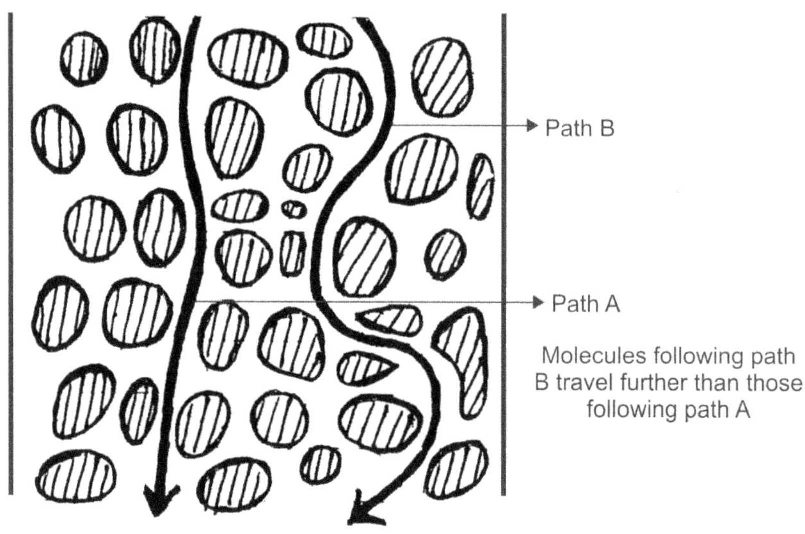

Fig. 1.22

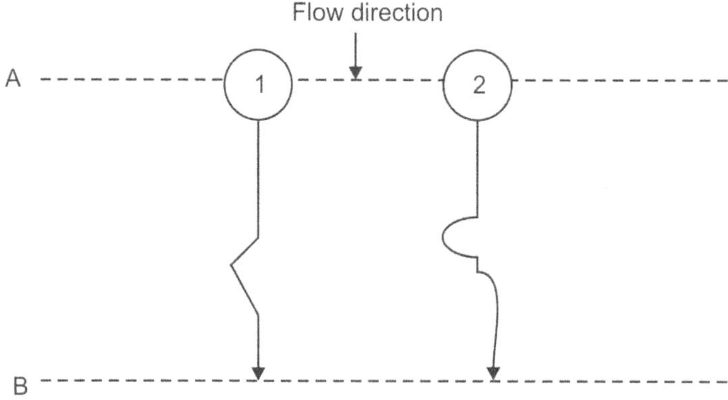

Fig. 1.22 (a)

Typical pathways of two solute molecules during elution. Note that distance travelled by molecule 2 is greater than the travelled by molecule 1. Thus, molecule 2 would arrive at B later than molecule 1.

Eddy Diffusion

Zone broadening from eddy diffusion is the result of the multitude of pathways by which a molecule can find its way through a packed column. As shown in above figure, the length of these pathways differ, thus, the residence times in the column for molecules of the same species are also variable. Solute molecules thus do not emerge simultaneously from the column; a broadening of the elution band results.

So, it is directly related to flow of mobile phase.

Mobile phase can flow in two types

(i) Turbulent flow [turbulent: uncontrolled/violent]

(ii) Laminar flow / streamline flow

In chromatography, laminar flow of mobile phase is seen.

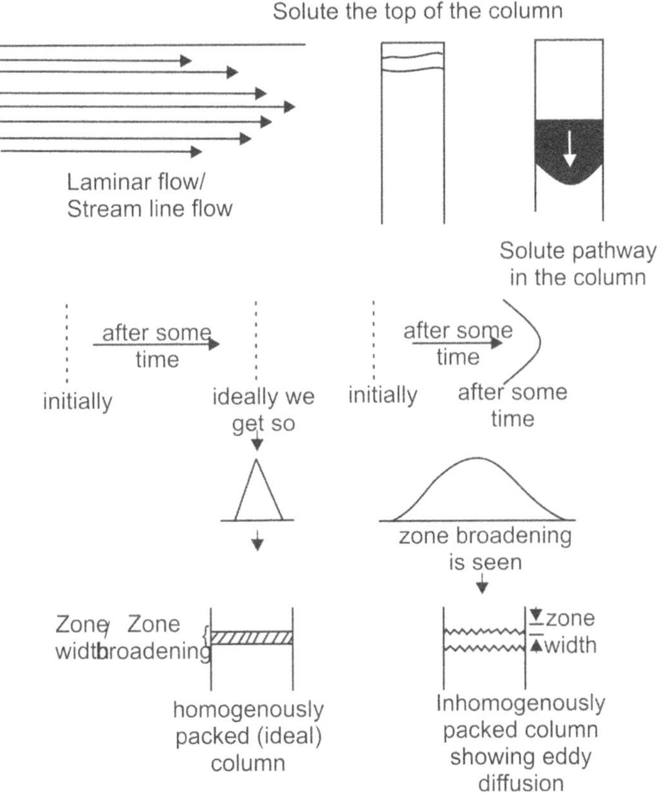

Fig. 1.23

In the stream line flow, mobile phase molecules at periphery move slower and molecules at the middle/centre moves faster than those at the periphery.

A is common in chromatography.

It is independent of the velocity of the mobile phase (μ)

So due to $A \rightarrow A \uparrow increases \rightarrow HETP \uparrow increases$

Zone broadening/band broadening occurs and so → separation efficiency decreases.

Here solute molecules are carried by solvent so we don't get an ideal peak such as ∧, instead we get such inhomogeneous peak due to such flow, so that H increases and separation efficiency decreases.

The quantity A in equation describes the effect of eddy diffusion and can be related to particle size, geometry and tightness of packing of the stationary phase. As a first approximation A is independent of flow rate.

Logitudinal diffusion / Normal / Natural Diffusion Factor

Diffusion is natural property of substance which spread in all direction and is directly proportional to concentration gradient

Spreading of solute from higher concentration to lower concentration is generally called the natural or normal diffusion.

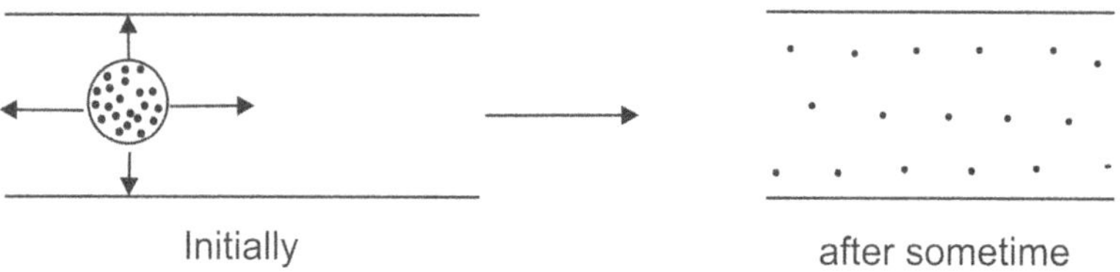

Fig. 1.24

Diffusion occurs generally in all directions.

Diffusion α time

If time is more, diffusion/spreading will be more.

Because of diffusion, we have zone broadening.

If the velocity of mobile phase (μ) increases

$\Downarrow$

Available time with solute is less

$\Downarrow$

Spreading or longitudinal diffusion is less

$\Downarrow$

H/h is less and hence B is less

$\Downarrow$

Zone broadening is less

$\Downarrow$

Separation efficiency increases

And if the velocity of mobile phase $\downarrow$ *decreases*

$\Downarrow$

Available time with solute is more

$\Downarrow$

Spreading is more

$\Downarrow$

B is more

$\Downarrow$

h/H is more

$\Downarrow$

Zone broadening is more

$\Downarrow$

Separation efficiency is less

Thus, with reference to longitudinal diffusion factor i.e., B;

Separation efficiency α velocity of mobile phase (μ)

Logitudinal diffusion results from the tendency of molecules to migrate from the concentrated center part of a band toward more dilute regions on either side. This type of diffusion, which can occur in both the mobile and stationary phase, causes further band broadening. Logitudinal diffusion is most important where the mobile phase is a gas, because diffusion rates in gases are several order of magnitude greater than those in liquids. The amount of diffusion increases with time; thus, the extent of broadening increases as the flow rate decreases.

So, the second term (the longitudinal term, is inversely proportional to flow rate.

$$\Rightarrow B \, \alpha \, \frac{1}{\mu}$$

Non-Equilibrium Mass Transfer

Chromatographic bands are also broadened because the flow of the mobile phase is ordinarily so rapid that true equilibrium between phases cannot be realised. For example, at the front of the zone, where the mobile phase encounters fresh stationary phase, equilibrium is not instantly achieved, and solute is therefore carried some what further down the column than would be expected under true equilibrium conditions. Similarly at the end of the zone, solutes in the stationary phase encounter fresh mobile phases. Again the rate of transfer of solute molecules is not instaneous; thus, the tail of zone is more drawn out than it would be if time existed for equilibrations. The net effect is a broadening at both ends of the solute band.

The effects of non-equilibrium mass transfer become smaller as the flow rate is decreased because more time is available for equilibrium to be approached. Further-more, a closer approach to true equilibrium is to be expected if the channels through which the mobile phase flows are narrow so that solute molecules do not have far to diffuse in order to reach the stationary phase. For the same reason, the layers of immobilised liquid on a stationary phase should be as thin as possible.

The last term is equation which is of considerable importance at high flow rates of a gaseous mobile phase, describes the effect of non-equilibrium on band broadening .

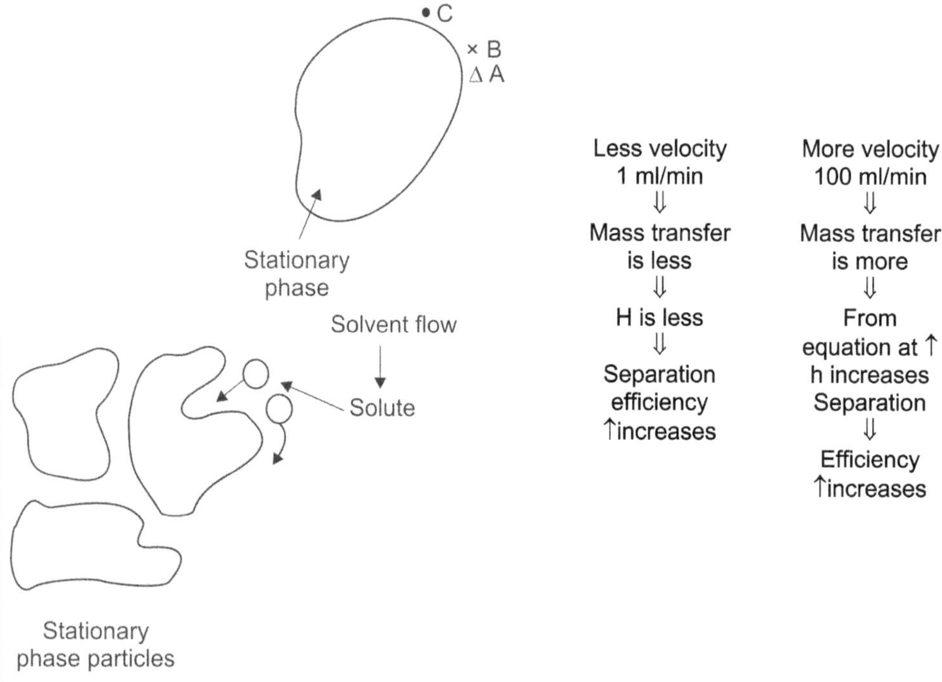

Fig. 1.25

So, as mass transfer increases ⇒ HETP/h/H also increases so zone broadening increases and so separation efficiency decreases.

Thus, with reference to mass transfer factor C,

$$C \propto \mu$$

$$\Rightarrow S.E \propto \frac{1}{C} \qquad [\because H \propto C \;\&\; S.E \propto \frac{1}{H}]$$

$$\Rightarrow S.E \propto \frac{1}{\mu}$$

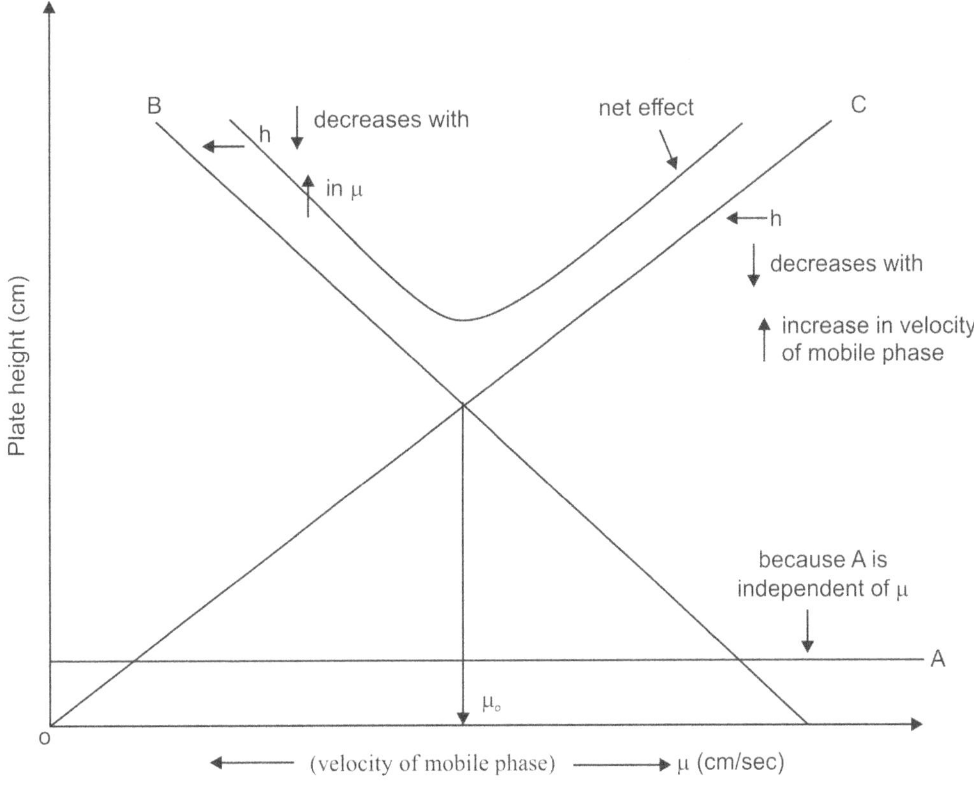

Fig. 1.26

Effect of variables in equation on plate height

So, from the graph,

A is independent of velocity of mobile phase so with reference to A → H remains constant.

B is inversely related to velocity of mobile phase. So, with reference to B, if μ ↑ *increases*, H ↓ *decreases* separation efficiency ↑ *increases.*

C is directly proportional to velocity of mobile phase. So, with reference to C, H ↑ *increases* with ↑ *increases* in μ. So, ↓ *decrease* in separation efficiency.

So, μ_o is the best to give highest separation efficiency.

Net effect of zone broadening

Graph shows the contribution of each term in the Van Deemter equation as a function of mobile phase velocity as well as their net effect on H. Clearly, the optimum efficiency is realised at a flow rate corresponding to the minimum is the solid curve. Experimental curves of this type permit evaluation of A, B, C for any column. Such data provide hints for improving the performance of a given type of packing.

The Van Deemter equation provides only a first approximation of plate height, and several modifications have been developed that give a more precise description of variables effecting column efficiency.

Separation on column

The discussion thus far has focused upon the efficiency of a chromatographic column, that is, how many plates it contains.

(III) Random-Walk Theory

OR

Non-Equillibrium Theory

OR

Gidding Theory

According to this theory solute molecules move randomly, so perfect equilibrium is not there.

Random walk of solute molecules make the spreading (and increase zone broadening).

More the distance travelled by the molecules, more will be the spreading.

$$\sigma = \sqrt{hL} \quad \text{Gidding equation.}$$

where

h = HETP

L = Total length of chromatographic system

σ = Standard deviation of infinite obstacles (measurement of spreading)

If H is more → σ is more → spreading more → separation efficiency is less.

Because σ is more

⇓

Zone broadening is high

If σ is less → zone broadening less → separation effi ciency will be high.

If σ value is very low, compounds can be separated easily.

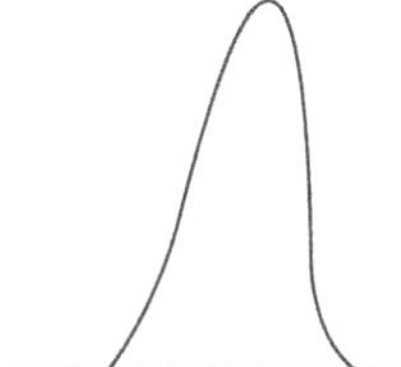

If σ value is very high, then 10 or more compounds can't be separated easily.

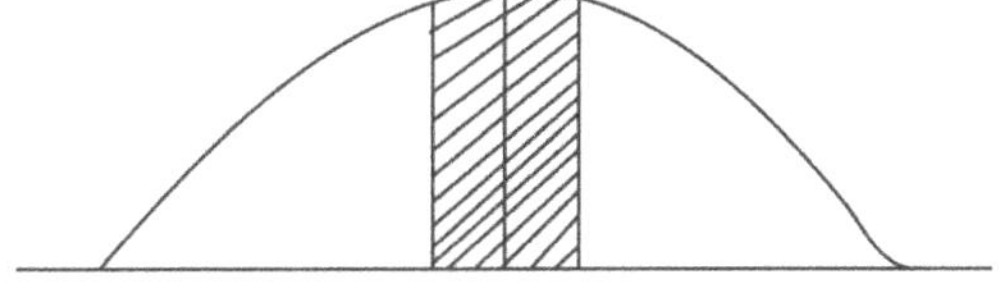

Fig. 1.27

Our aim is to cover 68% area of the curve.

Retention Mechanism

It indicates how different solutes are retained by stationary phase

Mobile phase moves ahead and stationary phase binds different solute with different strength.

i.e., more tightly bound solute moves slowly.

Due to differential migration, we achieve separation.

Partitioning

For this mechanism, both stationary and mobile phase must be in liquid form. Hence Liquid–liquid chromatography (LLC) takes place, because both the liquid phases must be immiscible with each other.

Liquid liquid chromatography is similar in principle to solvent extraction; it based upon the distribution of solute molecules between two immiscible liquid phases according to their relative solubilities. The separating medium consists of a finely divied inert support (e.g. Silica gel, Kieselguhr) holding a fixed (stationary) liquid phase, and separation is achieved by passing a mobile phase over the stationary phase. The stationary phase may be in form of a packed column, a thin layer on glass, or on a paper strip.

It is convenient to divide LLC into two categories, based on the relative polarities of the stationary and mobile phases.

***Normal LLC / Normal Phase / NP*:** The term 'normal LLC' is used when the stationary phase is polar and the mobile phase is non-polar.

Generally all organic solvents are non-polar and at the time of investigation there was an understanding that mobile phase must be organic liquid (non-polar). So, when mobile phase is any organic liquid, it is called the normal phase chromatography.

***The main principle of NP LLC*:** In this case the solute elution order is based on the principle that non-polar solutes prefer the mobile phase and elute earlier whereas polar solutes prefer the stationary phase and elute later.

***Reverse-phase chromatography*:** The term **'Reverse LLC'** is used when the stationary phase is non polar (organic solvent) and the mobile phase is polar (water).

***The main principle of RP-LLC/RPC*:** Here the solute elution order is commonly the reverse of that observed in LLC, i.e., polar compounds elute earlier and non-polar compounds elute later.

This (RPC) is a popular mode (mechanism) of operation due to its versatility and scope. It is more used and more advanced method.

Now-a-days, more than 70% analysis in pharcacopoiea are carried out by RP.

This is the popular mode of operation due to its versatility and Scope : the almost universal application of RPC arises because nearly all organic molecules have hydrophobic regions in their structure and are therefore capable of interacting with the non-polar stationary phase, means organic which is not containing or devoid of water so hydrobholic solute molecules will interact with it.

Since the mobile phase in RPC is polar and commonly contains water, the method is particularly suited to the separation of polar substances which are either insoluble in organic solvents or bind too strongly to solid adsorbents (LSC) for successful elution.

The table shows some typical stationary and mobile phases which are used in normal and reverse-phase chromatography.

Stationary Phases	*Mobile Phases*
Normal-phase	
B, β^1 – oxydipropionitrite	*Saturated hydrocarbons, e.g. hexane, heptane*
Cyanoethyl silicone Carbowax (400, 600, 750 etc)	*mixed with upto 10% dioxin, methanol, ethanol, chloroform, methylene chloride (dichloromethare)*
Glycols (ethylene, diethylenes)	
Reverse – phase	
Squalane	*water and alcohol-water mixtures, acetonitrite and acetonitrile water mixture.*
Zipax-HCP	
Cyanoethylsilicone	

Problem that occur with RPC: *Although the stationary and mobile phases in LLC are chosen to have as little solubility in one as possible, even slight solubility of the stationary phase in the mobile phase may result in the slow removal of the stationary phase as the mobile phase flows over the column support. For this reason the mobile phase must be presaturated with stationary phase before entering the column. The precolumn should contain a large-particle packing (e.g. 30-60 mesh silica gel) coated with a high percentage (30-40%) of the stationary phase to be used in the chromatographic column. As the mobile phase passes through the precolumn, it becomes saturated with stationary phase before entering the chromatographic column.*

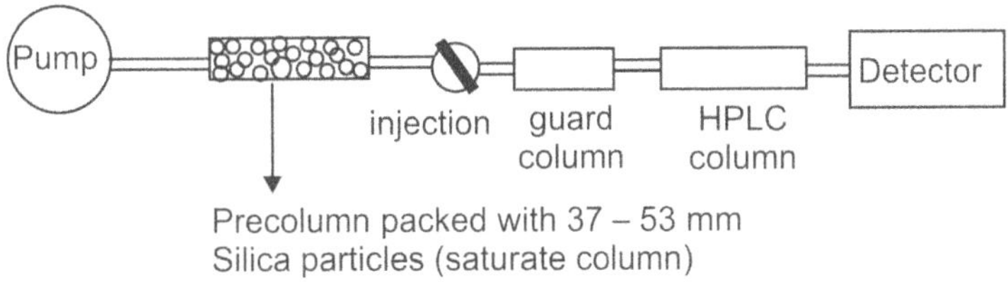

Fig. 1.28

The support materials for the stationary phase can be relatively inactive supports, e.g., glass beads, or absorbents similar to those in LSC. It is important that the support surface should not interact with the solute, as this can produce a mix mechanism (partition and adsorption) rather than true partition. This complicates the chromatographic process and may give non reproducible separations. For this reason, high loadings of liquid phase are required to cover the active sites when using porous adsorbents with a high surface area.

To overcome some of the problems associated with conventional LLC, such as loss of stationary phase from the support material, the stationary phase may be chemically bonded to support the material. This form of chromatography in which both monomeric and polymeric phases have been bonded to a wide range of support materials, is called bonded phase chromatography.

Silylation reactions have been widely used to prepare bonded phases. The silanol groups ($\rightarrow$ Si – OH) at the surface of silica gel are reacted with substituted chlorosilanes. A typical example is the reaction of silica with a dimethyl chlorosilane which produces a monomeric bonded phase, since each molecule of the silylating agent can react with only one silanol group:

$$\equiv Si{-}OH + Cl{-}Si(CH_3)_2{-}R \longrightarrow \equiv Si{-}O{-}Si(CH_3)_2{-}R + HCl$$

The use if di or tri chlorosilanes in the presence of moisture can cause a polymeric layer to be formed at the silica surface, i.e., a polymeric bonded phase. But monomeric bonded phases are preferred since they are easier to manufacture reproducibly than the polymeric type. The nature of the main chromatographic interaction can be varied by changing the characteristics of the functional group R ; in analytical HPLC the most important bonded phase is non-polar C-18 type in which the modifying group R is an Octadeayl hydro-carbon chain. Unreacted silanol groups are capable of absorbing polar molecules and will therefore affect the chromatographic properties of the bonded phase, sometimes producing underirable effects such as tailing in RPC. These effects can be minimised by the process of end-caping in which these silanol groups are rendered inactive by reaction with trimethylchlorosilane.

$$\equiv Si{-}OH + Cl{-}Si(CH_3)_2{-}CH_3 \longrightarrow \equiv Si{-}O{-}Si(CH_3)_2{-}CH_3$$

An important property of these siloxane phase in their stability under the conditions used in most chromatographic separations ; the siloxane bonds are attracted only in very acidic (pH < 2) or basic (pH > 9) conditions. A large number of commercial bonded phase packings are available in particle size suitable for HPLC.

Partitioning: ***(short)***

For this mechanism, mobile phase and stationary phase must be liquid and immiscible with each other.

For these two immiscible liquids one must be polar and other must be non-polar.

If mobile phase is non-polar/organic solvent and stationary phase is polar, the chromatographic system is known as "Non-polar phase".

- *In reverse phase*

  Mobile phase : Polar

  Stationary phase : Non – polar

- *Now-a-days, RP is more used in advanced method.*

  $V_R = V_M + KV_s$

  where $K = \dfrac{C_s}{C_M}$

  K = Partitioning co-efficient of solvent

  $K \uparrow$ *increases* $\Rightarrow V_R \uparrow$ *increases*

  $K \downarrow$ *decreases* $\Rightarrow V_R \downarrow$ *decreases* $\Rightarrow$ *comes first*

- *In partitioning mechanism, both phases are liquids.*
- *Liquid stationary phase can't itself be stable, so along with mobile phase it starts moving.*
- *To overcome this difficulty, we have made two approaches*

  (i) Solid support

  (ii) chemically bounded liquid

  (i) Solid support

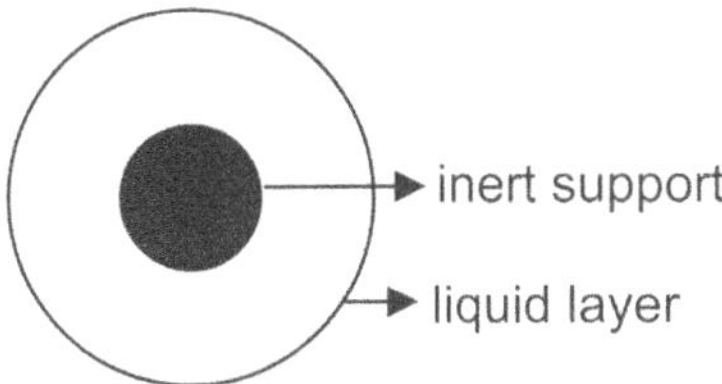

Fig. 1.29

- *Binding is simple physical binding*
- *Mobile phase is constantly moving so there is possibility that stationary phase can also start movement.*

- *Movement of stationary phase with mibile phase is called "leaching" or "bleeding".*
- *This is unwanted phenomena and it occurs more or less in all types of chromatographic systems.*
- *In HiLC, where pressure of mobile phase is extremely high, the process of leaching also becomes extremely high.*
- *This problem can be overcome by "Chemically bounded stationary phase" normally it is covalently bounded and so it is not possible to break them.*
- *Thus, chemically bonded liquid is stable and free from leaching.*

Advantages of chemically bonded stationary phase

Glass beads are taken and on glass, there are certain free hydroxyl groups are present.

Step I

glass —OH + Cl—Si(CH3)(CH3)—Cl

Step II $+ H_2O \downarrow - HCl$

glass—O—Si(CH3)(CH3)—OH

Step I

Cl—Si(R)(R)—Cl

Repeated n times

Step II H_2O

glass—O—Si(CH3)(CH3)—OH

↓ *–HCl*

$$Cl-Si(CH_3)_2-CH_3$$

$$\text{glass}-O-Si(CH_3)_2-O\quad -SP(R)_2-O\quad -Si(CH_3)_2-CH_3$$

Where R = any alkyl group. So, this is tailor made compound. Generally 18 c long chain compound is used.

Which is

C_{18} i.e. : $CH_2\,(CH_2)_{16}\,CH_3$

: Octadecyl stationary phase

- *This is very popular stationary phase used in drug analysis in pharmacopoiea.*
- *This is RP system, because C_{18} (stationary phase) is non polar so mobile phase is water.*

R can be C_8 also

Octachain

Another standard phase popular in pharmacopoeia

R =

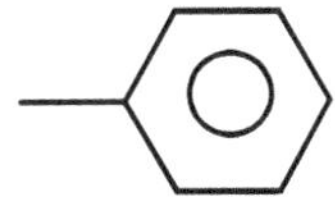

R = esters or ethers or amides

Thus, we can make any type of stationary phase by changing R. So, these are tailor molecules.

$$\left.\begin{array}{l} R = CH_3CH_2CH_2NH_2 \\ R = CH_3CH_2CH_2C = N \end{array}\right\} \text{highly polar}$$

As advanced analytical method,

RP chemical bonded stationary phase, in HPLC is used.

Characteristics of support

- *Support must be containing very fine particles for greater surface area.*
- *It should be insoluble in both stationary and mobile phase.*
- *it should be cololurless*
- *It should be chemically inert*
- *Characteristics of support is defined in terms of available surface area, say, ($5m^2/gm$).*
- *Mostly used support is "Diatomaceous Earth" which is the powder of skeleton of living system Diatomes (creatures). It has surface area of about $4m^2/gm$.*
- *Other support is "Silica gel" which is highly purified sand, it is manually made so we can ↑increase or ↓decrease its surface area as per our requirements.*

II Adsorption

- *Adsorption is a physical phenomenon.*
- *In this mechanism, stationary phase must be solid which must be an adsorbent and mobile phase must be liquid/gas.*

Ideal Requirements of solid stationary phase

(i) *Must have greater surface area.*

(ii) *It should adsorb different adsorbate differentially.*

(iii) *Adsorption of solute should be reversible (should adsorb and desorb the solute very easily).*

(iv) *It should be inert to mobile phase and also to the solute.*

(v) *Adsorbant should provide suitable flowrate to mobile phase.*

(vi) Adsorption property should be reproducible i.e., for long time, it should remain same.

- *The solute with low k value will not get adsorbed so much and so comes out first.*

From the fundamental equation of chromatography

$$V_R = V_o + KV_s$$

Where,

$$K = \text{adsorption co-efficient}$$

- *So, the solute with high K value will get absorbed more strongly and hence will come out lastly.*
- *Where as the solute with low K value will not get adsorbed so much and so it will come out first.*

Types of Adsorption isotherm

(i) Linear adsorption isotherm

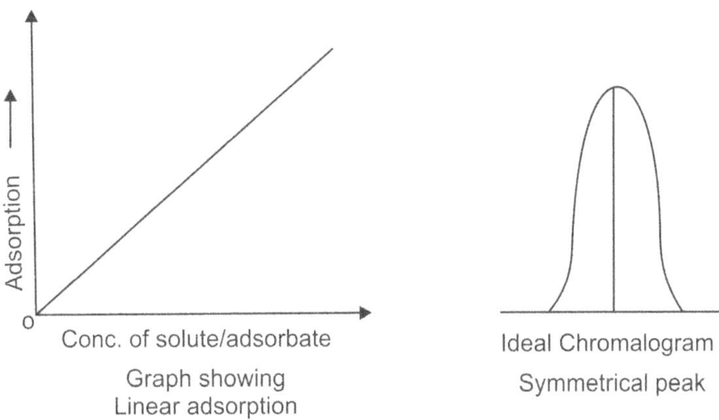

Fig. 1.30

Adsorption: *It is defined as amount of adsorbate adsorbed per unit quantity of adsorbent.*

Here Adsorption $\propto$ Concentration of adsorbate.

(ii) Langomuir adsorption isotherm

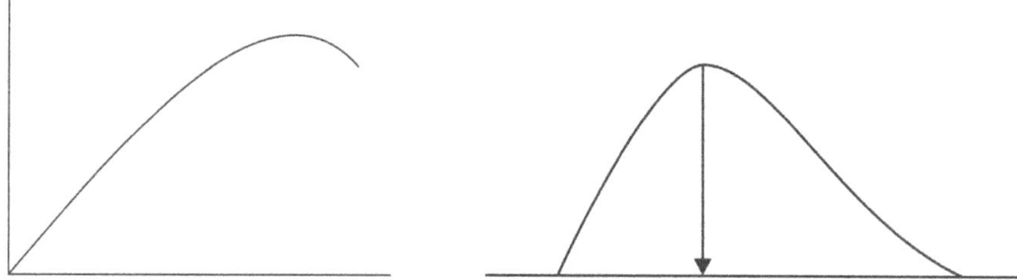

Asymmetrical Chromatogram is obtained

Fig. 1.31

- *It is very common practically*
- *After certain limit of concentration of solute, linearity is not seen ⇒ insufficient separation.*

(iii) Freundlich adsorption isotherm

- *There is no linear relationship between concentration of adsorbate and its adsorption, so asymmetrical chromatogram is observed.*

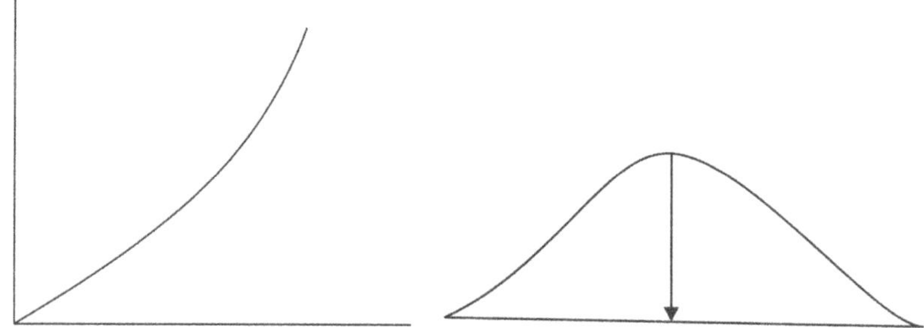

Asymmetrical Chromatography.

Fig. 1.32

To minimise this asymetricity, modified mobile phase is used.

The most important requirements for efficient chromatography in different mechanisms are :

(A) Adsorption mechanism

(i) It should have high surface area

- *as all interactions are directly related to surface area, if particle size is small higher will be the surface area.*

- *in modern chromatography, particles of few μm size is used.*
- *in ultrahigh pressure chromatography ⇒ < 1 μm particle size is used.*

(ii) Adsorption should be reversible and differentially: *not desired if all solute get adsorbed permanently and firmly.*

(iii) Adsorbent should be chemically inert, means it should not interact with solute molecules and change its properties.

(iv) It should be colourless and give reproducibility.

List of adsorbents in order of decreasing adsorption strength

I Diatomaceous earth

II Fuller's earth

III Activated charcoal

IV Activated alumina

V Activated salicylic acid

VI Magnesium oxide

VII $CaCO_3$

VIII K_2CO_3

IX Talc

X Starch weakly bounded (minimum adsorption power)

Limitations of adsorption mechanism

(i) Number of adsorbents are found which modify drug molecules.

Eg: *Alumina is weakly basic so it causes hydrolysis of number of drugs specially of ester.*

(ii) Number of drugs get decomposed or neutralized.

Eg : *Activated charcoal causes oxidation of some solute molecules.*

So adsorption mechanism is very rarely used.

It is popular in the analysis of gaseous compounds i.e., O_2*, laughing gas.*

B. Mobile Phase

- *Solvents are classified on the bases of two parameters.*
  - *(i) Strength*
  - *(ii) Selectivity*

(i) **Strength:** *It refers to capacity of solvent to take ahead solute for longer distance. This property is termed as elution power.*

Poor solvent → not making solute to move easily.

Polarity of solvent and strength.

$$Strength \propto Polarity$$

(ii) **Selectivity:** *It refers to capacity of solvent to separate closely related solutes*

If solute is highly polar → selectivity is less.

$$Selectivity \propto \frac{1}{\text{Polarity}}$$

Classification of solvents on selectivity – (Lowest Selectivity and Highest Strength)

↓ Decreasing order:

(i) *Petroleum ether*

(ii) CCl_4

(iii) CS_2

(iv) *Acetone*

(v) *Benzene*

(vi) *Toluene*

(vii) *Diethyl ether*

(viii) $CHCl_3$

(ix) *Ethanol*

(x) *Water*

(xi) *Pyridine*

(xii) *Carboxylic acid*

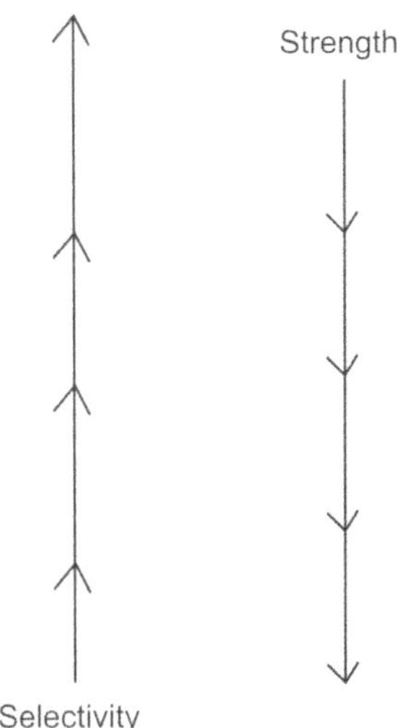

Fig. 1.33

- *Liquid–Solid Chromatography, often called adsoption chromatography, is based on interaction between, the solute and fixed active sites on a finely divided solid adsorbent used as the stationary phase.*
- *The adsorbent may be packed in a column or spread on a plate (as in TLC); it is generally an active solid with a high surface area, e.g., alumina, charcoal or silica gel, silica gel is the most widely used.*
- *A practical consideration is that highly active absorbents may give rise to irreversible solute adsorption; silica gel, which is slightly acidic may strongly retain basic compounds, whereas alumina (non-acid washed) is basic and should not be used for the chromatography of base sensitive compounds. Adsorbents of varying particle size perhaps down to 5 μm for HPLC, may be purchased commercially.*

The role of the solvent in LSC is clearly vital since mobile phase molecules (solvent) compete with solute molecules for polar adsorption sites. The stronger the interaction between the mobile phase and the stationary phase, the wernt the solute adsoption, and vice versa. The classification of solvents according to their strength of adsorption is called an eluotropic series, which may be used as a guide to find the optimum solvent strength for a particular separation; a trial-and error approach however, required and this is done more rapidly by TLC than by using a column technique. Solvent purity is very important in LSC since water and other polar impurities may significantly affect column performance, and the presence of UV-type detectors.

In general, the compounds best separated by LSC are those which are soluble in organic solvents and are non-ionic. Water soluble non-ionic compounds are better separated using either reverse phase or bonded-phase chromatography.

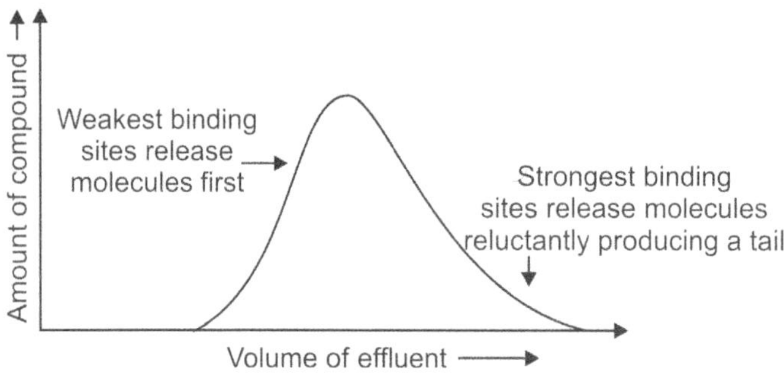

Fig. 1.34

"Tailing" observed in the elution of a compound from an adsorption column.

- *Adsorbent may be described as a solid which has property of holding molecules at its surface, particularly when it is porous and finely divided.*

CHAPTER 2

COLUMN CHROMATOGRAPHY

When a column of stationary phase is used, the technique is called as column chromatography, the oldest method discovered by Russian scientist Tswett.

- Based on the nature of stationary phase, i.e whether it is solid or liquid, it is called adsorption chromatography or column chromatography.
- Most of the discussions here will be devoted to column adsorption chromatography, since column partition chromatography is not being used widely.

Principle

A solid stationary phase and a liquid mobile phase is used and the principle of separation is adsorption. When a mixture of components dissolved in the mobile phase is introduced into the column, the individual components move with different rates depending upon their relative affinities. The compound with lesser affinity towards the stationary phase (adsorbent) moves faster and hence is eluted out of the column first. The one with greater affinity toward the stationary phase (adsorbent) moves slower down the coloumn and hence it is eluted later. Thus the compounds are separated. The type of interaction between the stationary phase (adsorbent) and the solute is reversible in nature. The rate of movement of a component (R) is given as follows:

$$R = \frac{\text{Rate of movement of a component in stationary phase}}{\text{Distance moved by the solvent}}$$

This equation can be simplified as follows.

$$R = \frac{\text{Distance moved by the solute}}{\text{Distance moved by the solvent}}$$

When a liquid mobile phase is used, the equation is written as

$$R = \frac{A_m}{A_m + \alpha A_s}$$

where α is the partition co-efficient

$$\alpha = \frac{\text{Concentration in stationary phase}}{\text{Concentration in mobile phase}}$$

A_m is the average cross section of mobile phase

A_s is the average cross section of stationary phase

Types of adsorbents

Based upon their adsorbent activity, they can be classified as weak, medium and strong adsorbents.

Weak	Medium	Strong
Sucrose	$CaCO_3$	Activated Mg Silicate (Silica gel)
Starch	$Ca_3(PO_4)_2$	Activated alumina
Inulin	$MgCO_3$	Activated charcoal
Talc	MgO	Activated Magnesia
Na_2CO_3	$Ca(OH)_2$	Fuller's earth

The most commonly used adsorbent is silica gel of 80-100 mesh or 100-200 mesh size which has a particle size of 60-200 μ.

Selection of Stationary phase

The success of chromatography depends upon the proper selection of stationary phase. The selection of stationary phase in column chromatography depends on the following:

(i) ***Removal of impurities*:** When a small quantity of impurity is present and there is difference in affinity when compared to major component, a weak adsorbent is sufficient.

(ii) ***No. of components to be separated*:** When few components are to be separated, weak adsorbent is used. When more components are to be separated a strong adsorbent is selected.

(iii) ***Affinity differences between components*:** When components have similar affinities, a strong absorbent will be effective. When there is more difference in affinities, a weak adsorbent is selected.

(iv) ***Length of the column used*:** When a shorter column is used, strong adsorbate has to be used. When a longer column is used, a weak adsorbent can be used.

(v) ***Quantity of adsorbent used*:** 20 or 30 times the weight of the adsorbate is used for effective separation.

Adsorbate : adsorbent ratio = 1 : 20 or 1 : 30.

Mobile Phase

Mobile phase is very important and they serve several functions. They act as solvent, developer and as eluent. The function of a mobile phase are :

- To introduce the mixture into the column – as solvent.
- To develop the zones for separation.
- As developing agent.
- To remove pure component out of the column – as eluent.

***Different mobile phases used*:** (in increasing order of polarity or elution strength).

Petrolium ether, carbon tetrachloride, Cyclohexane, carbondisulphide, ether, Acetone, Benzene, Toluene, esters (ethyl acetate), water, pyridine, organic acids (Acitic acid etc.), mixture of acids or bases with ethanol or pyridine etc.

These solvents can be used in either pure form or as mixtures of solvents of varying compositions.

Column Characteristics

The material of the column is mostly good quality neutral glass since it should not be affected by solvents, acids or alkalies. An ordinary burette can also be used as column for separation.

- The column dimensions are important for effective column dimensions are important for effective column separations. The length : diameter ratio ranges from 10 : 1 to 30 : 1.
- For more efficiency, the length : diameter ratio can be 100 : 1.
- The length of the column depends upon:

  Affinity of compounds towards the adsorbent used.

  Number of compounds to be separated.

  Type of adsorbent used

  Quatity of the sample.

- Better separation will be obtained with a long, narrow column than short thick column because number of plates will be more. But if the column is too long, flow rate is affected.

Preparation of the Column

The bottom portion of the column is packed with cotton wool or glass wool or may contain an asbestos pad, above which the column of adsorbent is packed.

- The Whatman filter paper disc can also be used.
- After packing the column with the adsorbent, a similar paper disc is kept on the top, so that the adsorbent layer is not disturbed during the introduction of sample or mobile phase. Disturbance in the layer of adsorbent will lead to irregular bands in separation.
- There are two types of preparing the column, which are called as packing techniques. They are :
  (i) Dry filling/packing technique
  (ii) wet filling/packing technique
- Column should be free from any impurity, so before using column, it should be washed properly and then dry it completely.
- Before filling column with stationary phase, support of cotton/glass wool is kept.
- Filling should not have air gaps.
- It should be uniformly filled/not uneven.

(i) ***Dry Packing technique*:** In this technique, the required quantity of adsorbent is packed in the column in dry form and the solvent allowed to flow through the column till equilibrium is reached.

- The demerit with this technique is that air bubbles are entrapped between the solvent and the stationary phase and the column may not be uniformly packed.
- Cracks appear in the adsorbent present in the column. Hence uniformity in flow characteristic and clear bond of the separated component may not be obtained.
- After filling tapping can be done to remove void spaces.

(ii) ***Wet packing techniques*:** This is the ideal technique.

- The required quantity of the adsorbent is mixed with the mobile phase solvent in a beaker in the form of suspension/slurry and then is poured into the column.

- The stationary phase settles uniformly in the column and there is no entrapment of air bubbles. There will not be any crack in the column of adsorbent.
- So, here solid settle down while the solvent remains upward.
- This solvent is removed then again cotton plug is placed.
- Now the column is ready for separation and the band eluted from the column will be ideal for separation.
- generally, wet filling technique is preferred as there is no entrapment of air bubbles and no crack in the column of adsorbent.

Introduction of the Sample

The sample which is usually a mixture of components is dissolved in minimum quantity of the mobile phase used for preparing the column or a solvent of minimum polarity. The entire sample is introduced into the column at once and gets adsorbed on the top portion of the column. From this zone, the individual sample can be separated by a process of elution.

Definitions

(i) ***Elution*:** Passing of mobile phase through a stationary phase for separation.

(ii) ***Eluent*:** It is the solvent used to separate mixture of components (mobile phase).

(iii) ***Elute*:** Desired solute taken out from the chromatographic column using elution.

Development Technique (Elution)

After the introduction of the sample, by elution techniques, the individual components are separated out from the column. The two techniques are :

(i) *Isocratic elution technique* : (iso means same or similar)

(ii) *Gradient elution technique* : (Gradient means gradually).

(i) ***Isocratic elution technique*:** (iso means same or similar) : In this elution technique, the same solvent amposition or solvent of the same polarity is used throughout the process of separation.

e.g: Chloroform only, petroleum ether : Benzene = 1 : 1 only, etc.

(ii) ***Gradient elution technique*: (Gradent means gradually) :** In this elution technique, solvents gradually increasing polarity or increasing elution strength are used during the process of separation. Initially low polar solvent is used followed by gradually increasing the polarity to a more polar solvent.

e.g.: Initially Benzene, then chloroform, the Ethyl acetate, then to Methanol, etc.

Other techniques like frontal analysis and displacement analysis where a graph of concentration of elute Vs volume of eluate will give an idea how compounds are eluted out from the column.

Detection of Components

The detection of coloured components can be done visually. Different coloured bands are seen moving down the column which can be collected separately. But for colourless compounds, the technique depends upon the properties of the components. Different properties which can be used are.

(i) Adsorption of light (UV/Vis)

(ii) Flourescence or light emission characteristics : using fluorescence detector.

(iii) By using flame ionisation detector.

(iv) Evaporation of solvent and weighing the residue.

(v) By monitoring the fractions by thin layer chromatography.

Any of the above techniques can be used for detection of compounds and hence it can be used for qualitative analysis and for isolation of compounds.

Recovery of Components

Earlier, recovery of the components was done by cutting the column into several distinct zones. Later, extrusion of the column into zones was done by using plunger.

- The best technique is to recover the components by a process called as elution. The components are called as eluate, the solvent called as eluent and the process of removing the components from the column is called as elution.
- Recovery is done by collecting as different fractions of mobile phase of equal volume like 10 ml, 20 ml, etc., or unequal volume.
- They can also be collected time wise i.e., a fraction every 10 or 20 minutes etc.
- The recovered fractions are detected by using the techniques discussed earlier.
- Similar fractions are mixed so that the bulk of the compound of each type is obtained in a pure form.
- If a fraction, still contains several components, it can be resolved by using another column.

***Factors affecting column efficiency*:** For any separation, efficiency of the column is important. Unless the factors affecting the column efficiency are known, efficiency cannot be improved. They are :

(i) ***Dimensions of the column*:** A length : diameter ratio of 20: 1 or 30 : 1 are ideal. But for improving the efficiency, 100 : 1 may be more satisfactory.

(ii) ***Particle size of the adsorbent*:** Adsorbent activity depends on the surface area of adsorbent. For increasing the surface area, particle size can be reduced and hence the adsorbent activity increases.

(iii) ***Nature of the Solvent*:** The flow rate of solvent is affected by its viscosity. The flow rate in inversely proportional to viscosity. Hence less viscous solvents are better efficient than more viscous solvents.

(iv) ***Temperature of the Column*:** Speed of elution is increased at higher temperature. But adsorbent power is decreased at higher temperatures. Hence a compromise is made between speed of elution and adsorbent power. Normally room temperature is used for all samples. Difficult solvents are separated at higher temperatures.

(v) ***Pressure*:** High pressure above the column and low pressure below th column increases the efficiency of separation. High pressure above the column is achieved by maintaining a column of liquid on the top of the column (reservoir) or by using pressure devices (pumps). Pressure below the column is decreased, by applying vacuum using vacuum pump.

Applications

(i) ***Separation of mixture of compounds*:** Column chromatography can be used for the separation of several classes of drugs and constituents like alkaloids, glycosides, amino acids, plant extracts, drugs and formulations etc.

(ii) ***Removal of impurities or purification process*:** Impurities present in a compound can be removed by using appropriate stationary and mobile phase.

(iii) ***Isolation of active constituents*:** From plant extracts or crude extracts or formulations, active constituents or required constituents can be isolated.

(iv) ***Isolation of metabolites from biological fluids*:** eg: 17 – Ketosteroids from urine, cortisol, other drugs etc., from biological fluids like blood, plasma or serum etc.

(v) ***Estimation of drugs in formulation or crude extracts*:**

(i) Determination of % w/v of strychnine in syrup of ferrous phosphate with quinine and strychnine.

(ii) Determination of primary and secondary glycoside in digitalis leaf.

(iii) Determination of phytomenacdine injection and tablets.

(iv) Determination of flucinolone actonide or Betamethasone 17 – valerate in formulated products.

(v) Separation of geometrical isomers Cis and transforms of bixin and crocetin dimethyl ether using alumina

(vi) Separation of diastereomers :

(vii) Separation of inorganic ions like copper, cobalt, nickel etc.

(viii) Separation of tautomers and racemates.

Advantages of Column chromatography

(i) Any type of mixture can be separated by column chromatography.

(ii) Any quantity of the mixture can be separated (μg to mg of substances).

(iii) Wider choice of mobile phase.

(iv) in preparative type, the sample can be separated and reused.

(v) Automation is possible.

Disadvantages of column chromatography

(i) time consuming method.

(ii) More amount of solvents are required which are expensive.

(iii) Automation makes the technique more complicated and expensive.

Partition column chromatography

The technique is similar to column adsorption chromatography except that, the stationary phase is liquid. A solid support like silica gel or cellulose is used to hold the liquid stationary phases like water, aqueous buffer solutions, etc., as thin film on the surface. Mobile phase is similar to that of column chromatography, but gradient elution technique is not used, since the equilibrium will be disturbed. All the other requirements and the technique is similar to column adsorption chromatography. Column partition chromatography is not being used widely.

CHAPTER 3

THIN LAYER CHROMATOGRAPHY (TLC)

Introduction

The history of thin layer Chromatography dates back to 1938 when Izmailov and Shraiber separated plant extracts using 2 mm thick and firm layer of the alumina set on glass plate. In 1944, Consden, Gorden and Martin used filter papers for separating amino acids.

- In 1950, Kirchner identified terpenes on filter paper and later glass fibre paper coated with alumina.
- Only in 1958, Stah developed standard equipment for analysing by thin layer chromatography.

Principle

The principle of separation is adsorption. One or more compounds are spotted on a thin layer of adsorbent coated on a chromatographic plate. The mobile phase solvent flour through because of capillary action (against gravitational force). The components move according to their affinities towards the adsorbent. The component with more affinity towards the stationary phase travels slower. The component with lesser affinity towards the stationary phase travels faster. Thus the components are separated on a thin layer chromatographic plate based on the affinity of the components towards the stationary phase.

Advantages of TLC

(i) Simple method and cost for the equipment is low.

(ii) Rapid technique and not time consuming like column chromatography.

(iii) Separation of μg of the substances can be achieved.

(iv) Any type of compound can be analysed.

(v) *Efficiency of separation*: very small particle size can be used which increases the efficiency of separation. Flow rate is not altered because of the particle size since it is not a closed column it is a planer type having thin layer of adsorbent.

(vi) Detection is easy and not tedious

(vii) Capacity of the thin layer can be altered. Hence analytical and preparative separations can be made.

(viii) Corrosive spray reagents can be used without damaging the plates.

(ix) Needs less solvent, stationary phase and time for every separation compared to column chromatography.

Practical Requirements

(i) Stationary phases

(ii) Glass plates

(iii) Preparation and activation of TLC plates

(iv) Application of sample

(v) Development tank

(vi) Mobile phase

(vii) Development technique

(viii) Detecting or visualising agents

(i) Stationary phases

There are several adsorbents which can be used as stationary phases. Some of the stationary phases, their composition and the ratio in which they have to be mixed with water or other solvents to form a slurry for preparing thin layer chromatographic plates are given in the following table:

Name	Composition	Adsorbent : water ratio
Silicagel H	Silicagel without binder	1 : 1.5
Silicagel G	Silicagel + $CuSO_4$	1 : 2
Silica GF	Silicagel + Binder + fluorescent – indicator	1 :2
Alumina		
Neutral	AL_2O_3 without binder	1 : 1 . 1
Basic		
Acidic		
Al_2O_3 G	Al_2O_3 + binder	1 : 2
Cellulose powder	Cellulose without binder	1 : 5
Cellulose powder	Cellulose with binder	1:6
Kieselguhr G	Diatomaceous earth + binder	1:2
Polymide powder	Polymide	1 : 9 $CCHCl_3 : CH_3OH = 2 : 3$

(ii) Glass plates

Glass plates which are specific dimensions like 20 cm × 20 cm (full plate), 20 cm × 10 cm (Half plate), 20 cm × 5 cm. (Quarter plate) can be used. These dimensions are used since the width of the commercially available TLC spreder is 20 cm.

Microscopic slides can also be used for some applications like monitoring the progress of a chemical reaction. The development time is much shorter like 5 minutes.

Glass plates of different dimensions are also be used when the TLC plates are prepared without the use of TLC spreader. In general the glass plates should be of good quality and should withstand temperatures used for drying the plates.

(iii) Preparation and activation of TLC plates

The slurry which is a mixture of stationary phase and water is prepared by using the ratio mentioned earlier. After preparing the slurry, the TLC plates can be prepared by using any one of the following techniques:
pouring, dipping, spraying and spreading.

In *pouring technique*, the slurry is prepared and poured on to a glass plate which is maintained on a levelled surface. The slurry is spread uniformly on the surface of the glass plate. After setting, the plates are dried in an oven. The disadvantage is that uniformity in thickness cannot be ensured.

In *dipping technique*, two plates (either of standard dimensions or microscopic slides) are dipped into the slurry and are separated after removing from slurry and later dried. The disadvantage is that a larger quantity of slurry is required even for preparing fewer plates.

Spraying technique resembles that of using a perfume spray or a cloth. The suspension of adsorbent or slurry is sprayed on a glass plate using a sprayer. The disadvantage is that the layer thickness cannot be maintained uniformly all over the plate.

Spreading is the best technique where a TLC spreader is used. The glass plates of specific dimensions (20 cm × 20 cm / 10 cm / 5 cm) are stacked on a base plate. The slurry after preparation is poured inside the reservoir of TLC spreader. The thickness of the adsorbent layer is adjusted by using a knob in the spreader. Normally a thickness of 0.25 mm is used for analytical purpose and 2 mm thickness for preparative purpose. Then the spreader is rolled only once on the plates. The plates are allowed for setting (air drying). This is done to avoid cracks on the surface of adsorbent. After setting, the plates are activated by keeping in an oven at 100^0C to 180°C for 1 hour.

Activation of TLC plates is nothing but removing water / moisture and other adsorbed substances from the surface of any adsorbent, by heating at high temperature. So that adsorbent activity is retained. The activated plates can be stored in thermostatically controlled oven or in desicator and can be used whenever required.

(iv) Application of sample

Usually to get good spots, the concentration of the sample or standard solution has to be minimum. 2-5 μl of a 1% solution of either standard or test sample is spotted using a capillary tube or micropipette. The spots can be placed at random or equidistant from each other by using a template, with markings. The spot should be kept atleast 2 cm above the base of the plate and the spotting area should not be immersed in the mobile in the development tank. Atleast 4 spots can be spotted conveniently on a quarter plate (20 cm × 5 cm).

(vi) Development Tank

For the purpose of development, a developing tank or chamber of different sizes to hold TLC plates of standard dimensions are used. These require more solvents for developing the chromatogram. When a new method is developed, it is better to develop in glass beakers, specimen jars, etc., to avoid more wastage of solvents. When developed method or standard method is used, it is better to use development tank. New types of development tanks (figure 2) have hump in the middle, which require less solvent. The development chamber or tank should be lined inside with filter paper moistened with the mobile phase so as to saturate the atmosphere. If this kind of saturation of the atmosphere is not done, "edge effect" occurs where the solvent front in the middle of TLC plate moves faster than that of the edge. Therefore the spots are distorted and not regular.

(vi) Mobile Phase

The solvent or the mobile phase used depends upon various factors as mentioned in column chromatography. Some of the factors are:

(i) Nature of the substance to be spread.

(ii) Nature of the stationary phase used.

(iii) Mode of chromatography (Normal phase or reverse phase).

(vi) Separation to be achieved – analytical or preparative.

Pure solvents or mixtures of solvents are used. The following gives a list of solvents (of increasing polarity).

Petrolium ether, carbon tetrachloride, Cyclohescane, Carbondisulphide, Ether, Acetone, Benzene, Toluene, Ethyl acetate, chloroform, Alcohols, (methanol, ethanol), water, pyridine, organic acids, mixtures of acids or bases with pyridine or alcohols, etc. The solvent composition is done by trial and error method only but with a review of literature and other logical considerations like solubility of the substance, polar or non-polar character of the samples, etc. Some examples of solvent compositions are given in the applications of TLC.

(vii) Development Technique

Different development techniques are used for efficient separations.

They are:

(a) One dimensional development

(b) Two dimensional development

(c) Horizontal development

(d) Multiple development

(a) ***One Dimensional Development (vertical)*****:** In this technique, the plates are kept vertical and the solvent flows against gravity, because of capillary action. Most separations done practically are of this type only.

(b) ***Two Dimensional Technique*****:** Although one dimensional technique is sufficient for most samples, for complex mixtures two dimensional technique is used. First, the plates are developed in one axis and the plates after drying are developed in the other axis. When large number of compounds cannot be separated by using one dimensional technique, this technique is followed. Figure given below explains the two dimensional development of separation of mixture of several amino acids.

(viii) Detecting or visualising agents

After the development of TLC plates, the spots should be visualised. Detecting coloured spots can be done visually. But for detecting colourless spots, any one of the following techniques can be used.

(a) ***Non specific methods*****:** Where the number of spots can be detected, but not the exact nature or type of compound.

Examples

(i) ***Iodine chamber method*****:** Where brown or amber spots are observed. Detecting coloured sports can be done visually. But for detecting colourless spots, any one of the following techniques can be used.

Examples

(i) ***Iodine Chamber method*****:** Where brown or amber spots are observed when the TLC plates are kept in a tank with few iodine crystals at the bottom.

(ii) ***Sulphuric acid spray reagent*****:** 70-80% V/V of sulphuric acid with few mg of either potassium dichromate or potassium permanganate or few ml of nitric acid as oxidising agent is used. This reagent after spraying on TLC plates is heated in an oven. Black spots are seen due to charring of compounds.

(iii) ***UV chamber for fluorescent compounds*****:** When compounds are viewed under UV chamber at 254 nm, (short λ) or at 365 nm (long λ) or at 365 nm (long λ), fluorescent compounds can be detected. Bright spots are seen under a dark background.

(iv) ***Using fluorescent stationary phase*****:** When the compounds are not fluorescent, a fluorescent stationary phase is used. When the plates are viewed under UV chamber, dark spots are seen on a fluorescent background. Example of such stationary phase is silica gel GF.

(b) ***Specific methods*****:** Specific spray reagents or visualising agents are used to find out the nature of compounds or for identification purposes. Examples are:

- **(i)** ***Ferric chloride*****:** For phenolic compounds and tannins.
- **(ii)** ***Ninhydrin in acetone*****:** For amino acids.
- **(iii)** ***Dragendroff's reagent*****:** for alkaloids
- **(iv)** ***3,5 – Dinitro benzoic acids*****:** for cardiglycosides.
- **(v)** ***2, 4 – Dinitrophenyl hydrazine*****:** For aldehydes and ketones

CHAPTER 4

PAPER CHROMATOGRAPHY

Introduction

Paper chromatography is defined as the technique in which the analysis of unknown substances is carried out mainly by the flow of solvents on specially designed filter paper. There are two types of paper chromatography, they are:

Paper adsorption chromatography**:** in which paper impregnated with silica or alumina acts as adsorbent (stationary phase) and solvent as mobile phase.

Paper partition chromatography: in which moisture/water present in the pores of cellulose fibres present in filter paper acts as stationary phase and another mobile phase is used as solvent.

In general, paper chromatography refers to paper partition chromatography only since most separations are based on partition type only.

Principle of Separation

The **principle of separation** is mainly **partition** rather than adsorption cellulose layers in filter paper contains moisture which acts as stationary phase. Organic solvents or buffers are used as mobile phases. Instead of water as stationary phase, other organic solvents can be used by suitable modification.

Practical Requirements

1. Stationary phase and papers used
2. Application of sample

3. Mobile phase
4. Development technique
5. Detecting or visualising agents

1. Stationary Phase and Papers Used

Paper of chromatographic grade consists of α-cellulose 98-99%, β-cellulose 0.3-1% pentosans 0.4-0.3%, ether soluble matter 0.015-15-2 C.02% - 0.01 – 0.17%. Whatman filter papers of different grade like No.1, No.2, No.3, No.4, No.17, No.20 etc are used. These papers differ in sizes, shapes, porosities and thickness.

- Choice of filter paper depends upon thickness, flow rate, purity, technique, etc.
- Modified papers: Acid or base washed filter paper, glass fibre type paper.
- Hydrophilic papers: Papers modified with methanol, formamide, glycol, glycerol etc.
- *Hydrophobic papers*: Acetylation of OH groups leads to hydrophobic nature, hence can be used for reverse phase chromatography. Silicone pre-treatment and organic non-polar polymers can also be impregnated to give reverse phase chromatographic mode.
- Impregnation of silica, alumina or ion exchange resins can also be made.
- Size of the paper used: Paper of any size can be used. Paper should be kept in a chamber of suitable size.

2. Application of Sample

The sample to be applied is dissolved in the mobile phase and applied using capillary tube or using micropipette. Very low concentration is used to avoid larger zone.

3. Mobile phase

Pure solvents, buffer solutions, or misture of solvents are used. Some of the examples of Hydrophilic mobile phases :

Isopropanol : Ammonia : water	-	9 : 1 : 2
n-Butanol : glacial acetic acid : water	-	4 : 1 : 5
Methanol : water	-	3 : 1 or 4 : 1
t-Butanol : water : Formic acid	-	40 : 20 : 5

Examples of Hydrophobic mobile phases

Kerosene : 70% Isopropanol

Dimethyl ether : cyclohexane

(Single/two phase or three phase solvent systems are also used.)

4. Development Technique

Since paper is flexible when compared to glass plate used in TLC, several types of development are possible which increases the ease and efficiency of operation.

They are:

(i) ***Ascending development*:** Like conventional type, the solvent flows against gravity. The spots are kept at the bottom portion of paper and kept in a chamber with mobile phase solvent at the bottom. (same as Fig 14.2 and 14.3 in TLC chapter).

(ii) ***Descending development*:** This is carried out in a special chamber where the solvent holder is at the top. The spot is kept at the top and the solvent flows down the paper. The advantage is that the flow of solvent is assisted by gravity and hence the development is faster.

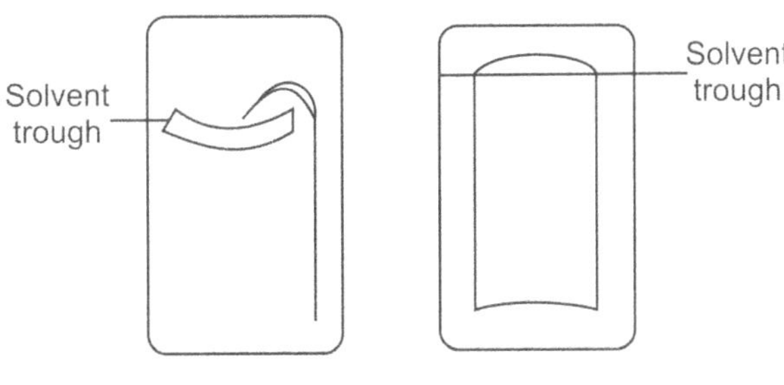

Development chamber
(Internal and posterior view)

(iii) ***Ascending-Descending development*:** This is a combination of ascending and descending type. Only the length of separation is increased by using a combination of techniques. First ascending takes place followed by descending development.

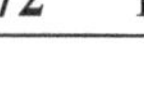

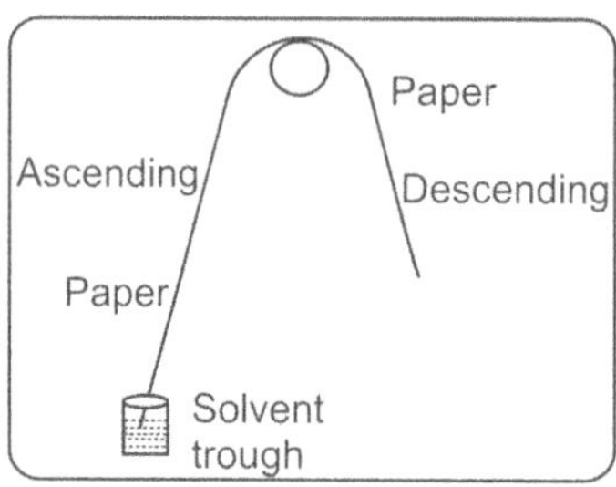

Ascending cum descending development

(iv) ***Circular/radial development (Horizontal)***: Here, the spot is kept at the centre of a circular paper. The solvent flows through a wick at the centre and spreads in all directions uniformly. Hence the individual spots after development look like concentric circles. By making perforations radially, number of quadrants can be created allowing more number of samples to be spoited.

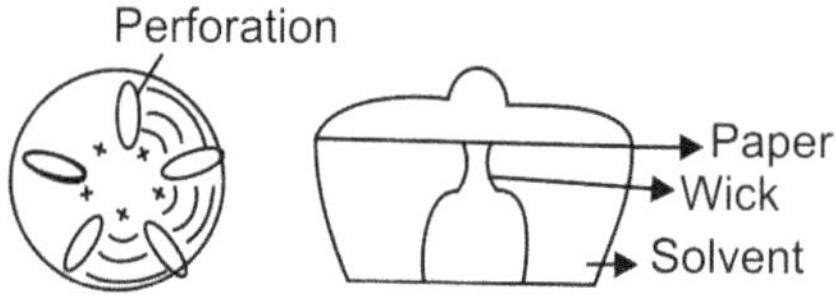

Radial development
(top view and side view)

(v) ***Two dimensional development***: This technique is similar to 2-Dimensional TLC. The paper is developed in one direction and after development, the paper is developed in the second direction allowing more compounds or complex mistures to be separated into individual spots. In the second direction, either the same solvent system or different solvent system can be used for development.

5. Detecting or Visualising Agents

After the development of chromatogram, the spots should be visualised. Detecting coloured spots can be done visually. But for detecting colourless spots, any one of the following techniques can be used.

(a) ***Non specific methods:*** Where the number of spots can be detected, but not the exact nature or type of compound.

Examples

(i) ***Iodine chamber method*:** where brown or amber spots are observed when the TLC plates are kept in a tank with few iodine crystals at the bottom.

(ii) ***UV Chamber for fluorescent compounds*:** When compounds are viewed under UV chamber at 254nm (short λ) or at 365nm (long λ), fluorescent compounds can be detected. Bright spots are seen against a dark background.

(b) Specific methods**:** Specific spray reagents or detecting agents or visualising agents are used to find out the nature of compounds or for identification purposes.

Examples

(i) Ferric chloride – for phenolic compounds and tannins

(ii) Ninhydrin in acetone – for alkaloids

(iii) Dragendroffs reagent – for alkaloids

(iv) 3.5 – Dinitro benzoic acid – for cardiac glycosides

(v) 2, 4 - Dinitrophenyl hydrazine – for aldehydes and ketones

The detecting techniques can also be categorised as

(i) *Destructive technique*: e.g. Specific spray reagents, etc where the samples are destroyed before detection. E.g. Ninhydrin reagent.

(ii) *Non-Destructive techniques*: Like UV chamber method. Iodine chamber method, densitometric method, etc., where the sample is not destroyed even after detection.

For radioactive materials, detection is by using autoradiography or Geiger muller counter.

For antibiotics, the chromatogram is layed on nutrient agar inoculated with appropriate strain and the zone of inhibition is compared.

Quantitative Analysis: (Direct and Indirect techniques)

***Direct technique*:** Densitometer is an instrument which measures quantitatively the density of the spots. When the optical density of the spots for the standard and test solution are determined, the quantity of the substance can be calculated. The papers are neither destroyed nor eluted with solvents to get the compounds. This method is also called as in-situ method.

***Indirect technique*:** In this technique, the spots are cut into portions and eluted with solvents. This solution can be analysied by any conventional techniques of analysis like spectrophotometry, electrochemical methods, etc.

Qualitative Analysis

R_f Value

The R_f value (Retardation factor) is calculated for identifying the spots i.e., in Qualitative analysis. R_f value is the ratio of distance travelled by the solute to the distance travelled by the solvent front.

$$R_f = \frac{\text{Distance travelled by solute}}{\text{Distance travelled by solvent front}}$$

The R_f value ranges from 0 10 1. But ideal values are from 0.3 to 0.8. R_f value is constant for every compound in a particular combination of stationary and mobile phase. When the R_f value of a sample and reference compound is same, the compound is identified by its standard. When the R_f value differs, the compound may be different from its reference standard.

R_x Values

R_x value is nothing but the ratio of distance travelled by the sample and the distance travelled by standard. R_x value is always closer to 1.

R_m Values

R_m value is used in qualitative analysis to find out whether the compounds belong to a homologous series. If they belong to a homologous series, the ΔR_m values are constant. The ΔR_m values are constant. The ΔR_m values for a pair of adjacent member of a homologous series is determined by using the formula:

$$R_m = \log\left(\frac{1}{R_f} - 1\right)$$

Applications

The applications are wider and there is no limitation to the compounds that can be analysed by paper chromatography. Paper chromatography is more useful for the analysis of polar compounds like amino acids, sugars, natural products, etc. The different types of applications are listed below.

1. Separation of mixtures of drugs of chemical or biological origin, plant extracts, etc.
2. Separation of carbohydrates (sugars), vitamins, antibiotics, proteins, alkaloids, glycosides, amino acids etc.
3. Identification of drugs

Drug	Mobile phase	Detecting agent
Erythromycin estolate	Isobutyl methyl ketone	Nutrient agar containing Bacillus pumilus
Gentamycin	Chloroform : Methanol : Ammonia : water (10 : 5 : 3 : 2)	Ninhydrin in pyridine – acetone mixture
Vancomycin	t-Amyl alcohol : Acetone : water (2 : 1 : 2)	Nutrient agar containing Bacillus subtilis

4. Identification of impurities

Drug	Mobile phase	Detecting agent
Hydroxocobalamin	s-Butyl alcohol : aceticv acid : Potassium cyanide	Elution and measurement of absorbance at 361 nm

5. Identification of related compounds

Drug	Mobile phase	Detecting agent
Phenformin HCl	Ethyl acetate : ethanol : water (6 : 3 : 1)	Potassium ferryicyanide, Sodium nitroprusside & NaOH
Ergotamine injection	Chloroform : methanol	p-dimethyl amino benzaldehyde reagent –
Vitamin A	Dioxan : methanol : water with BHA (70 : 15 : 5)	UV 366nm

6. Identification of foreign substances in drugs
7. Identification of decomposition products
8. Analysis of metabolites of drugs in blood, urine etc.

CHAPTER 5

ION EXCHANGE CHROMATOGRAPHY (IEC)

Introduction

Ion exchange chromatography is the process by which a mixture of similar charged ions can be separated by using an ion exchange resin which exchanges ions according to their relative affinities. There is a **reversible exchange of similar charged ions.** Mostly similar charged ions like cations or anions can be conveniently separated by this technique. Many drugs and pharmaceutical agents are weakly or strongly acidic or basic in nature. Hence a mixture of similar charged substances can also be separated into pure components.

Principle of Separation

The principle of separation is by **reversible exhange of ions** between the **ions present in the solution** and those present in the **ion exchange resin.**

Cation exchange

Let us consider the separation of cations using cation exchange resin. The cations to be separated are present in solution and exchanges for similar ions present in cation exchange resin, a solid matrix. The exchange can be represented by the following equation:

$$\text{Solid} - H^{+} + \underset{\text{(Solution)}}{M^{+}} \rightarrow \text{Solid} - M^{+} + \underset{\text{(Solution)}}{H^{+}}$$

The cations retained by the solid matrix of ion exchange resin can be eluted by using buffers of different strength and hence separation of cations can be effected.

Anion exchange

Similarly, separation of anions using anion exchange resin can be carried out. The anions to be separated are present in solution and exchanges for similar ions present in anion exchange resin, a solid matrix. The exchange can be represented by the following equation:

$$\text{Solid} - OH^- + \underset{\text{(Solution)}}{A^-} \rightarrow \text{Solid} - A^- + \underset{\text{(Solution)}}{OH-}$$

The anions retained by the solid matrix of ion exchange resin can eluted by using buffers of different strength and hence separation of anions can be effected.

The technique of ion exchange chromatography can be studied with respect to the following headings:

(i) Ion exchange resins – Classification of resins

(ii) Practical requirements

(iii) Factors affecting ion exchange separations

1. Classification of Resins

According to the chemical nature they can be classified as:

1. Strong cation exchange resin
2. Weak cation exchange resin
3. Strong anion exchange resin
4. Weak anion exchange resin

According to the source they can be classified as:

***Natural*:** cation – Zeolytes, clay, etc

Anion – Dolomite

***Synthetic*:** Inorganic and Organic resins

Of the above types, organic resins are the most widely used and hence they will be discussed in detail.

Organic ion exchange resins are polymeric resin matrix containing exchange sites. The resin is composed of Polystyrene and Divinyl benzene. Polystyrene contains sites for exchangeable functional groups. Divinyl benzene acts as a cross linkinga agent and offers adequate strength i.e., mechanical stability.

Structure of Styrene and Divinyl benzene

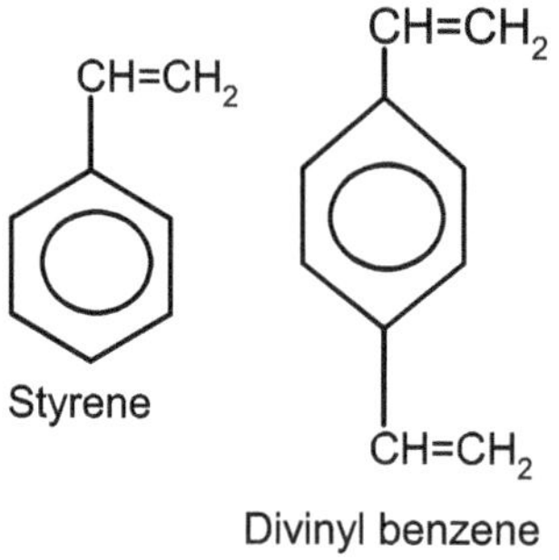

$CH=CH_2$

Styrene

$CH=CH_2$

$CH=CH_2$

Divinyl benzene

Functional groups present in different ion exchange resins

Strong Cation exchange resin – SO_3H

Weak cation exchange resin – COOH, OH, SH, PO_3H_2

Strong anion, exchange resin – N^+R_3, NR_2

Weak anion exchange resin - NHR, NH_2

The following tabular column gives a list of the ion exchange resins, the pH range to be used, nature and applications of the resins in different separations.

Class of resin	Nature	pH range	Applications
Cation – Strong	Sulfonated polystyrene	1-14	- fractionation of cations - inorganic separations (lanthanids) - peptides, amino acids, B vitamins
Cation – Weak	Carboxylic methcrylate	5 – 14	- fractionation of cations - biochemical separations - organic bases, antibiotics
Anion – Strong	Quaternary ammonium	0 – 12	- fractionation of anions - fractionation of anions complexes - anions of different valency - vitamins, amino acids
Anion – Strong	Polystyrene or phenol	0 – 9	
Anion – Strong	Formaldehyde	-	

Structural types of ion exchange resins

Pellicular type with ion exchange film**:** The particles have a size of 30 – 40μ with 1 – 2μ film thickness. These have very low exchange capacity to separate the ions. Their ion exchange efficiency is 0.01 – 0.1 meq/g of ion exchange resin.

(b) ***Porous resin coated with exchanger beads*****:** The size ranges from 5 – 10μ. They aretotally porous and highly efficient. Their exchange capacities are from 0.5 – 2 meq/g of ion exchange resin.

(c) ***Macroreticular resin bead*****:** A reticular network of the resin is seen superficially on the resin beads. They are not highly efficient and have very low exchange capacities.

(d) ***Surface sulfonated and bonded electrostationally with anion exchanger*****:** The particles are sulfonated and they are bonded electrostatically with anion exchanger resin. They are less efficient and have low exchange capacity. Their exchange capacity is 0.02meq/g of exchange resin.

The Physical structure of different resins are given in the following diagram:

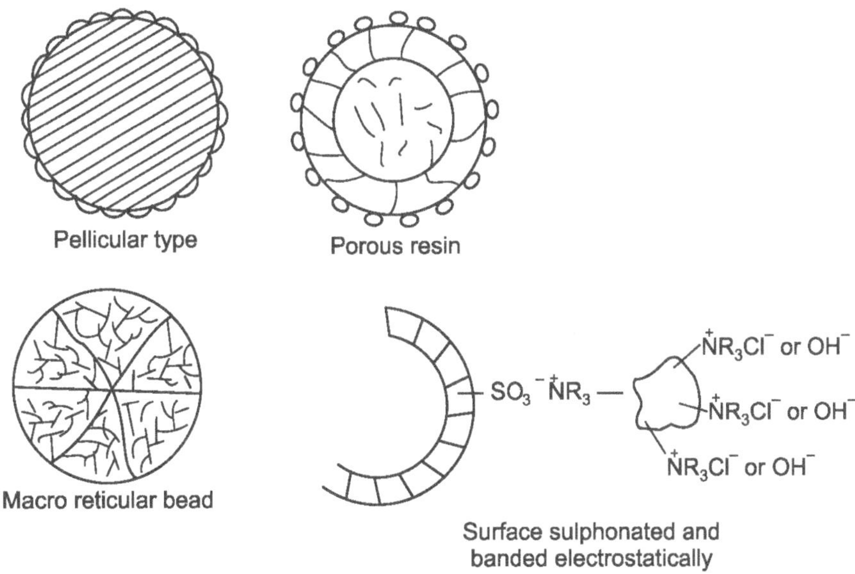

Fig. 5.1

Physical properties of Resins

1. ***Particle size***: They are available as fine powder of uniform particle size from 50-200 mesh. They should allow free and uniform flow of mobile phase. They should contain more exchangeable functional groups.

2. ***Cross linking and swelling***: When more cross linking agent is present, they are more rigid, but swells less. When swelling is less, separation of ions of different sizes is difficult as they cannot pass through the pores present.

   When less cross linking agent is present, they are less rigid but swell more. When swelling is more, separation will not be efficient as exchange of functional groups does not take place due to wide pore. Hence an optimum quantity of cross linking agent should be added to the polymeric ion exchange resin for the separation to be effective.

Chemical structure of resins

The chemical structure of different resins are given in the following diagram :

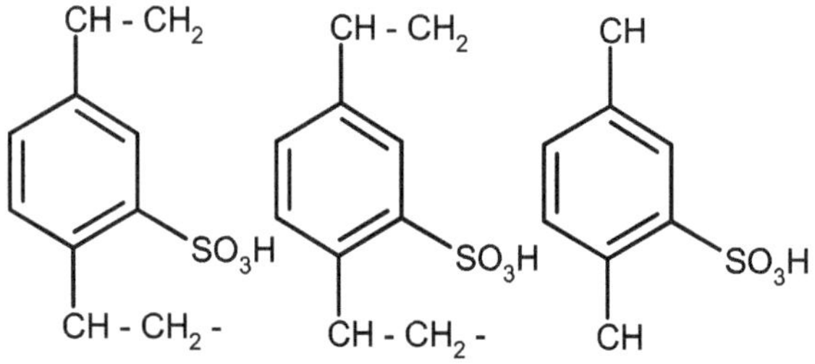

Strong acidic cation exchange
(Sulfonic acid group)

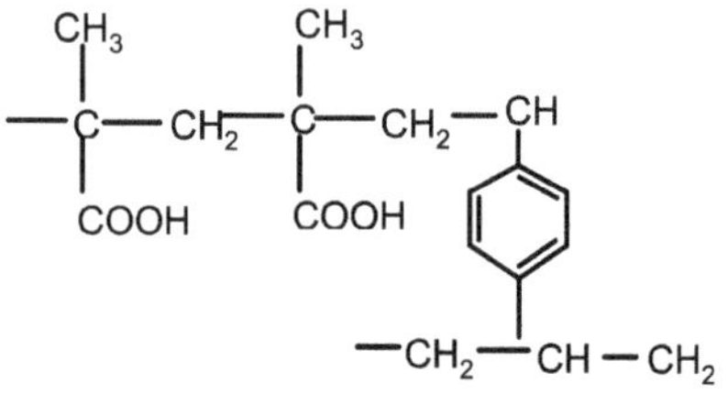

Weakly acidic cation exchange
(Methacrylate polymer)

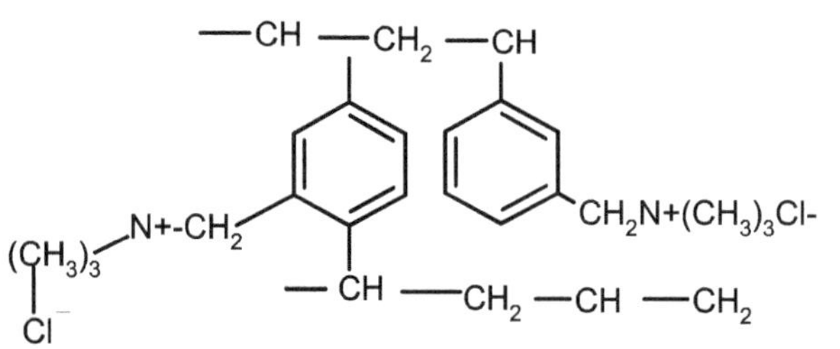

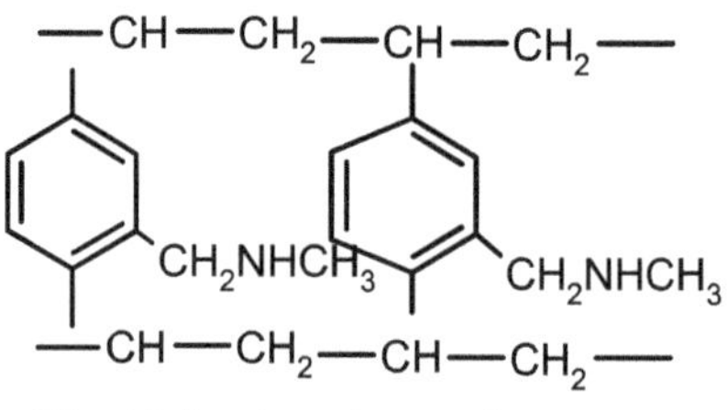

Weakly basic anion exchange
(Methyl Amino)

(II) Practical Requirements

(i) ***Column material and dimensions*:** Columns used in the laboratories are made up of glass. But those used in industries are made up of either high quality stainless steel or polymers which are resistant to strong acids and alkalis. The column dimensions are also important and a length : diameter ratio of 20 : 1 to 100 : 1 for higher efficiency can be used.

(ii) *Type of ion exchange resin and physical characteristics*: The selection of ion exchange resin depends upon the following properties :

1. Type of the ions to be separated – cations or anions.
2. Nature of the ions to be separated – Strong or weak.
3. ***Efficiency of the resin*** – it is measured by ion exchange capacity. Ion exchange capacity is the total ion exchange capacity in terms of the exchangeable functional groups expressed as milli equivalents per gram of the ion exchange resin.

$$\text{m.eq/g} = \frac{1000}{\text{eq.wt}}$$

4. Particle size of the resin – 50-100 mesh or 100-200 mesh is used.
5. Structural type of the resin – porous, pellicular, etc.
6. Amount of cross linking agent present – which decides swelling of the resin.

(iii) *Packing of the column*: Wet packing method is used. The resin is mixed with the mobile phase and packed in the column uniformly. The sample to be separated is dissolved in the mobile phase and introduced all at once into the column.

(iv) *Mobile phase*: Organic solvents are less useful and they are not used at all. Only different strengths of acids, alkalis and buffers are used as eluting solvents.

E.g. 0.1 N HCl, 1N NaOH, phosphate buffer, acetate buffer, borate buffer, phthalate buffer etc.

(v) *Development of the chromatogram and elution*: After introduction of the sample development of the chromatogram is done by using different mobile phases. As mentioned earlier, organic solvents are less useful and only acids, alkalis and buffers of different pH are used. There are two elution techniques. They are isocratic elution technique and gradient elution technique. In isocratic elution technique, the same solvent composition is uded. i.e. same strength of acid or alkali or buffer. In gradient elution technique, initially less acidic or basic character is used followed by increasing the acidity or basicity of the mobile phase. Gradient elution is usually used for complex mixtures. The different fractions of the eluent is collected volume wise or time wise and analysed.

(vi) *Analysis of the elute*: Different fractions collected with respect to volume or time is analysed for their contents. Several methods of analysis can be used which depends upon the nature and quantity of the sample. They are spectrophotometric method. Polarographic method, conductometric method, ampertometric method, flame photometric method, radiochemical methods (using Geiger Muller counter, ionisation chamber method) etc. After analysing, similar fractions are mixed in order to get pure ion or compound of each type.

(vii) *Regeneration of the ion exchange resin*: The ion exchange resin after separation may not be useful for next separation as exchangeable functional groups are lost. But due to the cost of the ion exchange resins, they cannot be disposed off. Hence like reactivation, regeneration of the resin is most important. Regeneration makes the used ion exchange resin to be as efficient as a virgin resin.

Regeneration refers to the replacement of the exchangeable cations or anions present in the original resin. Hence regeneration of the cation exchange resin is done by the charging the column with strong acid like hydrochloric acid. Regeneration of anion exchange resin is done by using strong alkali like sodium hydroxide or porassium hydroxide.

(iii) Factors Affecting Ion Exchange Separations

The factors affecting ion exchange separations are

A Nature and properties of ion exchange resins

B. Nature of exchanging ions

A. *Nature of ion exchange resin*: Cross linking and swelling is important factor which depends on the proportion of cross linking agent (divinyl benzene) and polystyrene. When more cross linking agent is present, they are more rigid, but swells less. When swelling is less, separation of ions of different sizes is difficult as they cannot pass through the pores present and it becomes selective to ions of different sizes. When cross linking agent is present, they are less rigid, but swell more. When swelling is more, separation will not be efficient as exchange of functional groups does not take place due to wide pore. Hence an optimum quantity of cross linking agent should be added to the polymeric ion exchange resins for the separation to be effective.

B. Nature of exchanging ions

(i) *Valency of ions*: At low concentrations and at ordinary temperatures, extent of exchange increases with increase in valency.

$$Na^{+} < Ca^{2+} < Al^{3+} < Th^{4+}$$

(ii) *Size of ions*: For similar charged ions, exchange increases with decrease in the size of hydrated ion.

$$Li^{+} < H^{+} < Na^{+} < NH^{4+} < K^{+} < Rb^{+} < Cs^{+}$$

(iii) *Polarizability*: Exchange is preferred for greater polarizable ion eg.

$$I^{-} < Br^{-} < Cl^{-} < F^{-}$$

(iv) *Concentration of solution*: in dilute solution, polyvalent anions are generally adsorbed preferentially.

(v) *Concentration and charge of ions*: If resin has higher +ve charge and solution has lower +ve charge, exchange is favoured at higher concentration. If the resin has lower +ve charge and solution has high +ve charge, then exchange is favoured at low concentration.

Applications

1. *Softening of Water*: Removal of monovalent and divalent ions like sodium, potassium, calcium, magnesium, etc.
2. *Demineralisation or deionisation of water*: Removal of different ions to get demineralised water.
3. Purification of some solutions to be free from ionic impurities.
4. *Separation of inorganic ions*: Cations and anions.
5. *Organic separations*: Most of the pharmaceutical compounds are either strongly or weakly acidic or basic in nature. Hence a mixture of those compounds can be separated by using ion exchange resins. Some classes of compounds which can be separated are amino acids, proteins, antibiotics, vitamis, fatty acids, etc.

   For example, a mixture of acidic, neutral and basic amino acids can be separated using ion exchange column. Similarly a mixture of vitamins like vitamin B1, B2, B6, Nicotinic acid, folic acid, cyanocobalamin etc., can be separated using ion exchange technique.

6. Biochemical separations like isolation of some drugs or metabolites from blood, urine etc.
7. *Concentration of ionic solutions*: A cation or anion from a bulk of solution can be adsorbed onto ion exchange resin. After adsorption, it can be eluted by using small volume of eluent.
8. *Ion exchange column in HPLC*: For separation of compounds of mixed nature like acidic and basic substances, ion exchange column is used in HPLC (High performance liquid chromatography).

CHAPTER 6

GAS CHROMATOGRAPHY

Introduction

Gas chromatography - specifically gas-liquid chromatography - involves a sample being vapourised and injected onto the head of the chromatographic column. The sample is transported through the column by the flow of inert, gaseous mobile phase. The column itself contains a liquid stationary phase which is adsorbed onto the surface of an inert solid

Gas Chromatography (GC) is a commonly used analytic technique in many research and industrial laboratories. A broad variety of samples can be analyzed as long as the compounds are sufficiently thermal stable and volatile enough.

Historical Perspectives

Chromatography, in one of its several forms, is the most commonly used procedure in contemporary chemical analysis and the first configuration of chromatography equipment to be produced in a single composite unit and made commercially available was the gas chromatograph. Gas chromatography was invented by A. J. P. Martin who, with R. L. M. Synge, suggested its possibility in a paper on liquid chromatography published in 1941. Martin and Synge recommended that the liquid mobile phase used in liquid chromatography could be replaced by a suitable gas. The basis for this recommendation was that, due to much higher diffusivities of solutes in gases compared with liquids, the equilibrium processes involved in a chromatographic process would be much faster and thus, the columns much more efficient and separation times much shorter. So the concept of *gas chromatography* was envisioned more than fifty years ago, but unfortunately, little notice was taken of the suggestion and it was left to Martin himself and his coworker A.T. James to bring the concept to practical reality some years later in 1951, when they published their epic paper describing the first gas chromatograph.

The first published gas chromatographic separation was that of a series of fatty acids, a titration procedure being used, in conjunction with a micro burette, as the detector. The micro burette was eventually automated providing a very effective in-line detector with an integral response. After its introduction by James and Martin, the technique of GC developed at a phenomenal rate, growing from a simple research novelty to a highly sophisticated instrument. The gas chromatograph was also one of the first analytical instruments to be associated with a computer which controlled the analysis, processed the data and reported the results.

A more sophisticated form of the gas chromatograph was constructed by James and Martin and described by James in 1955. The instrument was a somewhat bulky device with a straight packed column, 3 ft long, that was held vertically and thermostatted in a vapour jacket. Initially, the detector was situated at the base of the column and consisted of the automatic titrating device, the separation was presented as a chromatogram in the form of a series of steps, the height of each step being proportional to the mass of solute eluted. The apparatus was successfully used to separate some fatty acids, but the limited capability of the device to sense only ionic material motivated Martin to develop a more versatile detector, the Gas Density Balance. The gas density balance, was the first detector with a truly catholic response that was linearly related to the vapor density of the solute and consequently its molecular weight. The gas density balance had a maximum sensitivity (minimum detectable concentration) of about 10-6 g/ml at a signal to noise ratio of two. This detector inspired the invention of a wide range of detectors over the next decade providing both higher sensitivity and selective response. The modern gas chromatograph is a fairly complex instrument mostly computer controlled. The samples are mechanically injected, the analytical results are automatically calculated and the results printed out, together with the pertinent operating conditions in a standard format.

The Modern Gas Chromatograph

Most gas chromatographs consist of four chromatography units, supported by three temperature controllers and 2 micro processors systems. In some instruments, a single microprocessor unit is employed to service the entire chromatograph but this tends to restrict the choice available for the different parts of the chromatograph.

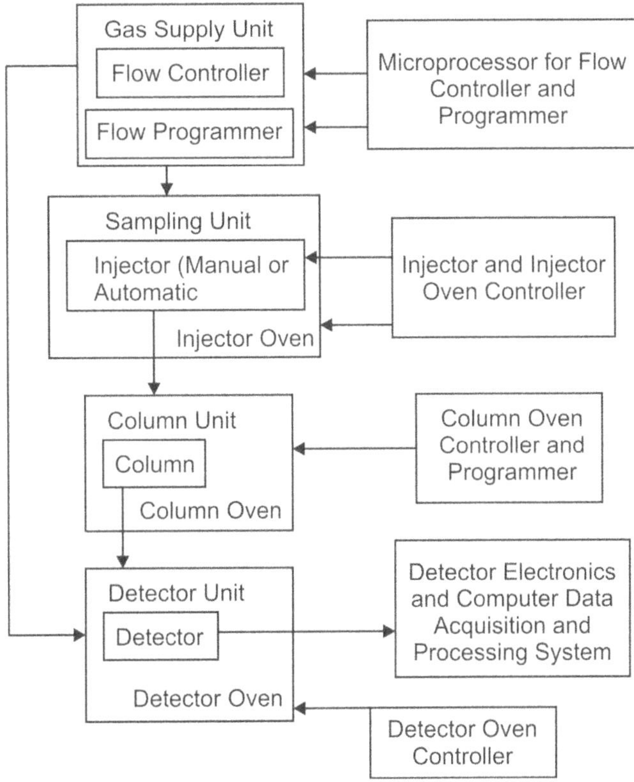

The Design of a Modern Gas Chromatograph.

The first unit, the gas supply unit, provides all the necessary gas supplies which may involve a number of different gases, depending on the type of detector that is chosen. For example, a flame ionization detector will require hydrogen or some other combustible gas mixture, air or oxygen to support combustion and a mobile phase supply that could be nitrogen, helium or some other appropriately inert gas. Thus, for the detector postulated, a minimum of three different gases would be required which will also involve the use of three flow controllers, three flow monitors and possibly a flow programmer. In addition the gas supply unit would be serviced by a microprocessor to monitor flow rates, adjust individual gas flows and, when and if necessary, program the mobile phase flow rate.

The second unit is the sampling unit which contains an automatic injector which is situated inside a thermostatically controlled enclosure. The injector usually has its own oven, but sometimes shares the column oven for temperature control. The injector oven, if separate from the column oven, is serviced by its own temperature controller which both monitors and controls the temperature. There is normally a separate controller, usually a microprocessor that controls the injector itself. The injector can range in complexity from a simple sample valve, or mechanically actuated syringe to an automatic multi sampler that is microprocessor controlled. It can have a complex transport system (such as a carousel) that can take samples, wash containers, prepare derivatives and, if necessary, carry out a very complex series of sample preparation procedures before injecting the sample onto the column.

The third unit is the column unit which contains the column, the essential device that actually achieves the necessary separation, and an oven to control the column temperature. It is interesting to note that despite the complexity of the apparatus, and its impressive appearance, the actual separation is achieved either in a relatively short length of packed tube or a simple wall-coated open tube. The rest of the apparatus is merely there to support this relatively trivial, but critical device. The oven also will contain a temperature sensor and if necessary an appropriate temperature programmer. As the mobile phase is a gas, there are virtually no interactions between the sample components and the mobile phase and thus the elution time can not be controlled by techniques such as solvent programming or gradient elution. The counterpart to gradient elution in gas chromatography is temperature programming. The column temperature is raised continuously during development to elute the more retained peaks in a reasonable time. It is a similar technique to flow programming but decreases the retention exponentially with temperature as opposed to linearly with flow rate.

The fourth unit contains the detector which is situated in its own oven. There is a wide range of detectors available each having unique operating parameters and its own performance characteristics. The detector, and the conduit connecting the column to the detector, must be maintained at a temperature at least 15°C above that of the maximum temperature the oven will reach during analysis to ensure no sample condenses in the conduits or detector, consequently, separate conduit heaters are necessary. Any condensation introduces serious detector noise into the system and also reduces the detector response thus affecting both the detector sensitivity and the accuracy and precision of the results. The detector oven is set at a user defined temperature and is operated isothermally, controlled by its own detector-oven temperature controller. The output from the detector is usually electronically modified and then acquired by the data processing computer which processes the data and prints out an appropriate report.

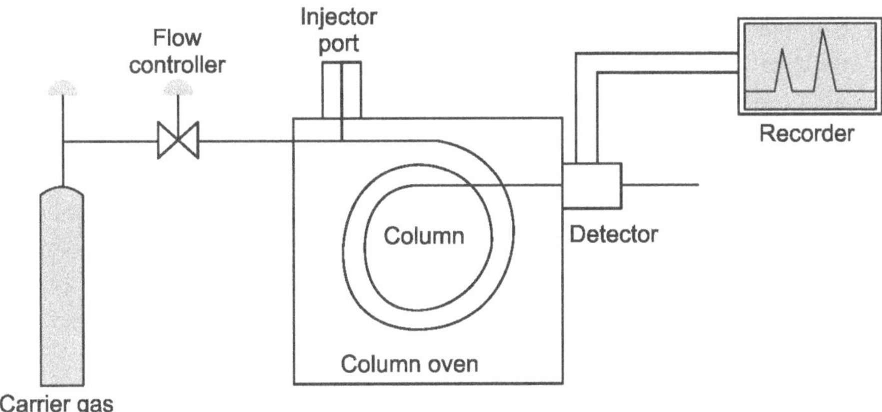

Schematic Diagram of a Gas Chromatography System.

Working of Gas Chromatograph

Like for all other chromatographic techniques, a mobile and a stationary phase are required. The mobile phase (=carrier gas) is comprised of an inert gas e.g. helium, argon, nitrogen, etc. The stationary phase consists of a packed column where the packing or solid support itself acts as stationary phase, or is coated with the liquid stationary phase (=high boiling polymer). More commonly used in many instruments are capillary columns, where the stationary phase coats the walls of a small-diameter tube directly (e.g. 0.25 mm film in a 0.32 mm tube).

The main reason why different compounds can be separated this way is the interaction of the compound with the stationary phase“(like-dissolves-like”-rule). The stronger the interaction is the longer the compound remains attached to the stationary phase, and the more time it takes to go through the column (=longer retention time).

Factors influencing the separation

1. ***Polarity of the stationary phase***: Polar compounds interact strongly with a polar stationary phase, hence have a longer retention time than non-polar columns. Chiral stationary phases based on amino acid derivatives, cyclodextrins, chiral silanes, etc are capable to separate enantiomers, because one form is slightly stronger bonded than the other one, often due to steric effects.
2. ***Temperature*:** The higher the temperature, the more of the compound is in the gas phase. It does interact less with the stationary phase, hence the retention time is shorter, but the quality of separation deteriorates.
3. ***Carrier gas flow***: If the carrier gas flow is high, the molecules do not have a chance to interact with the stationary phase. The result is the same as above.

4. ***Column length***: The longer the column is the better the separation usually is. The trade-off is that the retention time increases proportionally to the column length. There is also a significant broadening of peaks observed, because of increased back diffusion inside the column.
5. ***Amount of material injected***: If too much of the sample is injected, the peaks show a significant tailing, which causes a poorer separation. Most detectors are relatively sensitive and do not need a lot of material. High temperatures and high flow rates decrease the retention time, but also deteriorate the quality of the separation.

Carrier gas

The carrier gas must be chemically inert. Commonly used gases include nitrogen, helium, argon, and carbon dioxide. The choice of carrier gas is often dependant upon the type of detector which is used. The carrier gas system also contains a molecular sieve to remove water and other impurities.

Gas Supplies

Gases for use with the gas chromatograph were originally all obtained from gas tanks or gas cylinders. However, over the past decade the use of gas generators have become more popular as it avoids having gases at high pressure in the laboratory which is perceived by some as potentially dangerous. In addition, the use of a hydrogen generator avoids the use of a cylinder of hydrogen at high pressure which is also perceived by some as a serious fire hazard despite the fact that they have been used in laboratories, quite safely for nearly a century.

Supplies from Gas Tanks

Gasses are stored in large cylindrical tanks fitted with reducing valves that are set to supply the gas to the instrument at the recommended pressure defined by the manufacturers. The cylinders are often situated outside and away from the chromatograph for safety purposes and the gasses are passed to the chromatograph through copper or stainless steel conduits at relatively low pressure. The main disadvantage of gas tanks is their size and weight which makes them difficult to move and replace.

Pure Air Generators

Air generators require an air supply from air tanks or directly from the laboratory compressed air supply. The Packard Zero Air Generator passes the gas through a 0.5 μ filter to remove oil and water and finally over a catalyst to remove hydrocarbons. The hydrocarbon free air is then passed through a 0.01 μ cellulose fiber filter to remove any residual particulate matter that may be present.

Pure Nitrogen Generators

The nitrogen generator can also operate directly from the laboratory compressed air supply. General contaminants are first removed with appropriate filters and adsorbents and the purified air passes over layers of polymeric hollow fiber membranes through which nitrogen selectively permeates. The residual nitrogen-depleted air containing about 30% oxygen is vented to atmosphere.

Hydrogen Generators

In the Packard Hydrogen Generator, hydrogen is generated electrolytically from pure deionized water. Unfortunately, the technology used in hydrogen generators is largely proprietary and technical details are not readily available. The electrolysis unit uses a solid polymer electrolyte and thus does not need to be supplied with electrolytes, only the deionized water. The oxygen, produced simultaneously with hydrogen at half the flow rate, is vented to air.

Pressure Controllers

The first control on any gas line is afforded by a simple pressure controller. There are a number of pressure controllers associated with a gas chromatograph. The reducing valves on the gas tanks are examples of simple pressure controllers and the flow controllers that are used for detector and column flow control often involve devices based on the same principles.

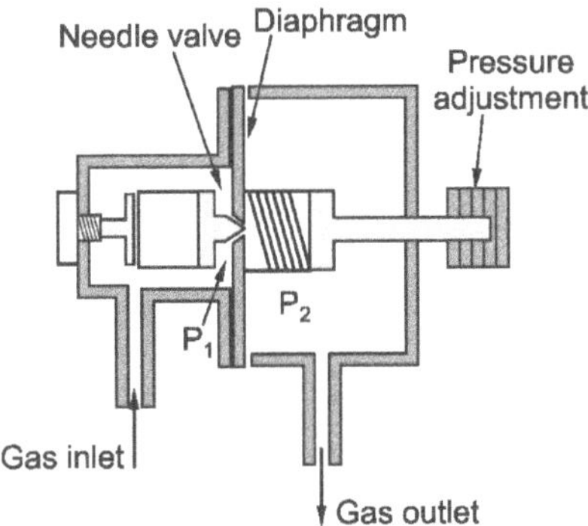

The Pressure Controller.

The pressure controller consists essentially of two chambers separated by a diaphragm, in the center of which is a needle valve that is actuated by the diaphragm. The diaphragm is held down by a spring that is adjustable so that the pressure in the second chamber, and thus the outlet flow, can be set at any chosen value. When gas enters the lower chamber, the pressure on the lower part of the diaphragm acts against the spring setting, and opens the valve. Gas then passes into the upper chamber and pressure is built up in the upper chamber to the value that has been set at which time the diaphragm moves downward closing the valve. If the pressure falls in the upper cylinder, the diaphragm again moves upward due to the pressure in the lower chamber, which opens the valve and the pressure in the upper chamber is brought back to its set value.

Flow Controllers

A constant pressure applied to a column does not ensure a constant flow of mobile phase though the chromatographic system, particularly if the column is being temperature programmed. Raising the temperature of a gas causes the viscosity to increase, and at a constant inlet pressure, the flow rate will fall. The reduction in flow rate will be related to the temperature program limits and to a certain extent on the temperature gradient. To obviate the flow rate change, mass controllers are used which ensure a constant mass of mobile passes through the column in unit time irrespective of the system temperature.

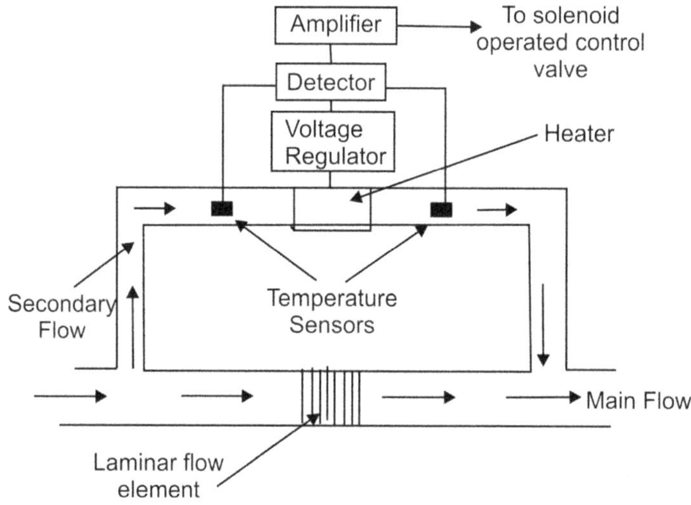

The Mass Flow Controller

The sensing system consists of a bypass tube with a heater situated at the center. Precision temperature sensors are placed equidistant up stream and down stream of the heater. A proprietary set of baffles situated in the main conduit creates a pressure drop that causes a fixed proportion of the flow to be diverted through the sensor tube. At zero flow rate both sensors are at the same temperature. At a finite flow rate, the down stream sensor is heated, producing a differential temperature across the sensors. The temperature of the gas will be proportional to the product of mass flowing and its specific heat and so the differential temperature that will be proportional to the mass flow rate. The differential voltage from the two sensors is compared to a set voltage and the difference used to generate a signal that actuates a valve controlling the flow. Thus, a closed loop control system is formed that maintains the mass flow rate set by the reference voltage. The device can be made extremely compact, is highly reliable and affords accurate control of the carrier gas flow rate irrespective of gas viscosity changes due to temperature programming.

Injection Devices

In gas chromatography two basic types of sampling system are used, those suitable for packed columns and those designed for open tubular columns. In addition, different sample injectors are necessary that will be appropriate for alternative column configurations. It must be stressed, however, that irrespective of the design of the associated equipment, the precision and accuracy of a GC analysis will only be as good as that provided by the sample injector. The sample injector is a very critical part of the chromatographic equipment and needs to be well designed and well maintained.

Packed Column Injectors

In general, the sample injected onto a packed GC column ranges in volume from 0.5 l to 5 l and usually contains the materials of interest at concentrations ranging from 5%v/v to 10%w/v. The sample is injected by a hypodermic syringe, through a silicone rubber septum directly into the column packing or into a flash heater. Although the latter tends to produce broader peaks it also disperses the sample radially across the column.

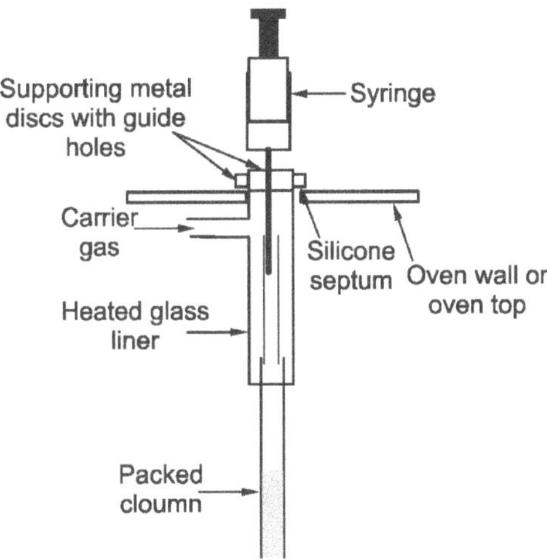

A Packed Column Injector

Direct injection into the packing constrains the sample into a small volume, but can cool the front of the packing. The silicone septum is compressed between made to penetrate past the liner and discharge its contents directly into the column packing. This procedure is called 'on-column injection' and, as it reduces peak dispersion on injection and thus, provides higher column efficiencies, is often the preferred procedure.

Direct injection into the packing constrains the sample into a small volume, but can cool the front of the packing. The silicone septum is compressed between metal surfaces in such a manner that a hypodermic needle can pierce it, but when it is withdrawn the hole is closed as a result of the septum compression and there is no gas leak. The glass liner prevents the sample coming in contact with the heated metal wall and thus, reduces the chance of thermal decomposition. The glass liner can be fitted with a separate heater and the volatilization temperature can, thus, be controlled. This "flash heater" system is available in most chromatographs. By using a syringe with a long needle, the tip can be made to penetrate past the liner and discharge its contents directly into the column packing. This procedure is called 'on-column injection' and, as it reduces peak dispersion on injection and thus, provides higher column efficiencies, is often the preferred procedure.

Open Tubular Column Injection Systems

Due to the very small sample size that must be placed on narrow bore capillary columns, a split injection system is necessary. The basic difference between the two types of injection systems is that the capillary column now projects into the glass liner and a portion of the carrier gas sweeps past the column inlet to waste. As the sample passes the column opening, a small fraction is split off and flows directly into the capillary column, *ipso facto* this device is called a split injector. The split ratio is changed by regulating the portion of the carrier gas that flows to waste which is achieved by an adjustable flow resistance in the waste flow line. This device is only used for small diameter capillary columns where the charge size is critical. The device has certain disadvantages due to component differentiation and the sample placed on the column may not be truly representative. The solutes with the higher diffusivities (low molecular weight) are lost preferentially to those with lower diffusivities (higher molecular weights). Consequently, quantitative analyses carried out using the high efficiency small diameter capillary columns may have limited accuracy and precision, depending on the nature of the sample.

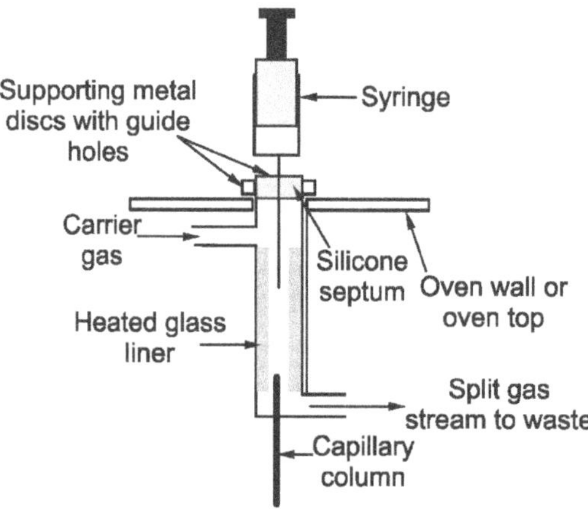

The Split Injection System

This problem was partially solved by using larger diameter columns that would permit *on-column* injection. The columns are constructed to have an I.D. of about 0.056 in; which is slightly greater than the diameter of a certain hypodermic needles.

However, there are also difficulties associated with this type of injector. On injection, the sample breaks up into separate portions, and bubbles form at the beginning of the column causing the sample to be deposited at different positions along the open tube as the solvent evaporates. On starting to develop the separation, each local concentration of sample acts as a separate injection. As a consequence, a chromatogram containing very wide or multiple peaks is produced. Procedures have been introduced in an attempt to eliminate sample splitting in this manner.

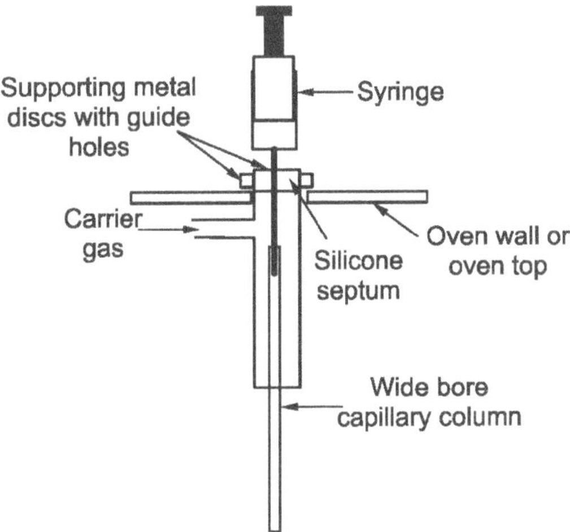

On-Column Injector for large bore open tubular columns.

Adsorbents

There are two types of packing employed in GC, the adsorbents and the supports, on which the stationary phase is coated. There are both inorganic and organic types of GSC adsorbents, each of which have specific areas of application. All are ground and screened to provide a range of particle sizes that extend from about 30/40 mesh to 100/120 mesh. In general, the smaller the particle size the higher the column efficiency, but the packing procedure is more difficult. It is also essential that the particle size *range* should be as narrow as possible. Packing materials that have a wide size range not only produce columns with poor efficiencies, but again, are also far more difficult to pack.

Alumina, in an activated form, is used to separate the permanent gases and hydrocarbons up to about pentane. Alumina is usually activated by heating to 200°C for about an hour. A common particle size is about 100/120 mesh and the pore size range from about 1 Å to 100,000Å. Silica gel in spherical form (prepared by spraying a neutralized silicate solution (a colloidal silica sol) into fine droplets, allowing the silica gel to be formed, and subsequently drying the droplets in a stream of hot air).

Silica is produced with a wide choice of surface areas and porosity's, which can range from about 750 m2/g and a mean pore size of 22 Å, to a material having a surface area of only 100m2/g and a mean pore diameter of 300 Å. It is used for the separation of the lower molecular weight gases and some of the smaller hydrocarbons. In a specially prepared form, silica can be used for the separation of the sulfur gases, hydrogen sulfide, sulfur dioxide and carbon disulfide.

Molecular sieves are used for the separation of small molecular weight gases largely by exclusion. The naturally occurring aluminosilicates are called zeolites, the *synthetic* zeolites are the Linde Molecular Sieves of which there are a number of different types available for specific applications. The zeolites have a crystalline structure which does not collapse when dehydrated. When water is removed from the crystals, channels of uniform dimensions are left within the structure which becomes very porous and the size of the channels changes only slightly with temperature.

Molecular sieves are used to separate substances of different molecular size and shape, *e.g.* straight chain hydrocarbons can be separated from their branched chain isomers. The molecular sieves designated 5A and 13X are commonly used for the separation of hydrogen, oxygen, nitrogen, methane and carbon monoxide and also argon, neon and the other rare gasses. Carbon is also used as an adsorbent of which there are two types. The high surface area active carbon and the graphitized carbon (surface areas ranging from 5 m2/g to about 100 m2/g).

The high surface area carbon, (*ca* 1000 m2/g) is used for the separation of the permanent gases and may need special treatment to modify its activity. The graphitized carbon adsorbents are much less active and separations appear to be based largely on exclusion. Macroporous Polymers such as the packings founded on the co-polymerization of polystyrene and divinylbenzene are also popular GC adsorbents. The extent of cross-linking determines its rigidity and the greater the cross-linking the harder the resin becomes until, at the extreme, the resin formed is very brittle.

The macro-porous resin consists of resin particles a few microns in diameter, which in turn are composed of a fused mass of polymer micro-spheres, a few Angstroms in diameter. Consequently, the resin polymer has a relatively high surface area as well as high porosity. They exhibit strong dispersive type interaction with solvents and solutes with some polarizability arising from the aromatic nuclei in the polymer.

Supports for GLC

There have been a number of materials used as supports for packed GC columns including, Celite (a proprietary form of a diatomaceous earth), fire-brick (calcined Celite), fire-brick coated with metallic silver or gold, glass beads, Teflon chips and polymer beads. Today however, the vast majority of contemporary packed GLC columns are filled with materials that are either based on of Celtic or polystyrene beads as a support. Diatomaceous supports comprise the silica skeletons of microscopic animals that lived many millions of years ago in ancient seas and lakes. As food transfer through the cells could only occur by diffusion, the supporting structure had to contain many apertures through which the cell nutrients could diffuse. This type of structure is ideal for a gas chromatography support, as rapid transfer by diffusion through the mobile and stationary phases is an essential requisite for the efficient operation of the column.

The original Celite material is too friable and the brickdust too active, and thus a series of modified Celites had to be introduced. There are two processes used to modify Celite. One was to crush, blend and press the Celite into the form of a brick and then calcine it at a temperature of about 900°C. Under these conditions some of the silica is changed into cristobalite and traces of iron and other heavy metals interact with the silica causing the material to become pink in color. This material is sold under the trade name of Chromosorb P. The second process involves mixing the Celite with sodium carbonate and fluxing the material at 900°C. This causes the structure of the Celite to be disrupted and the fragments adhere to one another by means of glass formed from the silica and the sodium carbonate. As the original Celite structure is disrupted, the material exhibits a wide range of pore sizes which differs significantly from the material that was calcined in the absence of sodium carbonate. This materials is sold under the name of Chromosorb W together with two similar materials called Chromosorb G and Chromosorb S. The residual deleterious adsorptive properties of the support are due to silanol groups on the surface and these can be removed by silanization. The support is treated with hexamethyldisilazane which replaces the hydrogen of the silanol group with a trimethylsilyl radical.

Glass beads have also been used as supports for packed GC columns and, if silanized, have little adsorption properties. Being non-porous, all the stationery phase must reside on the surface of the beads which gives them limited loading capacity. If the loading is increased, the stationary phase collects at the contact points of the spheres and form relatively thick accumulations, producing a high resistance to mass transfer and consequently low column efficiency. Glass beads appears to be the worst compromise between a column packed with modified Celite and a wall coated glass ,or fused silica, capillary column.

The macroporous polymer beads are used as supports as well as adsorbents. They exhibit significant adsorption as the support itself acts as a stationary phase and makes a substantial contribution to retention. However, with normal sample loads, the adsorption isotherm is linear and so the eluted peaks are symmetrical. Only stationary phases that do not affect the polymer in any way can be used with such beads, which is a distinct disadvantage. They also have relatively poor temperature stability.

Coating the Supports

It is important to have an accurate measure of the amount of stationary phase that has been placed on a support to ensure retention time reproducibility and qualitative accuracy. The reproducibility of the coating procedure may have particular significance when the analytical results are to be used for forensic purposes.

The material can be coated by the direct addition of the stationary phase to the support, by the filtration method or by the slurry method. The slurry method of coating is the one that is recommended. Coating by direct addition would appear to be the ideal quantitative method of preparing the column packings. A weighed amount of stationary phase is added directly to a known mass of support contained in a glass flask. The material is well mixed by rotating the flask for several hours, but even with extensive mixing, the stationary phase being is still irregularly distributed throughout the packing.

As a result, the efficiency of the column slowly increases with use, as the stationary phase distributes itself more evenly throughout the packing. It may take several weeks of use for the column to give a constant maximum efficiency. In the slurry method of coating, a weighed amount of the support is placed in the flask of a rotary evaporator and the required mass of stationary phase added. An appropriate volatile solvent is then added in sufficient quantity to produce free flowing slurry. The flask is then rotated at room temperature for ten minutes to ensure complete mixing. The rotating flask is then heated and the solvent removed by evaporation. When the packing appears dry, the material is then heated to about 150°C in and oven to remove the final traces of solvent. This method of coating gives an extremely homogeneous surface distribution of stationary phase throughout the support and an accurate value for the stationary phase loading.

GC Detectors

Detectors

There are many detectors which can be used in gas chromatography. Different detectors will give different types of selectivity. A *non-selective* detector responds to all compounds except the carrier gas, a *selective detector* responds to a range of compounds with a common physical or chemical property and a *specific detector* responds to a single chemical compound. Detectors can also be grouped into *concentration dependant detectors* and *mass flow dependant detectors*. The signal from a concentration dependant detector is related to the concentration of solute in the detector, and does not usually destroy the sample Dilution of with make-up gas will lower the detectors response. Mass flow dependant detectors usually destroy the sample, and the signal is related to the rate at which solute molecules enter the detector. The response of a mass flow dependant detector is unaffected by make-up gas. Have a look at this tabular summary of common GC detectors:

Detector	Type	Support gases	Selectivity	Detectability	Dynamic range
Flame ionization (FID)	Mass flow	Hydrogen and air	Most organic cpds.	100 pg	10^7
Thermal conductivity (TCD)	Concentration	Reference	Universal	1 ng	10^7
Electron capture (ECD)	Concentration	Make-up	Halides, nitrates, nitriles, peroxides, anhydrides, organometallics	50 fg	10^5
Nitrogen-phosphorus	Mass flow	Hydrogen and air	Nitrogen, phosphorus	10 pg	10^6
Flame photometric (FPD)	Mass flow	Hydrogen and air possibly oxygen	Sulphur, phosphorus, tin, boron, arsenic, germanium, selenium, chromium	100 pg	10^3
Photo-ionization (PID)	Concentration	Make-up	Aliphatics, aromatics, ketones, esters, aldehydes, amines, heterocyclics, organosulphurs, some organometallics	2 pg	10^7
Hall electrolytic conductivity	Mass flow	Hydrogen, oxygen	Halide, nitrogen, nitrosamine, sulphur		

Flame Ionisation Detector

The effluent from the column is mixed with hydrogen and air, and ignited. Organic compounds burning in the flame produce ions and electrons which can conduct electricity through the flame. A large electrical potential is applied at the burner tip, and a collector electrode is located above the flame. The current resulting from the pyrolysis of any organic compounds is measured. FIDs are mass sensitive rather than concentration sensitive; this gives the advantage that changes in mobile phase flow rate do not affect the detector's response. The FID is a useful general detector for the analysis of organic compounds; it has high sensitivity, a large linear response range, and low noise. It is also robust and easy to use, but unfortunately, it destroys the sample.

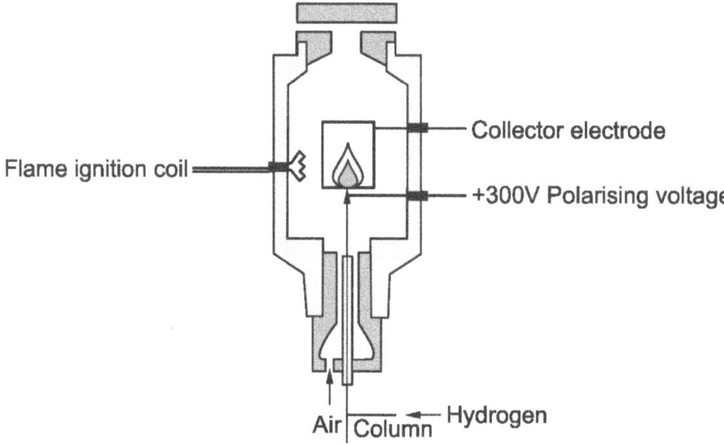

Thermal Conductivity Detector (TCD)

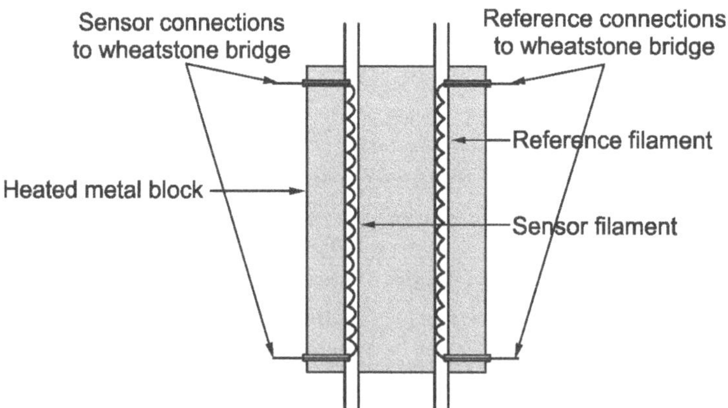

This detector is less sensitive than the FID (10^{-5}-10^{-6}g/s, linear range: 10^{3}-10^{4}), but is well suited for preparative applications, because the sample is not destroyed. It is based on the comparison of two gas streams, one containing only the carrier gas, the other one the carrier gas and the compound. Naturally, a carrier gas with a high thermal conductivity e.g. helium or hydrogen is used in order to maximize the temperature difference (and therefore the difference in resistance) between two thin tungsten wires. The large surface-to-mass ratio permits a fast equilibration to a steady state. The temperature difference between the reference cell and the sample cell filaments is monitored by a Wheatstone bridge circuit.

Electron Capture Detector (ECD)

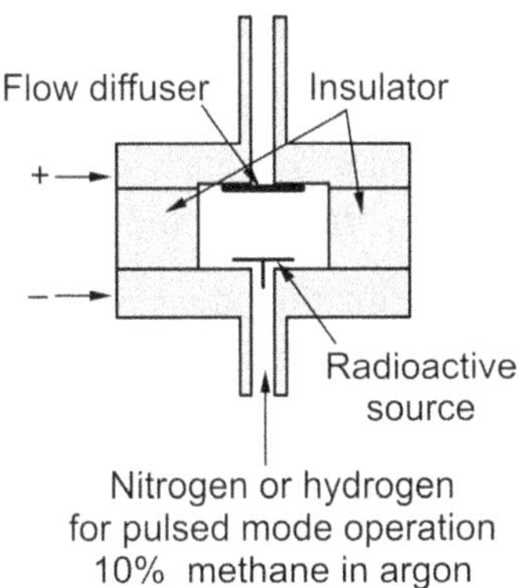

The detector consists of a cavity that contains two electrodes and a radiation source that emits β-radiation (e.g. ^{63}Ni, ^{3}H). The collision between electrons and the carrier gas (methane plus an inert gas) produces a plasma containing electrons and positive ions. If a compound is present that contains electronegative atoms, those electrons are "captured" and negative ions are formed, and the rate of electron collection decreases. The detector is extremely selective for compounds with atoms of high electron affinity (10^{-14} g/s), but has a relatively small linear range ($\sim 10^{2}$-10^{3}). This detector is frequently used in the analysis of chlorinated compounds e.g. pesticides, polychlorinated biphenyls, which show are very high sensitivity.

Parameters Used in Gas Chromatography

Retention time **(R_t):** Retention time is the difference in time between the *point of injection* and appearance of *peak maxima*. Retention time is the time required for 50% of a component to be eluted from a column. Retention time is measured in minutes or seconds. Retention time is also proportional to the distance moved on a chart paper, which can be measured in cm or mm.

Retention Volume **(Vr):** Retention volume is the volume of carrier gas required to elute 50% of the component from the column. It is the product of retention time and flow rate.

Retention volume = Retention time x flow rate

Separation factor (S)**:** Separation factor is the ratio of partition co-efficient of the two components to be separated. It can be expressed and determined by using the following equation:

$$S = K_b/K_a = K`_a/K`_b = (t_b\text{-}t_o)/(t_a\text{-}t_o)$$

where t_o = Retention time of unretained substance

K_b, K_a = Partition coefficients of b and a

t_b, t_a = Retention time of substance b and a

S = Depends on liquid phase, column temperature

If there is more difference in partition coefficient between two compounds, the peaks are far apart and the separation factor is more. If the partition coefficients of two compounds are similar, then the peaks are closer and the separation factor is less.

Resolution: Resolution is a measure of the extent of separation of two components and the baseline separation achieved. It can be determined by using the following formula:

$$Rs = 2(Rt_1 - Rt_2) / w_1 + w_2$$

Theoretical Plate (Plate theory)

A theoretical plate is an imaginary or hypothetical unit of a column where equilibrium has been established between stationary phase and mobile phase. A theoretical plate can also be called as a functional unit of the column.

HETP – Height Equivalent to a Theoretical Plate

A theoretical plate can be of any height, which decides the efficiency of separation. If HETP is more, the column is less efficient. HETP can be calculated by using the following formula:

$$HETP = \text{length of the column / no. of theoretical plates}$$

HETP is given by the Van Deemter equation

$$HETP = A + B/u + Cu$$

where A = Eddy diffusion term or multiple path diffusion which arises due to packing of the column. This is unaffected by carrier gas velocity of flow rate. This can be minimized by uniformity in packing.

B = Longitudinal diffusion term or molecular diffusion which depends on flow rate

C = Effect of mass transfer which depends on flow rate

U = flow rate or velocity of the mobile phase

A column is efficient only when HETP is minimum. Hence, an ideal flow rate corresponding to the minimum value of HETP is used.

Efficiency (No. of theoretical plates)

Efficiency of a column is expressed by the number of theoretical plates. It can be determined by using the formula:

$$n = 16\, x^2/y^2$$

where n = no. of theoretical plates

x = retention time

y = peak width

x and y are measured in common units (mm or cm or minutes or seconds) and are proportional to the distances marked on chart paper.

If the number of theoretical plates is high, the column is said to be highly efficient. If the number of theoretical plates is low, the column is said to be less efficient. For gas chromatographic column, a value of 600/metre is sufficient. But in HPLC, high values like 40,000 to 70,000/metre are recommended.

Asymmetry factor

A chromatographic peak should be symmetrical about its centre and said to follow Gaussian distribution. In such cases, the peak will be like an isosceles triangle. But in practice, due to some factors, the peak is not symmetrical and shows tailing or fronting.

Fronting is due to saturation of stationary phase and can be avoided by using less quantity of sample. Tailing is due to more active absorption sites and can be eliminated by support pretreatment, more polar mobile phased increasing the amount of liquid phase.

Asymmetry factor (0.95 to 1.05) can be calculated by using the formula: $AF = b/a$ (b and a calculated at 5% or 10% of the peak height)

Applications of Gas Chromatography

1. ***Qualitative analysis***: It is nothing but identification of compound. This is done by comparing the retention time of the sample as well as the standard. Under identical conditions, the retention time of the standard and the sample are same. If there is a deviation, then they are not the same compound.
2. ***Checking the purity of a compound***: by comparing the chromatogram of the standard and that of the sample, the purity of the compound can be reported. If additional peaks are obtained, impurities are present and hence the compound is not pure. From the percentage area of the peaks obtained, the percentage purity can also be reported.
3. ***Presence of impurities***: This can be seen by the presence of additional peaks when compared with a standard or reference material. The percentage of impurities may also be calculated from peak areas.

4. ***Quantitative analysis***: the quantity of a component can be determined by several methods like.
   (a) *Direct comparison method:* by injecting a sample and standard separately and comparing their peak areas, the quantity of the sample can be determined.

   Area of the peak = peak height x width of peak at the half height

   $$A_1/A_2 = \alpha \, W_1/W_2$$

   (b) *Calibration curve method:* In calibration curve method, standards of varying concentrations are used to determine their peak areas. A graph of peak area vs concentration of the drug is plotted. From the peak area of the unknown sample, by intrapolation, the concentration of the sample can be determined. This method has the advantage that errors, if any are minimized.
   (c) *Internal standard method:* in this method, a compound with similar retention characteristics is used. A known concentration of the internal standard is added to the sample solution whose concentration is not known. The chromatogram is recorded and their peak areas are determined. By using formula, the concentration of the unknown solution is determined.
5. ***Multi-component analysis or Determination of mixture of drugs***: Similar to the quantification of a single drug, multi-component analysis can also be done easily. The quantity of each component is determined by using any one of the above methods. Marketed formulations are available which contain several drugs and each component can be determined quantitatively.
6. ***Isolation and identification of drugs:*** Isolation and identification of drugs or metabolites in urine, plasma, serum etc can be carried out.
7. ***Isolation and identification of mixture of components:*** Isolation and identification of mixture of components like amino acids, plant extracts, volatile oils etc.

Some of the Pharmaceutical applications are described below:

1. Purity of compounds

Drug	Column	Temperature	Internal Standards
Atropine sulphate tablets	Phenylmethyl silicone	230°C	Homatropine hydrobromide
Fenfluramine tablets	Carboxwax 20 (10%) KOH (2%)	200°C	n-tetradecane
Scopolamine hydrobromide	Phenylmethyl silicone	230°C	Atropine sulphate

2. Presence of foreign or related substances

Drug	Purpose	Column	Temp	Internal Standard
Ethyloestrenol tablets	17 α-ethylestran-17 β-ol	Phenylmethyl silicone	200°C	Arachidic alcohol
Cimetidine	Residiual solvent	Porapak Q	135°C	n-Butyl alcohol
Tranylcypromine sulphate tablets	Cis isomer	OS 124 (10%)	220°C	4-bromo aniline HCl
Novobiocin sodium	Residiual solvent	Polyethylene glycol (10%)	100°C	Propanol

3. Assay of drugs

Drug	Column	Temperature
Diphenhydramine HCl	Carbowax	230°C
Antazoline HCl	Carbowax	230°C
Triprolidine HCl	Carbowax	230°C
Trifluoro acetyl methyl esters of amino acids • Alanine • Valine • Glycerine	Neopentyl glycol succinate	137°C

CHAPTER 7

HIGH PERFORMANCE LIQUID CHROMATOGRAPHY

Historical Perspective

- Russian botanist Tswett is credited with the discovery of chromatography.
- In 1903 he succeeded in separating leaf pigments using a solid polar stationary phase.
- It was not until the 1930's that this technique was followed up by Kuhn and Lederer as well as Reichstein and Van Euw for the separation of natural products.
- Martin and Synge were awarded the Nobel Prize for their work in 1941 in which they described liquid-liquid partition chromatography.
- Martin and Synge applied the concept of theoretical plates as a measure of chromatographic efficiency.
- This concept laid the foundation for gas-liquid chromatography (GLC) and high-performance liquid chromatography (HPLC).
- The GLC technique rapidly developed after Martin and James published the first use of GLC in 1952.
- HPLC was derived from classical column chromatography and has found an important place in analytical techniques.
- The major advancement in HPLC was found by the use of efficient separators. These separators used small particles and high pumping pressures.

Introduction

- The high performance liquid chromatography is a method of separation in which stationary phase is contained in a column, one end of which is attached to a source of pressurized liquid eluent (mobile phase).
- It is called high performance liquid chromatography as performance is also improved when compared to classical column chromatography.
- It is also called as high pressure liquid chromatography since high pressure is used when compared to classical column chromatography.
- In HPLC, the particle sizes are very smaller compare to classical column chromatography.
- Smaller particle size is important since they offer more surface area over the conventional larger particle sizes. For example a porous particle of 5μ offers a surface area of 100-860 sq. meters/gram with an average of 400 m^2/g. These offer very high plate counts upto 1,00, 000 plates/meter.

Comparison of Classical Column Chromatography with HPLC

PARAMETER	Classical Column Chromatography	HPLC
Stationary phase- Particle size	Large 60-200 μ	Small 3-30 μ
Column size length * Internal diameter	Large 0.5-5m × 0.5-5 cm	Small 5-50cm × 1-10 mm
Column material	glass	Mostly metal
Column packing pressure	Slurry packed at low pressure – Often gravity	Slurry paked at high pressure > 5000 psi
Operating pressure	Low (< 20 psi)	High (500-3000 psi)
Flow rates	Low to very low	Medium –high (often > 3 ml/min)
Sample load	Low to medium (g/mg)	Low to very low
Column efficiency i.e. Resolving power	(Low) < 500 theoretical plates/meter	(High) often < 1,00,000 theoretical plates/meter
Cost	Low – few hundred	High – few lakhs
Detector flow cell value	Large – 300 -1000 μl	Low – 2 to 10 μl
Types of stationary phase available	Limited range	Wide range
Scale of operation	Preparative scale	Analytical and preparative scale

Types of HPLC Techniques

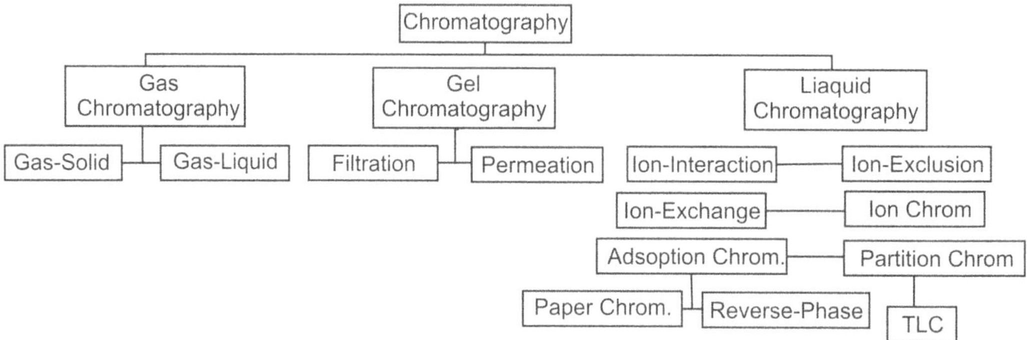

Types of Chromatography.

1. Based on mode of chromatography

- *There are two modes*: Normal phase mode and reverse phase mode
- These modes are based on the polarity of stationary and mobile phase.
- The interaction occurs between solute, stationary and mobile phase
  - (i) *Polar-polar*: Interaction or affinity is more
  - (ii) *Nonpolar-nonpolar*: Interaction or affinity is more
  - (iii) *Polar-nonpolar*: Interaction or affinity is less.

In the chromatography, the interaction is between solute and stationary phase or solute and mobile phase.

Normal phase mode

- In this, the stationary phase is polar and mobile phase is non-polar.
- In this technique, non-polar compound travel faster and eluted first. This is because less affinity between solute and stationary phase.
- Polar compound retained for longer time in the column because of more affinity towards stationary phase and take more time to eluted from the column.
- This is not advantageous in pharmaceutical applications as most of the drug molecules are polar in nature so takes longer time to eluted and detected.
- Hence this technique is not widely used in pharmacy.

Reverse phase mode

- In this, stationary phase is non polar and mobile phase is polar in nature.
- Hence polar component eluted first and non-polar are retained for longer time.

- Since most of the drug and pharmaceutical are polar in nature, they are not retained for longer time and eluted faster, which is advantageous.
- Different column used are ODS (Octadecyl silane) or C_{18}, C_8, C_4, etc.

2. **Based on the principle of separation**
    - Adsorption chromatography
    - Ion exchange chromatography
    - Ion Pair chromatography
    - Size exclusion or gel permeation chromatography
    - Affinity chromatography
    - Chiral phase chromatography

Each of the above technique is described in brief as follows:

(i) *Adsorption chromatography*

- The principle of separation is adsorption.
- Separation of component is done because of the difference in affinity of the compounds towards stationary phase.
- This principle is seen in normal phase as well as reverse phase mode, when adsorption take place.

(ii) *Ion exchange chromatography*

- The principle of separation is ion exchange which is reversible exchange of functional groups.
- In this, an ion exchange resin is used to separate the mixture of similar charged ion.
- For cations, a cation exchange resin is used and for anions, anion exchange resin is used.
- This technique is applicable to ion exchange chromatography by HPLC.

(iii) *Ion Pair chromatography*

- In this, a reverse phase column is converted temporarily into ion exchange column by using ion pairing agents like pentane, hexane, peptane or octane sulphonic acid sodium salt, Tetra methyl or tetra ethyl ammonium hydroxide, etc

(iv) *Size exclusion or gel permeation chromatography*

- In this, from mixture, components with different molecular sizes are separated by using gel.
- The gel used acts as a molecular sieve. Hence from mixture, components having different molecular sizes are separated.

- Soft gels like dextrose, agarose or Polyacrylamide are used.
- Semi rigid gels like polystyrene, alkyl dextran in non aqueous medium are also used.
- The mechanism of separation is steric and diffusion effects.

(v) ***Affinity chromatography***

- In this, Affinity of the sample with specific stationary phases is used.
- This technique is mostly used in field of biotechnology, microbiology and biochemistry, etc.

(vi) ***Chiral phase chromatography***

- Separation of optical isomer can be done by using chiral stationary phases.
- Different principles operate for different types of stationary phase and different kind of samples.
- The stationary phases used for this type of chromatography are mostly chemically bonded silica gel.

3. Based on elution technique

(i) ***Isocratic separation***

- In this same mobile phase combination is used through out the process of separation.
- The same polarity or elution strength is maintained throughout the process.

(ii) ***Gradient separation***

- In this, a mobile phase combination of lower polarity or elution strength is used followed by gradually increasing polarity or elution strength.

4. Based on the scale of the operation

- ***Analytical HPLC***
- Where only analysis of samples are done.
- Recovery of the sample for reusing is normally not done, since the sample used is very low. Eg. μg quantities.
- ***Preparative HPLC:***
- Where the individual fraction of pure compounds can be collected using fractional collector.
- The collected samples are reused.

e.g. Separation of few grams of mixtures by HPLC

5. **Based on the type of analysis**
   - ***Qualitative analysis***
     - It is used to identify the compound, detect the presence of impurities, to find out the number of components, etc.
     - This is done by using retention time values.
     - ***Quantitative analysi:***
     - It is done to determine the quantity of the individual or several components in the mixture.
     - This is done by comparing the peak area of the standard and sample.

Principle

- The principle of separation in normal phase mode and reverse phase mode is adsorption.
- When as a mixture, various components are introduced into a HPLC column; they travel according to their relative affinities toward the stationary phase.
- The component which has more affinity towards the absorbent travels slower.
- The component which has less affinity towards the stationary phase travels faster.
- Since none of the two components have the same affinity towards the stationary phase, the components are separated.

Parameters Involved in Chromatographic Separations

Capacity Factor

The capacity factor, k', of a compound indicates its retention behaviour on a column.

$$k' = \frac{k_d \times V_s}{V_m} = \frac{C_s \times V_m}{C_m \times V_s} \times \frac{t_{ms} - t_m}{t_m} = \frac{t_s}{t_m}$$

K_d: Distribution coefficient

V_s: Volume of stationary phase

V_m: Volume of mobile phase

C_s: Solute concentration in the stationary phase

C_m: Solute concentration in the mobile phase

- Small values of k' show that the compound is poorly retained and elutes near the void volume.
- Large k' values imply a good separation but downfalls of this are longer analysis times with peak broadening and decreases in sensitivity.
- Ideal separations occur with a capacity factor of between 1 and 5.

Resolution

- The aim of chromatography is to separate components in a mixture into bands or peaks as they migrate through the column.
- Resolution, R, provides a quantitative measure of the ability of a column to separate two analytes.
- This measurement is obtained by the retention times and peakwidths which are easily obtained directly from the chromatogram.

$$R = \frac{t_{ms_2} - t_{ms_1}}{\frac{w_1 + w_2}{2}} = \frac{2\Delta t}{w_1 + w_2}$$

t_{ms1} *and* t_{ms2}: Gross retention times for peaks 1 and 2 respectively

w_1 *and* w_2: Peak widths along the baseline of peak 1 and 2 respectively

$$R = \frac{t_{ms_2} - t_{ms_1}}{\frac{w_1 + w_2}{2}} = \frac{2\Delta t}{w_1 + w_2}$$

- For two peaks to be recognized as separate the resolution should be at least 0.5.
- Two peaks are seen as completely separate if R is greater than 1.5.
- The resolution can be improved by lengthening the column but this will also increase the analysis time.

Column Efficiency

- A chromatographic column is divided into N theoretical plates.
- A thermodynamic equilibrium of the analytes between the mobile and stationary phase occurs within each plate.
- The efficiency of the column is thus expressed as the number of theoretical plates.

$$N = \frac{L}{H}$$

L : Length of column packing (cm)

H : Plate height

- N is determined experimentally from a chromatogram using the equation:

$$N = 16\left(\frac{t_{ms}}{W}\right)^2$$

- Poor column efficiency results in band broadening.

Column Selectivity

- Column selectivity, α, is a measure of the relative separation of two peaks and is defined as the ratio of the net retention times of the two peaks.

$$\alpha = \frac{t_{ms_2} - t_m}{t_{ms_1} - t_m}$$

Distribution or Partition Coefficient

- The distribution coefficient, K_d, indicates the distribution of analytes between the resin and the eluent.
- It is defined as the ratio of the molar concentrations of the solute in the stationary and mobile phase.

$$K_d = \frac{\text{Mass of Compound on resin (g)} \times \text{Volume of resin (ml)}}{\text{mass of dry resin(g)} \times \text{volume of eluent (ml)}} = \frac{C_s}{C_m}$$

C_s *and* C_m : Molar concentrations of the solute in the stationary and mobile phases respectively

Factors Affecting Band Broadening

Various factors affect the peak variance, σ^2, and thus the bandwidth.

- It is important to consider these processes in the correct design of any chromatographic system so that the variance and thus peak width can be minimised and the efficiency can be maximised.
- The extent of band broadening can be expressed in terms of plate height as follows:

$$H = A + \frac{B}{u} + C_{stationary}\bar{u} + C_{mobile}\bar{u}$$

A. Eddy Diffusion

- The A term in the above equation is called eddy diffusion.
- This term describes the multitude of pathways that the solute molecules can follow in a packed column.

- Each of the paths is a different length and molecules will pass through at various rates thus leading to band broadening.
- Eddy diffusion can be minimised with a column that is uniformly packed with particles of constant size.
- Band broadening is independent of the flow rate of the eluent.

B. Longitudinal Diffusion

- Molecules in a sample band tend to diffuse out of this band during it passage through the chromatographic column.
- This process is known as longitudinal diffusion and is the B term in the above equation.
- Longitudinal diffusion occurs in both the direction of flow of the mobile phase as well as in the opposite direction.
- Longitudinal diffusion increases at low eluent flow rates, as diffusion is a time dependant process.

C. Mass Transfer

- The C term is due to mass transfer, which is the interchange of solute molecules between the mobile and stationary phases.
- In an ideal chromatographic system this process would occur instantaneously but this is not the case in practice.
- Hence different molecules spend varying amounts of time in the stationary and mobile phases, which leads to band broadening.
- Band broadening increases as the eluent flow rate increases although it can be minimised by using a stationary phase with a small diameter or one, which has an active layer that is confined to the outer surface of the particle.

HPLC Instrumentation

The main components of an HPLC system are:

- a high-pressure pump
- a column
- an injector system
- a detector
- *The system works as follows*: eluent is filtered and pumped through a chromatographic column, the sample is loaded and injected onto the column and the effluent is monitored using a detector and recorded as peaks.

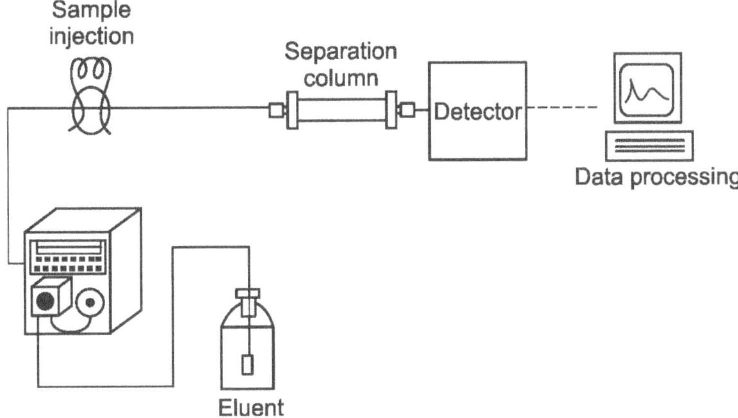

HPLC Instrumentation

Analytical Pumps (Solvent Delivery System)

The requirements for HPLC pumps are as follows

- They must be able to generate high pressures, have a pulse-free output, deliver flow rates ranging from 0.1 to 10 ml/min, have flow reproducibility's of 0.5 % relative or better and they must be resistant to corrosion by a variety of solvents.

Various types of pumping systems exist, these include:

A. *Direct Gas-pressure Systems*

- This system consists of a cylinder gas pressure, which is applied directly to the eluent in a holding coil.
- Advantages of this pump are that it is reliable and economical although solvent changing is found to be tedious.

B. Syringe-type Pumps

- In these pumps an electrically driven lead-screw moves a piston, which is able to pressurise a finite volume of solvent, and thus delivers a pulseless constant flow of solvent to the system.
- These pumps are found to be reliable although they are expensive, solvent changing is tedious and they have a finite capacity (~250 ml).

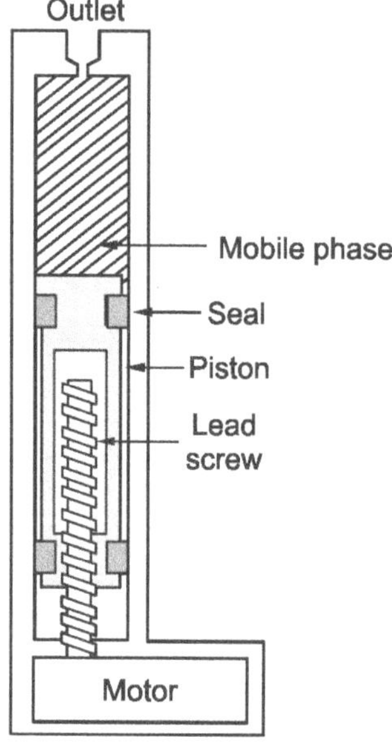

Syringe-type Pump

C. Pneumatic Intensifier (Constant Pressure) Pumps

- Pneumatic intensifier pumps are operated via gas pressure.
- A large area piston drives a small area piston when acted on by pressure from a gas line.
- The gas pressure is thus amplified in the ratio of the areas of the forces of the pistons and a high-pressure liquid at constant pressure is introduced into the system.
- If a partial blockage occurs in this system a drop in flow rate occurs but the pressure remains constant.
- The flow sensitivity of the detector cell will determine how much pulse damping is required in the system to suppress the detector signal caused when the flow stops during the return stroke.

D. Reciprocating (Constant Flow) Pumps

- A reciprocating pump is the most generally used, as it is economical and allows a wide range of flow rates.
- With this pump there is no limit on the reservoir size or operating time as is commonly found with other pumps.
- This type of pump is electrically driven by a motor, which moves back and forth within a hydraulic chamber.

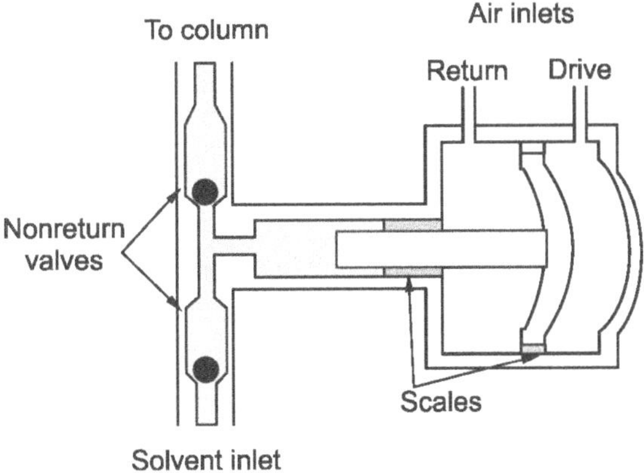

Constant Pressure Pump

- On the backward stroke the piston sucks in eluent from the reservoir and due to check valves the outlet to the separation column is closed.
- During the forward stroke the eluent is pushed onto the column and the inlet from the reservoir is closed.
- The pumping motion of the piston produces a pulsed flow that requires dampeni
- These pumps include a high output pressure with constant flow rates and the ability to be used for gradient elution.

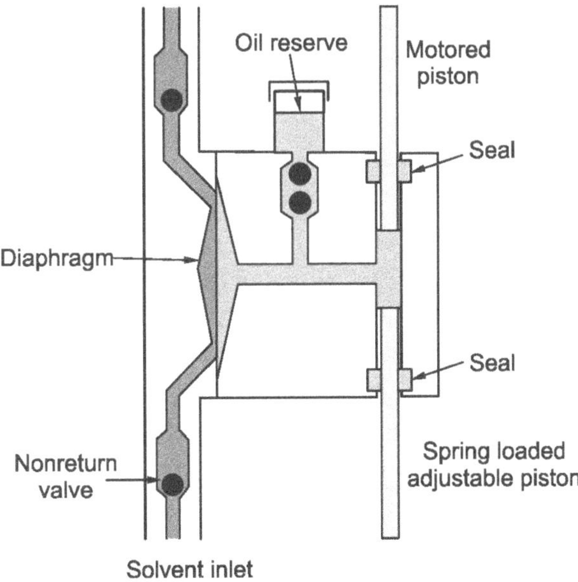

Reciprocating pump

HPLC Gradient Mixers

- HPLC gradient mixers must provide a very precise control of solvent composition to maintain a reproducible gradient profile.
- This can be complicated in HPLC by the small elution volumes required by many systems.
- It is much more difficult to produce a constant gradient when mixing small volumes then when mixing large volumes.
- For low pressure systems this requires great precision in the operation of the miniature mixing valves used and low dispersion flows throughout the mixer.
- For multi-pump high pressure systems, it requires a very precise control of the flow rate while making very small changes of the flow rate.

HPLC Sample Valves

Since sample valves come between the pump and the column it follows that HPLC sample valves must also tolerate pressures up to 10,000 p.s.i. (Pascals per Square Inch) For analytical HPLC, the sample volume should be selectable from sub- micro liter to a few micro liters, whereas in preparative HPLC the sample volume may be even greater than 10 ml. To maintain system efficiency the sample valve must be designed to have very low dispersion characteristics, this is true not only for flow dispersion but also for the less obvious problems of dispersion caused by sample adsorption/desorption on valve surfaces and diffusion of sample into and out of the mating surfaces between valve moving parts. It goes without saying that the valves must deliver a very constant sample size but this is usually attained by the use of a constant size sample loop.

Mobile Phase

- The mobile phase in HPLC refers to the solvent being continuously applied to the column, or stationary phase.
- The mobile phase acts as a carrier for the sample solution.
- A sample solution is injected into the mobile phase of an assay through the injector port.
- As a sample solution flows through a column with the mobile phase, the components of that solution migrate according to the non-covalent interactions of the compound with the column.
- The chemical interactions of the mobile phase and sample, with the column, determine the degree of migration and separation of components contained in the sample.

- For example, those samples which have stronger interactions with the mobile phase than with the stationary phase will elute from the column faster, and thus have a shorter retention time, while the reverse is also true.
- The mobile phase can be altered in order to manipulate the interactions of the sample and the stationary phase.
- There are several types of mobile phases, these include: Isocratic, gradient, and polytyptic.
- In isocratic elution compounds are eluted using constant mobile phase composition. The separation of compounds can be described using several equations:

Equations for Gradient Elution

Retention Time (s) 1. $t_g - t_o\bar{k}\ \log(2.3\ k_0/\bar{k})$

Bandwidth (ml) 2. $\sigma_g - V_m\,(1 + \bar{k})N^{-1/2}/2$

Resolution ($\Delta t_R/4\sigma$ or $\Delta t_g/4\sigma_g$) 3. $R_s - [(1/4)\,(\alpha - 1)^{N1/2}]\,[\bar{k}/(1 + \bar{k})]$

Capacity Factor 4. $\bar{k}\ - t_G/\Delta\phi S t_0$

$- t_G F/\Delta\phi S\ V_m$

- All compounds begin migration through the column at onset.
- However, each migrates at a different rate, resulting in faster or slower elution rate.
- This type of elution is both simple and inexpensive, but resolution of some compounds is questionable and elution may not be obtained in a reasonable amount of time.
- In gradient elution different compounds are eluted by increasing the strength of the organic solvent.
- The sample is injected while a weaker mobile phase is being applied to the system.
- The strength of the mobile phase is later increased in increments by raising the organic solvent fraction, which subsequently results in elution of retained components.
- This is usually done in a stepwise or linear fashion. There are several equations that describe gradient elution:

Equations for Gradient Elution

Retention Time (s) 1. $t_g - t_o\bar{k}\ \log(2.3\ k_0/\bar{k})$

Bandwidth (ml) 2. $\sigma_g - V_m\,(1 + \bar{k})N^{-1/2}/2$

Resolution ($\Delta t_R/4\sigma$ or $\Delta t_g/4\sigma_g$) 3. $R_s - [(1/4)(\alpha - 1)^{N1/2}] [\bar{k}/(1 + \bar{k})]$

Capacity Factor 4. $\bar{k} - t_G/\Delta\phi S t_0$

$- t_G F/\Delta\phi S\ V_m$

- At the onset of sample introduction, the compounds are initially retained at the inlet of the column.
- As the solute capacity, or k', for the compound decreases, the compound begins to migrate through the stationary phase.
- Each of the other compounds in the sample subsequently migrate as their k' values decrease.
- Compared with isocratic elution, resolution and separation are improved, and bandwidths are nearly equal.

Isocratic Vs. Gradient Elution

- The Knox equation describes column efficiency or plate number N in relation to certain experimental conditions, such as column length, column diameter, temperature, flow-rate, molecular weight, etc.
- Plate number N is equal to plate height value H divided by particle diameter (dp).
- Plate height value H is in turn equal to column length L divided by N.
- Two of the Knox coefficients, B and C, depend on k' and size of the compound.
- In the equations above, k' in the isocratic equations is replaced with average k' in the gradient equations.
- In fact, this is the only difference in the bandwidth and resolution equations between the two.
- Thus, separation and height of the peak are dictated by the exact same conditions for both isocratic and gradient elution
- From the equation for capacity factor in gradient elution, it can be seen that average k' value depends on flow-rate, gradient time, and column dead volume.
- This differs in isocratic elution where k' is not dependent on time of separation, flow- rate, or column dimensions.
- A special feature in gradient elution is linear-solvent strength (LSS) gradients.
- These give approximately equal values of average k' for samples eluting at different times during separation.
- This is the reason why gradient elution can yield constant bandwidths for different compounds and equal resolution for pairs of compounds which have similar alpha or separation factor values.

- Polytyptic Mobile Phase, sometimes referred to as mixed-mode chromatography, is a versatile method in which several types of chromatographic techniques, or modes, can be employed using the same column.
- These columns contain rigid macroporous hydrophobic resins covalently bonded to a hydrophilic organic layer.
- SEC, IEC, hydrophobic or affinity chromatography are some of the methods that may be utilized.
- By changing the mobile phase, the mode of separation is thereby changed which allows the chromatographer to achieve the desired selectivity in the separations.

Separation Columns

- There are various columns that are secondary to the separating column or stationary phase. They are: Guard, Derivatizing, Capillary, Fast, and Preparatory Columns.
- **Guard Columns**
  - They are placed anterior to the separating column.
  - This serves as a protective factor that prolongs the life and usefulness of the separation column.
  - They are dependable columns designed to filter or remove
    1. particles that clog the separation column.
    2. compounds and ions that could ultimately cause "baseline drift", decreased resolution, decreased sensitivity, and create false peaks.
    3. compounds that may cause precipitation upon contact with the stationary or mobile phase.
    4. compounds that might co-elute and cause extraneous peaks and interfere with detection and/or quantification.
    - These columns must be changed on a regular basis in order to optimize their protective function.
    - Size of the packing varies with the type of protection needed.

Derivatizing Columns

- Pre or post-primary column derivatization can be an important aspect of the sample analysis.

- Reducing or altering the parent compound to a chemically related daughter molecule or fragment elicits potentially tangible data which may complement other results or prior analysis.
- In few cases, the derivatization step can serve to cause data to become questionable, which is one reason why HPLC was advantageous over gas chromatography, or GC.
- Because GC requires volatile, thermally stabile, or nonpolar analytes, derivatization was usually required for those samples which did not contain these properties.
- Acetylation, silylation, or concentrated acid hydrolysis are a few derivatization techniques.

Capillary Columns

Advances in HPLC led to smaller analytical columns. Also known as microcolumns, capillary columns have a diameter much less than a millimeter and there are three types:

- open-tubular
- partially packed
- tightly packed
- They allow the user to work with nanoliter sample volumes, decreased flow rate, and decreased solvent volume usage which may lead to cost effectiveness.
- However, most conditions and instrumentation must be miniaturized, flow rate can be difficult to reproduce, gradient elution is not as efficient, and care must be taken when loading minute sample volumes.
- Microbore and small-bore columns are also used for analytical and small volumes assays.
- A typical diameter for a small-bore column is 1-2 mm. Like capillary columns, instruments must usually be modified to accommodate these smaller capacity columns (i.e., decreased flow rate).
- However, besides the advantage of smaller sample and mobile phase volume, there is a noted increase in mass sensitivity without significant loss in resolution.-- Capillary Electrophoresis

Fast Columns

- One of the primary reasons for using these columns is to obtain improved sample throughput (amount of compound per unit time).

- For many columns, increasing the flow or migration rate through the stationary phase will adversely affect the resolution and separation.
- Therefore, fast columns are designed to decrease time of the chromatographic analysis without forsaking significant deviations in results.
- These columns have the same internal diameter but much shorter length than most other columns, and they are packed with smaller particles that are typically 3 µm in diameter.

Advantages

- increased sensitivity
- decreased analysis time,
- decreased mobile phase usage, and
- increased reproducibility

Preparatory Columns

- These columns are utilized when the objective is to prepare bulk (milligrams) of sample for laboratory preparatory applications.
- A preparatory column usually has a large column diameter which is designed to facilitate large volume injections into the HPLC system.
- Accessories important to mention are the back-pressure regulator and the fraction collector.
- The back-pressure regulator is placed immediately posterior to the HPLC detector. It is designed to apply constant pressure to the detector outlet which prevents the formation of air bubbles within the system.
- This, in turn, improves chromatographic baseline stability. It is usually devised to operate regardless of flow rate, mobile phase, or viscosity.
- The fraction collector is an automated device that collects uniform increments of the HPLC output.
- Vials are placed in the carousel and the user programs the time interval in which the machine is to collect each fraction.
- Each vial contains mobile phase and sample fractions at the corresponding time of elution.
- Packings for columns are diverse since there are many modes of HPLC.
- They are available in different sizes, diameters, pore sizes, or they can have special materials attached (such as an antigen or antibody for immunoaffinity chromatography).

- Packings available range from those needed for specific applications (affinity, immunoaffinity, chiral, biological, etc.) to those for all-purpose applications.
- The packings are attached to the internal column hull by resins or supports, which include oxides, polymers, carbon, hydroxyapatite beads, agarose, or silica, the most common type.
- Heavy-wall glass, stainless steel and plastic are among materials that can withstand high pressures and are thus used to construct HPLC columns.
- They must also be able to resist the chemical action of the mobile phase.
- Wall irregularities will cause a well-packed column to channel near the wall or packing interface thus the tubing must have a smooth, precision bore internal diameter.
- Channels would cause peak broadening and a decrease in efficiency.
- Column connections are made with low dead-volume fittings, which prevent stagnant pockets of eluent.
- Usually a short guard column is placed in front of the analytical column.
- This serves to increase the life of the analytical column by removing particulate matter and contaminants from the solvents.

Column efficiency refers to the performance of the stationary phase to accomplish particular separations. This entails how well the column is packed and its kinetic performance. The efficiency of a column can be measured by several methods which may or may not be affected by chromatographic anomalies, such as "tailing" or appearance of a "front." This is important because many chromatographic peaks do not appear in the preferred shape of normal Gaussian distribution. For this reason efficiency can be an enigmatic value since manufacturers may use different methods in determining the efficiency of their columns.

Calculation of column efficiency value

All the following methods use this formula that measures N, or number of theoretical plates:

$$N = a\frac{t_r^2}{w^2}$$

a = constant dependent on height where peak width measured

t_r = retention time

w = peak width

***Inflection Method*:** Calculation is based upon inflection point which appears at 60.7% of the peak height for a normal Gaussian peak. At this point the width of the peak is equivalent to two standard deviation units. Any asymmetrical aspect of a peak should not affect this calculation since the width is measured above the anomalous occurrence (i.e., tailing or fronting).

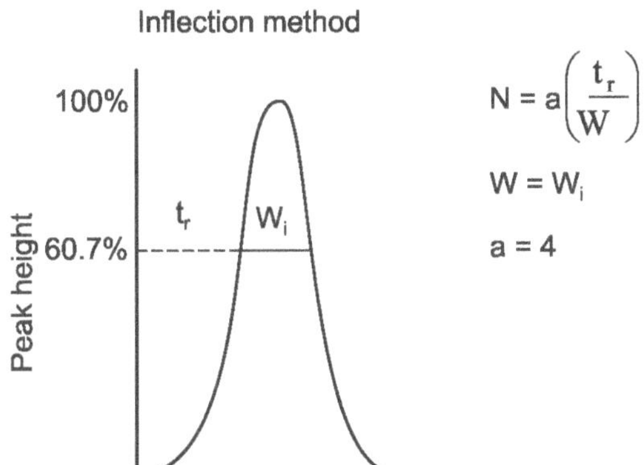

***Half-peak Height Method*:** As the name suggests, the measurement is based upon the width at 50% of peak height. For the same reason as inflection method, this measurement is not affected by asymmetry; however, this method is more reproducible from person to person since width at 50% peak height is less prone to be varied.

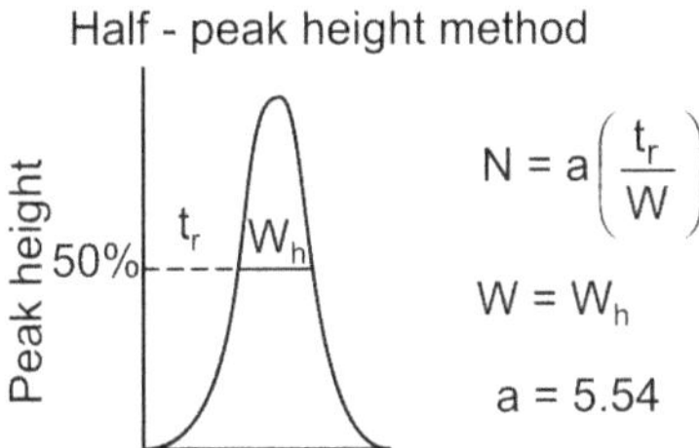

Tangent Method: Tangent lines are drawn on each side of the peak and the width is the distance between the two lines at the base of the peak. Therefore, it is more sensitive to asymmetrical peaks and variation in efficiency values is usually seen from user to user.

***Sigma Methods*:** These methods measure peak width at decreasing levels of peak height. Thus, the **three sigma method** measures width at 32.4% of peak height, the **four sigma method** measures at 13.4%, and the **five sigma method** measures at 4.4%. The five sigma method is most sensitive to asymmetry because the width is measured at the lowest point.

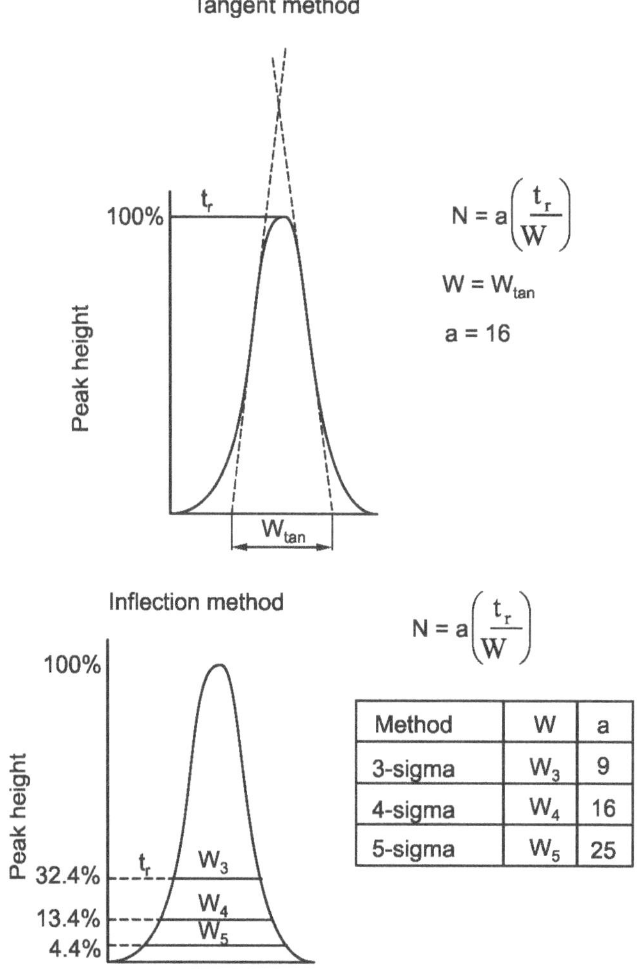

Height/Area Method: This method utilizes the fact that the area of a peak is a function of its height and standard deviation. To determine efficiency, values for peak height and area are used in a different formula.

$$N = \frac{2\pi(ht_r)^2}{A^2}$$

H = peak height; A = area

A computer is usually necessary to use this method in order to calculate the area and height.

***Moment Method*:** This method entails disregarding peak shape and expresses parameters of the peak in statistical moments. The zero moment, $\mu 0$, is the peak area. The first moment, $\mu 1$, is the mean and occurs at the center of the peak (which is the maximum peak height in normal Gaussian peaks). The second moment, $\mu 2$, is the variance of the peak. This is a detailed method where appropriate data systems are needed.

These methods were evaluated by computer simulation based on efficiency values obtained on a series of synthetically modified Gaussian peaks (i.e., increasing the 'tailing') and compared to the actual value based on the moment method (which was determined to be the most accurate). Briefly, the results were as follows:

Calculation Method – Accuracy

Inflection	Low
Half-peak height	Low
Tangent	Low
Height:Area ratio	Medium
Four Sigma	Medium
Five sigma	High
Asymmetry	High

Types of Stationary Phases

Various stationary phases are available for HPLC and are discussed below.

Polystyrene/Divinylbenzene – Based Resins

In ion chromatography, the support material is a polystyrene/divinylbenzene (PS/DVB) based resin that is relatively stable with respect to pH.

- The copolymerisation of PS with DVB is used to give the resin mechanical stability.
- The amount of DVB in the resin is denoted as "percent crosslinking". The percentage of crosslinking is directly related to the extent to which PS/DVB resin shrinks or swells in an aqueous media or in the presence of organic solvents.
- If the resin shrinks a loss in column efficiency occurs as a dead volume occurs at the beginning of the column.
- Swelling of the resin leads to higher column backpressures. The optimum degree of crosslinking is said to be 2-5%.

A. Anion-Exchange Resin

- The anion-exchange resins used by Dionex are composed of a surface sulphonated PS/DVB core (10-25 μm) and a totally porous latex particle (0.1 μm), which is completely aminated.
- Electrostatic and van der Waals interactions are used to agglomerate the latex particles onto the core particles.
- It is the latex particles that carry the actual ion exchange function.

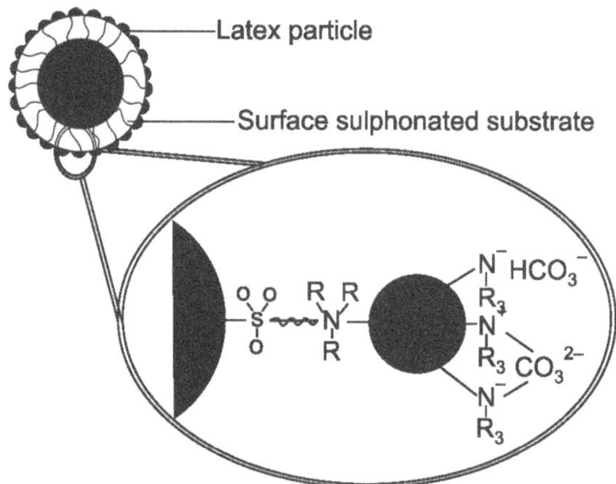

The structure of a latex anion exchange particle

- The length of the diffusion path as well as the rate of diffusion is determined by the particle size of the latex material.
- Advantages of this stationary phase include mechanical stability of the resin due to the inner core, which also ensures moderate backpressures.
- Rapid exchange processes and thus high efficiencies occur due to the small, totally porous, latex particles.
- Surface sulphonation greatly reduces swelling and shrinking of the material.
- The selectivity of the resin can be varied by making use of various quaternary ammonium bases.

B. Cation-Exchange Resins

- The stationary phase of a cation exchange column is based on inert, surface sulphonated, crosslinked polystyrene.

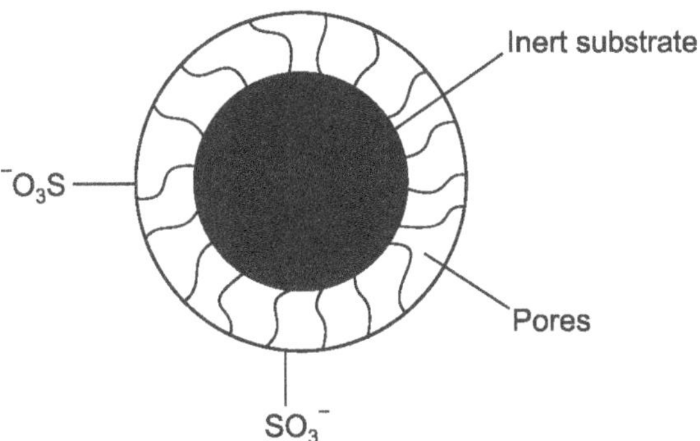

The structure of a latex cation exchange particle

- The exchange process for a cation, $\overset{+}{M}$, occurs as follows:

$$\sim SO_3\,H^+ + M + A^- \quad \leftrightarrow \quad \sim SO_3\,M^+ + \quad H^+\,A^-$$

Silica-Based Resins

- Silica-based resins make up one of the most important classes of ion-exchangers used in chromatography.
- There are two main groups of silica-based materials namely polymer-coated and functionalised silica materials.
- Polymer-coated materials consist of silica particles, which are coated, with a layer of polymer such as polystyrene, silicone or fluorocarbon and then derivitised to introduce functional groups.
- The advantage of polymer-coated materials is that diffusion in the thin layer of the polymer occurs more rapidly than it would in totally polymeric particles.
- Functionalised silica materials comprise a functional group, which is chemically bonded directly to a silica particle.
- The silica particles used in both groups can be either pellicular or microparticulate.
- A disadvantage of silica-based resins is that they can only be operated over a limited pH range.
- At a pH below 2 the covalent bond linking the ion-exchange functionality to the silica substrate becomes unstable.
- At high pH values dissolution of the silica matrix itself occurs.

Chelating Resins

- Chelating resins, which are able to separate metal ions, are made up of a suitable ligand immobilized onto a stationary phase.

- Many chelating resins have been synthesised using styrene-divinylbenzene polymers or silica as the support material.
- The ligands are chemically bound to the stationary phase by an appropriate reaction.
- Solute retention is altered by manipulating the eluent pH or by adding a competing ligand to the eluent.
- The success of using chelating resins is dependant on the rate at which the metal-ligand complex is formed and dissociated.
- Broad peaks are characteristic of slow formation and dissociation rates.

Sample Introduction

- The ideal method for sample introduction should enable the sample to be injected as a narrow plug onto the column so that peak broadening is negligible.
- The injection system should contain no void volume, as this would cause a loss of resolution.
- Syringe injection through an elastomeric septum is often used although it is not very reproducible and is constricted to low pressures.
- The most widely used methods are those based on sampling valves and loops. Here the sample loop is filled with sample by means of a syringe.
- A rotation of the valve rotor causes the eluent stream to pass through the sample loop thus injecting the sample onto the column without a noticeable change in flow.
- These valves have interchangeable loops and reproducibility is a few tenths of a percent relative.

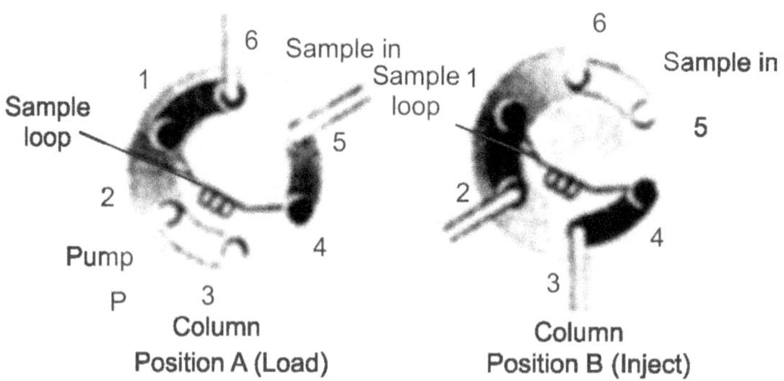

Flow Paths of the Load and Inject positions of an Injection Valve.

- In stopped-flow injection, the eluent flow is stopped and the sample is injected directly onto the head of the column by means of a syringe.
- The pump is then switched on again.

Detection Methods

There is no one highly sensitive, universal detector system used for HPLC.

- The system used is thus based on the requirements which need to be met such as detection limits, expense etc.
- A summary of detection methods, which are used with HPLC separation, and some methods are discussed below.

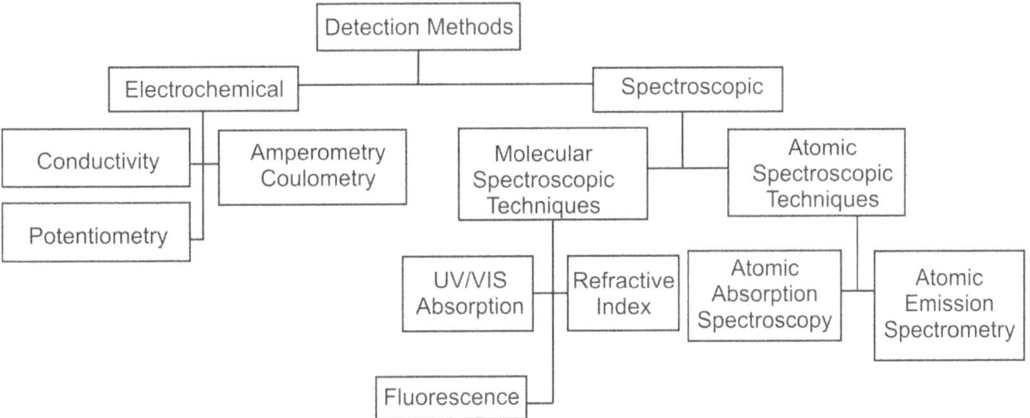

Summary of Detection Methods for HPLC.

Electrochemical Detection Methods

A. Conductivity Detection

- Conductivity is frequently used for detection purposes as all ions are electrically conducting thus conductivity detection should be universal in response.
- Conductivity detectors are also relatively simple to construct and operate, thus they find wide applicability.
- Conductivity detection is based on conductance of an eluent prior to and during elution of an analyte.
- The detector response equation for an anion-exchange system is

$$\Delta G = \frac{(\lambda_s - \lambda_s)C_s}{10^{-3}K}$$

ΔG: Conductance signal

λ_s – and λ_s : Limiting equivalent ionic conductances of the analyte and eluent anions respectively

C_s: Concentration of the analyte anion

K: Cell constant

- The above equation shows that when conductivity detection is used to monitor the effluent from an anion-exchange column the observed signal for an eluted solute is proportional to the solute concentration as well as the difference in the limiting equivalent ionic conductances between the eluent and solute ions.
- A similar equation can be derived for the conductimetric detection of a cation-exchange separation.
- It can be seen from the above equation that sensitive detection is possible as long as there is a considerable difference in the limiting equivalent ionic conductances of the solute and eluent ions.
- The resulting difference can be positive or negative depending on whether the eluent ion is weakly or strongly conducting resulting in direct or indirect detection respectively.

B. Amperometric Detection

- Amperometric detection is used for ions, which have a pK value of above 7 and thus cannot be detected by conductivity as the products formed are only slightly dissociated.
- Amperometric detectors usually consist of a three-electrode measuring cell, which contains a working electrode, a reference electrode and a counter electrode.
- The potential required for oxidation, or reduction of the species being analysed is applied between the working electrode and the Ag/AgCl reference electrode.
- A "glassy carbon" electrode acts as the counter electrode and functions to preserve the potential during operation as well as to prevent the destruction of the reference electrode.
- The detector functions as follows when an electrochemically active substance flows through the measuring cell it is partially oxidised or reduced.
- This produces an anodic or cathodic current, which is proportional to the concentration of the analyte.
- This signal is subsequently converted into a chromatographic peak.

C. Potentiometric Detection

- Potentiometry is the process by which potential changes at an indicator electrode are measured with respect to a reference electrode at a constant current.
- Potentiometry enables ion concentration determinations as the potential of the indicator electrode varies with the concentration of the ions in solution that come into contact with the electrode.
- Potentiometric detection has found wide applicability in aqueous solutions of which ion-selective electrodes are the most generally used.
- Potentiometry coupled with ion chromatography is however limited as it has moderate sensitivity as well as slow response and poor baseline stability on flowing solutions.

Spectroscopic Detection Methods

A. Molecular Spectroscopic Techniques

I. UV Detectors

- UV detectors measure the change in the UV absorption as the solute passes through a flow cell.
- In a UV transparent solvent UV detectors are concentration sensitive.
- Direct detection has a flaw as not all inorganic ions have appropriate chromophores but this can be compensated for by using the method of derivitisation.
- This is done by mixing the effluent with a chromogenic reagent in a post column reactor.
- The formed chelate complex subsequently absorbs at a particular wavelength.

II. Refractive Index Detectors

- The refractive index of a medium is the ratio of the speed of light in a vacuum to the speed in the medium.
- These detectors measure the change in refractive index in the eluent as the solute passes through the sample cell.
- This method of detection is less sensitive than UV detection although non-chromatographic compounds can be measured directly without derivitisation.

III Fluorometric Detection

- In this detection system the solute is excited by UV radiation at a particular wavelength and the emission wavelength is detected.

- Fluorometric detection has been used with naturally fluorescent compounds but compounds can be reacted to produce fluorescent derivatives.

B. Atomic Spectroscopic Techniques

- Atomic spectroscopy includes atomic absorption spectroscopy as well as atomic emission spectroscopy.
- The spectroscopic determination of atomic species can only be performed on a gaseous medium in which the individual atoms are well separated from one another.
- Thus the first step in atomic spectroscopic techniques is atomization, a process in which the sample is volatilised in such a manner as to produce an atomic gas.

Applications for HPLC

***Preparative HPLC*:** refers to the process of isolation and purification of compounds. Important is the degree of solute purity and the throughput, which is the amount of compound produced per unit time. This differs from **analytical HPLC**, where the focus is to obtain information about the sample compound. The information that can be obtained includes identification, quantification, and resolution of a compound.

***Chemical Separations*:** can be accomplished using HPLC by utilizing the fact that certain compounds have different migration rates given a particular column and mobile phase. Thus, the chromatographer can separate compounds from each other using HPLC; the extent or degree of separation is mostly determined by the choice of stationary phase and mobile phase.

***Purification*:** refers to the process of separating or extracting the target compound from other (possibly structurally related) compounds or contaminants. Each compound should have a characteristic peak under certain chromatographic conditions. Depending on what needs to be separated and how closely related the samples are, the chromatographer may choose the conditions, such as the proper mobile phase, to allow adequate separation in order to collect or extract the desired compound as it elutes from the stationary phase. The migration of the compounds and contaminants through the column need to differ enough so that the pure desired compound can be collected or extracted without incurring any other undesired compound.

***Identification*:** of compounds by HPLC is a crucial part of any HPLC assay. In order to identify any compound by HPLC a detector must first be selected. Once the detector is selected and is set to optimal detection settings, a separation assay must be developed. The parameters of this assay should be such that a clean peak of the known sample is observed from the chromatograph. The identifying peak should have a reasonable retention time and should be well separated from extraneous peaks at the detection levels which the assay will be performed. To alter the retention time of a compound, several parameters can be manipulated. The first is the choice of column, another is the choice of mobile phase, and last is the choice in flow rate. All of these topics are reviewed in detail in this document.

Identifying a compound by HPLC is accomplished by researching the literature and by trial and error. A sample of a known compound must be utilized in order to assure identification of the unknown compound. Identification of compounds can be assured by combining two or more detection methods.

***Quantification*:** of compounds by HPLC is the process of determining the unknown concentration of a compound in a known solution. It involves injecting a series of known concentrations of the standard compound solution onto the HPLC for detection. The chromatograph of these known concentrations will give a series of peaks that correlate to the concentration of the compound injected.

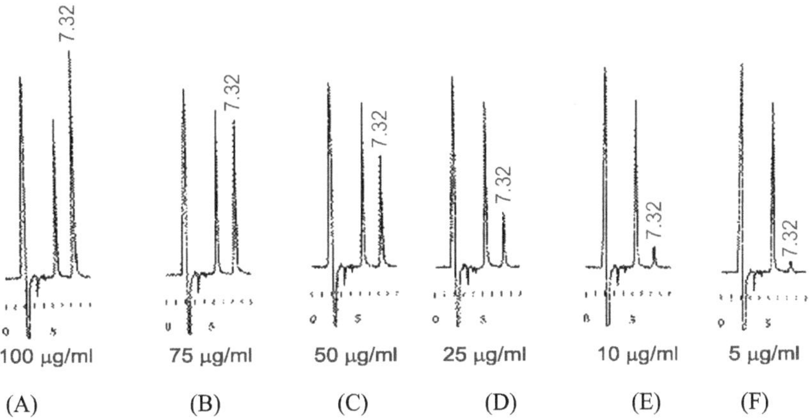

HPLC chromatogram of a standard solution (7.32) at decreasing concentrations
(A) 100 µg/mL, B) 75 µg/mL, (C) 50 µg/ml (D) 25 µg/ml (E) 10 µg/ml, and (F) 5 µg/mL

Using the area of a triangle equation (A=1/2b x h) to calculate the area under each peak, a set of data is generated to develop a calibration curve. This is done by graphing peak area vs. the concentration of the sample solution. Most graphs can be generated using a computer software program such as Excel or Cricketgraph. From this graphing software, a best-fit line can be derived, and the equation of that line can be determined. This equation of a line, $y = mx + b$, generated by the data, is the calibration curve equation.

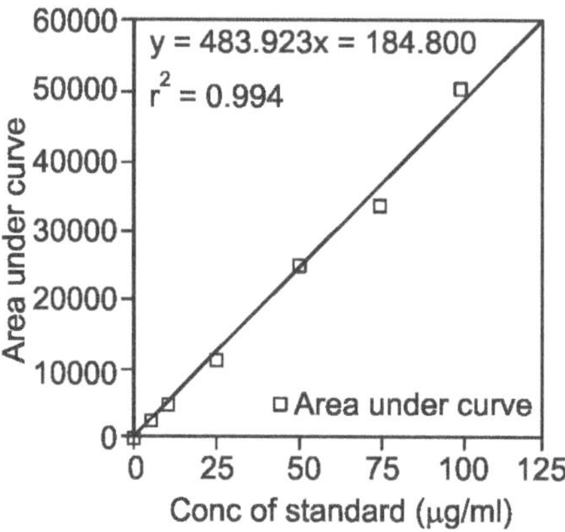

Standard Calibration graph of data generated by HPLC using Cricket Graph III™ to generate linear curve fit.

The equation of the line is then used in the following manner: A scientist injects a sample of unknown concentration x (x-axis of calibration curve) onto the HPLC; the chromatograph gives a peak output of area y (y-axis of the calibration curve). The area, y, is then in the equation of a line $y = mx + b$ from the calibration curve, and the concentration is found by solving the equation for x.

CHAPTER 8

HIGH PERFORMANCE THIN LAYER CHROMATOGRAPHY

Introduction

Chromatography is the science of separation used either for identification or quantification of chemical substances. Various modes of chromatographic techniques were developed based on the initial discovery by Michael T. Swett, a Russian Botanist. In the field of Pharmaceutical sciences, TLC enjoys a practical application status as it combines the art of chromatography with quickness at a moderato cost. High Performance Thin Layer Chromatography (HPTLC) is a major advancement introducing even shorter time with better resolution. The basic difference between TLC and HPTLC is only the particle and pore size of solvents. It can be considered a time that can speed up our work and allows us to do many things at a time usually not possible with other analytical techniques.

Main Difference of HPTLC and TLC - Particle and Pore size of Sorbents

Parameter	HPTLC	TLC
Layer of Sorbent	• 100 μm	• 250 μm
Efficiency	• High due to smaller particle size generated	• Less
Separations	• 3 - 5 cm	• 10 - 15 cm
Analysis Time	• Shorter migration distance and the analysis time is greatly reduced	• Slower

Contd...

Parameter	HPTLC	TLC
Solid support	• Wide choice of stationary phases like silica gel for normal phase and C8 , C18 for reversed phase modes	• Silica gel , Alumina & Kiesulguhr
Development chamber	• New type that require less amount of mobile phase	• More amount
Sample spotting	• Auto sampler	• Manual spotting
Scanning	• Use of UV/ Visible/ Fluorescence scanner scans the entire chromatogram qualitatively and quantitatively and the scanner is an advanced type of densitometer	• Not possible

Comparative Account of HPTLC and HPLC

Parameter of HPTLC	Parameter of HPLC
1. Sample preparation is simple	1. Sample preparation is laborious and time consuming. Even filtration through membrane filters may some times be needed
2. *In situ* derivatization is possible and routinely employed.	2. *In situ* derivatisation is not possible
3. Cannot be fully automated	3. Can be fully automated
4. Technically it is simple to learn and operate	4. Skilled and well trained personnel are required
5. Negligible wear and tear hence low maintenance cost	5. High maintenance cost
6. Low cost pre coated HPTLC plates are available	6. HPLC columns are very expensive
7. Solvents of analytical grades are suitable	7. Solvents of only HPLC grades are recommended for use
8. Simultaneous processing of sample and standard under similar conditions leads to better analytical precision and accuracy, less need for internal standard. Instability problems if any, can be detected immediately	8. Simultaneous processing of sample and standard not possible. Internal standard is frequently required for precision and accuracy of analysis

Contd...

Parameter of HPTLC	Parameter of HPLC
9. Extreme flexibility for various steps: stationary phase, mobile phase, developing technique, detection pre and post chromatographic derivatization	9. Limited flexibility
10. Co-chromatography (Co-TLC) possible and often practiced	10. Co-chromatography (Co-HPLC) usually not practiced
11. Several analysis either of the same laboratory or of different laboratories can simultaneously work on the system.	11. Only one analyst can work at a given time.
12. Solvents need no prior treatment like filtration and degassing	12. De-gassing and filtration of solvents essential.
13. Mobile phase consumption per sample is extremely low thus reducing the acquisition and disposal cost	13. Mobile phase consumption is very high. Increase of acquisition and disposal cost, an economic problem or impediments
14. Sample application (a) Variable volumes can be applied (b) Spot or band (c) Manual or automatic	14. Sample application Normally fixed volumes is selected Injected/introduced Manual as well as automatic
15. Chromatographic development (a) Vertical, horizontal, single or multiple, two-dimensional continuous, circular anticircular etc. (b) Variety of stationary phases including modified layers are commercially available (c) Wide combination of stationary, mobile phase is possible	15. Chromatographic development (a) Tubular elution by pressure (b) Limited No. of stationary phases are possible. (c) Limited combination of stationary mobile phases exist.
16. Corrosive and UV absorbing mobile phases can be used	16. Not possible
17. Mobile phases having pH 8 and above can be employed	17. Not recommended as stationary phase is unstable in highly alkaline media

Contd....

Parameter of HPTLC	Parameter of HPLC
18. No carry over. Hence no contamination	18. Possibility of carry over, hence contamination
19. System equilibrium time is small	19. Equilibrium time is much larger
20. Detection (a) Visible detection is possible being open system (b) Derivatization is simple and routinely used (c) Non UV absorbing compounds can easily be detected by post chromatographic derivatization	20. Detection (a) Visual detection is not possible (closed system) (b) Not possible (c) Difficult to detect
21. Stationary phase is usually not susceptible to sample poisoning	21. HPLC columns are susceptible to sample poisoning
22. Resolution is inferior to HPLC	22. Resolution is superior
23. Substances sensitive to light & O_2 can create problem being an open system	23. There are no problems in HPLC being a closed system
24. Quality of operation can be continuously monitored as the whole chromatogram has seen through a glass	24. Not possible
25. From starting time to solvent front almost every thing is detectable	25. It is difficult to ascertain whether all the components of an unknown sample have been eluted out or not
26. Low analytical requirements	26. High analytical requirements

Features of HPTLC

1. Simultaneous processing of sample and standard - better analytical precision and accuracy less need for Internal Standard
2. Several analysts work simultaneously
3. Lower analysis time and less cost per analysis
4. Low maintenance cost
5. Simple sample preparation - handle samples of divergent nature
6. No prior treatment for solvents like filtration and degassing
7. Low mobile phase consumption per sample
8. No interference from previous analysis - fresh stationary and mobile phases for each analysis - no contamination

9. Visual detection possible - open system
10. Non UV absorbing compounds detected by post-chromatographic derivatization

Steps Involved in HPTLC

1. Selection of HPTLC plates
2. Selection of chromatographic layer
3. Sample and standard preparation
4. Layer pre washing
5. Layer pre conditioning
6. Application of the sample and standard
7. Chromatographic development
8. Detection of spots
9. Scanning
10. Documentation of chromato plates

Selection of HPTLC Plates

(a) ***Hand made Plates*****:** The amount of each sorbent indicated is sufficient to coat five plates of 20 × 20 cm each. The used sorbent is

1. Cellulose
2. Cellulose with starch or binder
3. Micro crystalline cellulose
4. Silica gel or silica gel G
5. Silica gel with starch

(b) ***Pre coated Plates*****:** These are most commonly used plates. The pre coated plates with different support materials like glass, polyester (plastic), aluminum are used.

Plate size: pre coated HPTLC plates in size of 20 x 20 cm with aluminum or polyester support are usually procured mainly for economic reasons. These plates can be cut to size and shape to suit particular analysis by using general purpose scissors.

Pre washing of pre coated plates: Sorbants with large surface area absorb not only water vapours and other impurities from atmosphere but other volatile substances as well, which often condense particularly after the packing has been opened and exposed to laboratory atmosphere for a long time.

For these reasons, it is always recommended to clear the plates before actual chromatography. This process is called pre washing of plates. Ascending, dipping, continuous mode are the common methods of cleaning the plates. After washing, the plates must be dried for sufficient time to ensure complete removal of the washing liquids. The solvents used for this purpose are methanol, chloroform, chloroform : methanol (1:1), chloroform : methanol : ammonia (90:10:1), 1% acetic acid methylene chloride (1:1).

Activation of pre coated plates: HPTLC plates usually do not require activation. However, plates exposed to high humidity kept on hand for long time may have to be activated by placing in oven at 110-120°C for 30 minutes prior to sample spotting. This step removes water that has been physically absorbed on the surface of the sorbent. After the plates are removed from pre-wash chambers, they should always be dried in vertical position.

Selection of Chromatographic Layer

At present with the availability of precoated plates commercially the use of laboratory hand made plates is on decline. The precoated plates with different support material (i.e. glass, aluminium and plastic) and with different sorbent layers are available in different format and thickness by various manufacturers. Usually plates with sorbent thickness of 100-250μm are used for qualitative and quantitative analysis, however, for preparative work, TLC work plates with sorbent thickness of 1.0-2.0 mm are available in addition to chemically notified layers.

In general, the following is the selection of chromatographic layers in HPTLC.

1. 80% analysis-Silica gel GF.
2. Basic substances, alkaloids and steroids, aluminum oxide.
3. Aminoacids, Dipeptides, sugars and alkaloids cellulose.
4. Non polar substances, fatty acids, carotenoids, cholesterol, RP2, RP8 and RP18.
5. Preservatives, barbiturates, analgesics and phenothiazenes hybrid plates $RPWF_{254S}$

Sample and Standard Preparation

Proper sample and standard preparation is an important prerequisite for success of HPTLC. The idea of sample preparation is to dissolve the dosage form with complete recovery of intact compound(s) of interest and minimum of matrix with a suitable concentration of analyte(s) for direct application on the HPTLC plate. The following procedure is followed for sample and standard preparation.

1. Normal phase mode, non-polar solvent should be used for dissolving the sample and standard
2. Reverse phase mode, polar solvent should be used for dissolving the sample and standard.

Application of Sample and Standard

Sample application is the most critical step for obtaining good resolution for qualification by HPTLC. The sample should be completely transferred to the layer, however under no circumstances, the application process should damage the layer, as damaged layer results in unevenly shaped spots. Wherever possible, use of automatic application devices is recommended for quantitative analysis. In HPTLC, volume and concentration of sample and standard depend on the component under analysis and their sensitivity to various detection techniques. Application of 0.5-5.0 μl volume and 0.5-1.0 mm size in the concentration range of 0.1-1.0 μg/ml for HPTLC. The sample should be applied through clean upper end of the capillary for applying the sample. It is advantageous by applying the sample as band.

Advantages of applying sample as band are

1. Better separation because of rectangular area is which the compounds are present on the plate
2. Equal R_f value of the compounds from sample and reference solution.
3. Spot broadening and the direction of development is smaller in the case of band wise application.

Selection of mobile Phase

Mobile phase commonly called solvent system is traditionally selected by controlled process, by trial and error and also based on one's own experience in the field. Mobile phase should be chosen taking into consideration chemical properties of analytes and the sorbent layer.

Poor grade of solvent used in preparing mobile phase have been found to decrease resolution. Spot definition and R_f reproducibility. The following points should be remembered in the selection of mobile phase.

Normal Phase

- Stationary phase is polar and mobile phase is non polar
- Non polar compounds are selected first because of lower affinity with stationary phase
- Polar compounds are referred because of higher affinity with the stationary phase.

Reverse Phase

- Stationary phase is non-polar and mobile phase is polar.
- Polar compounds are eluted first because of lower affinity with the stationary phase.
- Non polar compounds are retained because of higher affinity with the stationary phase.

- 3-4 components mobile phase should be avoided
- Solvent composition is expressed by volumes (v/v) and sum of volumes is usually 100.
- Multi component mobile phase once used is not recommended for further use. Various component of mobile phase should be measured separately and then placed in the mixing vessel. These will not only prevent the contamination of solvent stock by evaporation from already partially filled mixing vessel but also any possible volumetric error arising due to volumes expansion on contraction on mixing.
- Laboratories equipped with complete HPTLC system usually use smaller development chamber such as twin trough chambers (10x10 cm) where comparatively smaller volumes of mobile phase usually 10-15 ml is required. It is advisable that different components of mobile phase should be measured with volumetric pipettes.
- Different components of mobile phase should be first mixed in mixing vessel and then introduced into the developing chamber.
- Solvent components which are relatively volatile at room temperature and may play significant role in final mobile phase such as pH of the solvent system should not be used for long time after the container is one opened, such as strong solution of NH_3, glacial acetic acid or diethylamide.

Pre Conditioning (Chamber Saturation)

Chamber saturation has pronounced influence on the separation profile. When the plate is introduced into unsaturated chamber, during the course of development, the solvent evaporates from the plate. Therefore larger quantity of the solvent is required for a given distance. If the tank is saturated prior to development, solvent vapors soon get uniformly distributed through out the chamber. As soon as the plate is placed in such a saturated chamber it soon gets pre-loaded with solvent vapors, hence less solvent shall be required to travel a particular distance, resulting in lower R_f Value.

Before and during development the components of the mobile phase are in equilibrium with the entire space. Inside of the chamber is lined with filter paper on three sides. Time required for saturation will depend on the nature and composition of mobile phase and layer thickness.

Chromatographic Development and Drying

Ascending, descending, two dimensional, horizontal, multiple over run (continuous) gradient radical (circular), anti-radial (anti-circular) multi model (multidimensional) traced flow planar chromatography are the most common modes of chromatographic development. Rectangular glass chamber, twin-trough chambers, ‘V’-shaped chambers, sandwich chambers, horizontal development chambers, circular and anti-circular U chambers and automated multiple development chambers are commonly used for carrying out different types of HPTLC development.

After development the plate is removed from the chamber and Mobile Phase is removed as completely and as quickly as possible. This step should preferably be performed in time to avoid contamination of laboratory atmosphere. The plates should always be laid horizontally, so that while mobile phase evaporates, the separate substances will migrate evenly to the surface where they can be easily detected.

Resolution

This is also called separation efficiency. Factors influencing HPTLC resolution of spots are:

1. Type of stationary phase [sorbent]
2. Type of precoated plates [HPTLC] for quantitative analysis, use of HPTLC pre coated plates is absolutely essential.
3. Layer thickness
4. Binder in the layer
5. Mobile phase (solvent system)
6. Solvent purity.
7. Size of the development chamber
8. Saturation of chamber (pre-equillibrium)
9. Sample volume to be spotted.
10. Size (diameter) of the initial spot.
11. Solvent level in the chamber.
12. Gradient
13. Relative humidity
14. Temperature (RF values usually increase with rise in temp.)
15. Flow rate of solvent
16. Separation distance
17. Mode of development

Retention factor is determined by

$$R_f = \frac{\text{Distance from Starting} > \text{Middle of spot}}{\text{Distance from starting line} > \text{Solvent front}}$$

Detection and Visualization

One of the most characteristic features of HPTLC is the possibility to utilize post chromatographic off-line derivatization. These visualization reactions are possible, for identification even if the separation is not optimal. The zones can be located by various physical, chemical, biological and physiological methods. There is apparently no difficulty in detection of colour substance or colourless substances absorbing in soft ware – ultraviolet (UV) region 254 nm or with intrinsic fluorescence such as riboflavin, guainine sulphate. The substances which do have above properties have to be transferred into detectable. Substances by means of chromatogenic or fluorogenic reagents. Iodine is the universal detection reagent. Detection under UV light is the first choice and is non-destructive in most of the cases and is commonly employed for densitometric scanning.

Derivatization reactions are essentially required for detection when individual compound does not respond to UV (or) does not have intrinsic fluorescence. In HPTLC, both pre and post chromatographic derivatizations are employed. Pre-chromatographic derivatization not only helps in detection but enhances the selectivity of the mobile phase or may even stabilize the otherwise labile or volatile compounds such as formaldehyde, in medicated toothpastes whereas in post-chromatographic derivatization, smaller the chromatographic zone, greater the concentration of the substance in particular area leading to increase in detection sensitivity. Other simple detection method is based on wetting and solubility phenomena.

Quantitation (Evaluation)

Requirement for various steps in HPTLC are more stringent for quantitative analysis. Accurate and precise application of samples is most critical.

***In situ densitometry*:** Densitometry is the in situ instrumental measurement of visible, UV, fluorescence of fluorescence quenching directly on the layer without resorting to scrapping and elution. The measurements are usually made by reflection from the plate using single beam, double beam or single beam dual wave length operation of scanning instruments.

To carry out a HPTLC densitometric analysis, three or four standard and purified samples are applied in the same plate. After development, detection, (if necessary) the chromatogram is scanned. A calibration curve consisting of scan area of standard versus amount of analyte is constructed and amount of analyte in the sample represented by scan area is interpolated from the standard curve.

Concentration of the analyte in the sample is calculated by considering the weight of the sample initially taken and dilution factors. Since contents of active ingredients in Pharmaceutical formulations are usually well defined, part of linearity curve falling in the range of 75-125% in a five points is adequate.

Documentation

To assist the analysts and researchers in practice of GLP/HPTLC, E. Merck has recently introduced HPTLC pre-coated plates with an imprinted identification code. The data needed for traceability according to GLP such as suppliers name, item number, batch and individual plate number are imprinted near the upper edge of the pre-coated plates. This will not only help in traceability of analytical data but will also avoid manipulation of data at any stage as coding will automatically get recorded during photo documentation.

Validation of HPTLC Procedure for Pharmaceutical Analysis

Validation Parameters are

1. Selectivity
2. Linearity sensitivity
3. Precision
4. Accuracy
5. Ruggedness
6. Robustness
7. Limit of detection (LOD)
8. Limit of quantitation (LOQ)
9. Stability

Applications of HPTLC

HPTLC is a well established, well-spread and versatile separation technique used for many applications in different areas. In 20th century, it is a wonderful analytical tool in the hands of analyst for :

1. Biochemical research
2. Clinical research
3. Cosmetics analysis
4. Environmental analysis
5. Food analysis
6. Natural products, plant ingredients
7. Toxicology, forensic analysis
8. Doping analysis
9. Metallurgy, electroplating etc.

Conclusion

High performance thin layer chromatography is most advanced technique nowadays. By this technique, accurate separation of sample takes place. It can be considered as a time machine that can speed up our work and do many things at a time usually not possible with other analytical techniques.

Applications of HPTLC

Sr. No.	Product Formulation	Plate	Mobile Phase	Quantitative
1	Propranolol Hydrochloride, Hydroflumethiazide	Reverse phase, HPTLC, Precoated plates silica get 60 RP-18 F_{254S} aluminum	0.3 M sodium chloride Methanol-Glacial acetic acid (12+8+0.1, v/v)	Densitometry at 254 nm (or) 275 nm
2	Paracetamol, caffeine, Ascorbic acid	HPTLC pre-coated plates, silica gel 60 F_{254} aluminum	Dichloro methane-Etheylacetate Ethanol (5+5+1, v/v)	Densitometry at 254 nm
3	Phenyl butazone, propyl butazone	HPTLC pre-coated plates, silica gel 60 F_{254} aluminum	Toluene-acetone-glacial acetic acid (8+2+0.1 v/v)	Densitometry at 272 (or) 245 nm
4	Ampicillin, Cloxacillin sodium	Reverse phase TLC coated with silica gel KC-18F (whatman) without pre-wash	Methanol-0.1 dipotassium hydrogen phosphate (5, 5+4.5 v/v)	Densitometry at 490 nm
5	Sulphadoxine, Pyramethamine	Reverse phase, plates, silica gel 60 HPTLC pre-coated RP-18 F_{45S} aluminum	0.5M sodium chloride-glacial acetic acid methanol acetonitrile (5+2+3+0.1) v/v	Densitometry at 235 nm (or) 260 nm
6	Alprazolam	TLC Plates coated with silica gel 60 F_{254}	Cyclohexane-chloroform diethylamide – (5+4 + 1.0 v/v)	Densitometry at 246 (or) 320 nm
7	Omeprazole	HPTLC pre-coated plates, silica gel GF_{254} – Glass (activated for 30 min at 110°C prior to u.c.	Methanol – water (40 + 20 v/v)	Densitometry at 320 nm
8	Norfloxacin, Tindazole	HPTLC pre-coated plates, silica gel 60 F_{254} Aluminum	Chloroform-methanol-toluene-diethylamide-water (4+4+2+1.4+0.8 v/v)	Densitometry at 290 nm
9	Metronidazole, Nalidixic acid	HPTLC precoated plates silica gel 60 F_{254} Aluminum	Ethyl acetate-chloroform-methanol-ammonia (2.5+2.5+1.5+0.5, v/v)	Densitometry at 320 nm
10	Pefloxacin	HPTLC precoated plates, silica gel 60 F_{254} Aluminum (prewash the plate with methanol dry at 105°C for 60 min prior to use	Chloroform-methanol ammonia (5+3.5+1.5 v/v)	Densitometry at 330 nm with K_{400} filter
11	Theophylline, etofylline	HPTLC precoated plate, silica gel 60 F_{254} Aluminum	1. Chloroform-acetone glacial acetic (8+2+0.2) 2. Chloroform Ethylalcohol-formic acid (19+1+2)	Densitometry at 275 nm

Contd....

Sr. No.	Product Formulation	Plate	Mobile Phase	Quantitative
12	Terbutaline Sulphate, Guaiphenesin	HPTLC precoated plates, silica gel 60 F_{254} Aluminum	1. Chloroform-acetone methanol-ammonia (8+2+1+0.2 v/v) 2. Toluene-methanol-ammonia (5+5+0.5 v/v)	Densitometry scanning wavelength TS = 205 nm TSLG 275 nm
13	Terfenadine, Terfenadinone	HPTLC precoated plates silica gel 60 F_{254} Aluminum	1. Chloroform-ethylacetate-methanol-3% ammonia (9+8+1+1, v/v) 2. Methanol-N-butanol-water-Toluene-glacial acetic acid (20+30+10+20+1, v.v)	Densitometry at 210 nm (or) 254 nm
14	Beclamethasone dipropionate, clotrimazole	HPTLC pre-coated plates, silica gel 60 F_{254} aluminum	Toluene-acetone, ammonia (7+3+0.5 v/v)	Densitometry at 254 nm
15	Salicylic acid, dithranol	HPTLC pre-coated plates, silica gel 60 F_{254} aluminum	N-hexane-ethyl acetate-glacial acetic acid (9.5+0.5+0.1. v/v)	Densitometry at 338 nm
16	Norgestrol Ethinylestradiol	HPTLC pre-coated plates, silica gel F_{254} glass (pre washed with methanol and dried)	Chloroform-methanol (9.6+0.4 v/v)	Densitometry at 240 nm, 360 nm and 400 nm
17	Vitamin – E (α – tocopherol)	HPTLC pre-coated plates, silica gel-60 F_{254} aluminum	1. Toluene 2. Toluene-acetone (9+1, v/v)	Densitometry at 272 nm

CHAPTER 9

INTRODUCTION TO SPECTROSCOPY

Introduction

Most of the optical techniques are described as Photometry. In short, photometry is the detection of light radiation and changes in radiation energy, usually within the visible spectrum.

In most practical applications, light is originated from a light source and it passes through a chemical compound with the sample placed in its path. The resultant light is then detected and analyzed. This form of measurement is called absorptiometry. Alternatively, the sample itself can act as a light source as in the case of bioluminescence.

Absorptiometry

Absorbance is the most common optical assay technique used in Instrumental analysis.

If a beam of light from a light source passes through a cuvette containing a chemical compound in solution, part of the beam can be absorbed. In formal terms one can say that some photons collide with ions or molecules in the solution and thus impart their energy to these. These apply only to those photons with precisely the correct energy level, i.e., only when light of a certain wavelength is absorbed.

The intensity of light leaving the sample will thus be less than its intensity when it entered. The loss of intensity is a function of the concentration of the compound.

Intensity is generally understood to mean a stream of radiation which is power and can thus be measured in units such as watts. Since measurements always relate to a ratio between two intensities, the actual units of measurement are, however, not important. Instead, convenient units such as readings on an arbitrary scale are normally used.

Colorimetry is the term applied to measurement of light in the visible portion of the spectral range. The extent to which light is absorbed by a compound in solution depends on the wavelength of the incident light and the colour of the solution. For clinical chemistry applications, the compound usually absorbs light in the visible range of the electromagnetic spectrum (400 to 700).

Colour	Complement
Violet	Green-Yellow
Blue	Red-Orange
Blue-Green	Red-Orange
Green-Blue	Red
Green	Red-Purple
Green-Yellow	Violet
Yellow	Blue
Red-Orange	Blue-Green
Red	Green-Blue
Red-Purple	Green

For certain applications, this range is extended into the ultraviolet (UV) region. Even though the human eye cannot detect UV radiation, it is still termed light.

Each absorbing compound has a typical absorption spectrum as detailed in the above table. If the absorbance peak of a compound is within the blue wavelength region, the eye will see the solution as a yellow colour since yellow is the complementary colour to blue. The more blue the light that is absorbed, the more yellow the solution will appear.

If the resultant yellow colour is compared with a given scale of yellow standards, the human eye can estimate the concentration of the compound in the solution.

When an electronic detector is substituted for the human eye, the decrease in light energy caused by an absorbing substance is easily registered and therefore be measured. In practice, monochromatic light (light is of single colour) used as the light source rather than polychromatic light (light of several colours).

Monochromatic light can be produced from white light by the use of such wavelength selection devices as filters, prisms or diffraction gratings.

Absorption Photometer

Simple photometers often use a simple meter or a chart recorder as a registering device while automated photometers use a microprocessor or computer on-line with the photometer.

The path length of each individual light ray through a cuvette must be identical. Hence a cuvette with parallel sides must receive a parallel light beam. If the cuvette is cylindrical, every light ray must pass through an imaginary point at its center, which is achieved by placing the cuvette between two cylindrical lenses.

Depending on the particular application, photometers can be divided into several groups.

Filter Photometers – where the wavelengths are selected by coloured filters or interference filters.

Spectral Line Photometers – where the light is supplied at discrete wavelengths using a spectral line source.

Spectrophotometers – where wavelengths are selected by a dispersing device, e.g., a prism or diffraction grating.

Light Sources

Two different types of light sources are used to produce light. One uses blackbody radiation such as the tungsten filament lamp and the other which uses radiation produced by specific energy. Such as a gas discharge lamp or LED.

Tungsten halogen lamps may also be used. These consist of a tungsten filament in a quartz envelope which also contains traces of a halogen such as iodine. These types of lamp give intense light in the visible and near UV range but, Tungsten lamps can only be usefully used for the production of light with wavelengths down to 340 nm. In order to work satisfactorily in the UV region, different light sources are therefore required. A gas discharge lamp is the most satisfactory.

It should be noted that for UV radiation below 340 nm the bulb/tube shall have atleast a window area made of quartz, since glass appears to be opaque to UV radiations.

Wavelength Selection

In absorbance chemistry it is often necessary to utilise narrow wavelength bands. In some instances a line source provides the narrow bands required, but more often it is desirable to select a band of wavelengths from a continuous source of radiation, such as the halogen lamp. This gives greater flexibility in choosing the wavelength bands.

There are two different methods of wavelength selection:

1. by using a filter or
2. by the use of a dispersing device such as a prism or a diffraction grating in a monochromator.

Filters

Glass Filter

The simplest and economically way to isolate a definite range of wavelengths is to use a filter of coloured glass or other coloured material which transmits some wavelengths and absorbs others.

The main disadvantage with these types of filters is that they allow a considerable amount of the radiation outside their pass band to be transmitted.

Interference Filters

The most common types of filters used in photometers based on electronics are interference filters. This type of filters is composed of a very thin, transparent plate with a semi-transplant metallic film on each side. The films are applied through evaporation in a vacuum.

The thickness of the plate determines the wavelength at which radiation can pass through the filter. When white light strikes the filter, at right angles to the surface, part is reflected off the first metallic film while the rest passes through. The light which passes through is similarly split when it strikes the second metallic mirror. If this second reflected part has the correct wavelength then it will be reflected again, off the inside of the first metallic mirror, in phase with the incoming light of the same wavelength. Therefore, light at those special wavelength is reinforced. Light at other wavelengths interfere destructively, so that essentially no energy passes through the filter. Reinforcement occurs according to the formula $\lambda = 2d/m$ where lamda is the wavelength of light, d is the effective thickness of the layer and m is an integer.

Prisms

To obtain better definition a prism can be used as an alternative to the filter. A prism separates white light into its components. The entrance slit acts as a monochromatic light source and is located at the focal point of the first lens, because the light beam must be parallel when it passes through the prism. On leaving the prisms all light rays with the same wavelengths are still parallel, but red rays have been deflected less than violet, etc. The lens following the prism concentrates these rays into one plane, the focal plane, where the exit slit is placed.

The part of the spectrum required can be selected by rotation of the prism. This technique produces monochromatic light, and the combined prism and mounting is called a monochromator.

Gratings

Diffraction grating provides an alternative means of producing monochromatic light. A grating comprises a large number of parallel lines or grooves etched closely together on a highly polished surface such as steel or glass.

In practice several spectra of different orders are produced and by using higher order spectra the dispersion can be increased.

The dispersion capability of a grating is determined by the total number of grating grooves and by the order number of the spectrum, but is not dependent on the light wavelength or the grating space.

The advantages of using a grating is that the dispersion of the different wavelengths is linear over the whole spectrum making it easier to calibrate a linear wavelength scale. By rotating the granting different parts of the spectrum can be made to pass through the exit slit.

Grating Mounting

There are many ways of mounting a grating in a monochromator. The most common method is the Ebert mounting. The required wavelength is selected by rotating the granting around its central axis. The position of the grating determines which wavelength reaches the exit slit.

Having obtained a narrow band of energy, a means of measuring the energy is required. This is accomplished by converting light energy into an electric current by means of a transducer. A transducer is a device which converts one form of energy into another. Two common transducers, also called photo-emissive devices, are the phototube and the photo-multiplier.

Phototube

The simplest type consists of two electrodes in a glass vacuum tube. The cathode is coated with an alkali metal oxide such as caesium oxide. When light strikes the electrode, some negatively charged electron are released. These electrons are attracted to the positively charged anode, causing an electric current, proportional to the incident light, to flow in the anode circuit. The anode current of the phototube causes an output voltage to be developed across the anode load resistor. This voltage requires amplification prior to measurement.

Photo-Multiplier

The second photo-emissive device is the photo-multiplier. The photo-multiplier contains a series of collecting dynodes (anodes) set at progressively increasing potentials. Light strikes the cathode and releases a few electrons, these accelerate towards a few electrons, these accelerate towards the first dynode and on impact, release a secondary emission are then accelerated towards the next dynode liberating even more electrons as they strike the dynode.

Measuring Cells or Cuvettes

In automated clinical analyser systems, the measuring cell is usually either a stopflow cell or a cuvette. The name stop-flow indicates that a flow of samples passes a cell but stops each time an absorbance measurement is taken. The cuvette may be discarded or alternatively washed after each measurement. In continuous flow systems, the absorption is continuously monitored.

In manual use, a cuvette is often a plain parallel container of glass or crystal with a volume ranging from a few micro-litres to several ml. Cylindrical cuvettes of polystyrene or acrylate are conveniently used in many photometers.

Some instruments use cuvettes arranged in circular trays allowing serial measurements to be interpreted by the analysers.

Slit Width

To obtain the best results, the absorbance should be measured using the narrowest possible slit, otherwise significant spectrum details can be lost. This applies particularly to quantitative analyses.

There are, however, a number of other factors which limit minimum bandwidth, principally the "radiant power" of the light source, and the sensitively of the detection system.

Detectors and Detection Limits

The detector for an HPLC is the component that emits a response due to the eluting sample compound and subsequently signals a peak on the chromatogram. It is positioned immediately posterior to the stationary phase in order to detect the compounds as they elute from the column. The bandwidth and height of the peaks may usually be adjusted using the coarse and fine tuning controls, and the detection and sensitivity parameters may also be controlled. There are may types of detectors that can be used with HPLC. Some of the more common detectors include: Refractive Index (RI), Ultra-Violet (UV), Fluorescent, Radiochemical, Electrochemical, Near-Infra Red (Near-IR), Mass Spectroscopy (MS), Nuclear Magnetic Resonance (NMR), and Light Scattering (LS).

Refractive Index (RI) detectors measure the ability of sample molecules to bend or refract light. This property for each molecule or compound is called its refractive index. For most RI detectors, light proceeds through a bi-modular flow-cell to a photodetector. One channel of the flow-cell directs the mobile phase passing through the column while the other directs only the mobile phase. Detection occurs when the light is bent due to samples eluting from the column, and this is read as a disparity between the two channels.

Laser-Based RI Detectors

Ultra-Violet (UV) detectors measure the ability of a sample to absorb light. This can be accomplished at one or several wavelengths.

(a) **Fixed Wavelength** measures at one wave length, usually 254 nm

(b) **Variable Wavelength** measures at one wave length at a time, but can detect over a wide range of wave lengths.

(c) **Diode Array** measures a spectrum of wave lengths simultaneously.

[More on Diode Detectors]

UV detectors have a sensitively to approximately 10^{-8} or 10^{-9} gm/ml.

Laser-Based Absorbance Detectors

Using Fourier Transformer in UV Spectrometry

Fluorescent detectors measure the ability of a compound to absorb the re-emitted light at given wavelengths. Each compound has a characteristic fluorescence. The excitation source passes through the flow-cell to a photodetector while a monochromator measure the emission wavelengths.

Sensitively limit of 10^{-9} to 10^{-11} gm/ml.

Laser-based fluorescence detectors

Radiochemical detection involves the use of radio labelled material, usually tritium (^3H) or carbon-14 (^{14}C). It operates by detection of fluorescence associated with beta-particle ionization, and it is most popular in metabolite research. Two detector types:

(a) ***Homogeneous*****:** Where addition of scintillation fluid to column effluent causes fluorescence.

(b) ***Heterogeneous*****:** Where lithium silicate and fluorescence caused by beta-particle emission interact with the detector cell.

Sensitivity limit up to 10^{-9} to 10^{-11} gm/ml.

Electrochemical

Electrochemical detectors measure compounds that undergo oxidation or reduction reactions. Usually accomplished by measuring gain or loss of electrons from migrating samples as they pass between electrodes at a given difference in electrical potential. Has sensitivity of 10^{-2} to 10^{-13} gm/ml.

Mass Spectroscopy (MS) Detectors

The sample compound or molecular is ionized, it is passed through a mass analyzer, and the ion current is detected. There are various methods for ionization:

(a) ***Electron Impact (EI)*****:** An electron current or beam created under high electric potential is used to ionize the sample migrating off the column.

(b) ***Chemical Ionization*****:** A less aggressive method which utilize ionized gas to remove electrons from the compounds eluting from the column.

(c) ***Fast Atom Bombarbment (FAB)*****:** Xenon atoms are propelled at high speed in order to ionize the eluents from the column. Has detection limit of 10^{-8} to 10^{-10} gm/ml.

Nuclear Magnetic Resonance (NMR) Detectors

Certain nuclei with odd-numbered masses, including H and ^{13}C, spin about an axis in a random fashion. However, when placed between poles of a strong magnet, the spins are aligned either parallel or anti-parallel to the magnetic field, with the parallel orientation favored since it is slightly lower in energy. The nuclei are then irradiated with electromagnetic radiation which is absorbed and places the parallel nuclei into a higher energy state; consequently, they are now in "resonance" with the radiation. Each H or C will produce different spectra depending on their location and adjacent molecules, or elements in the compound, because all nuclei in molecules are surrounded by electron clouds which change the encompassing magnetic field and thereby alter the absorption frequency.

***Light-Scattering (LS) Detectors*:** When a source emits a parallel beam of light which strikes particles in solution, some light is reflected, absorbed, transmitted, or scattered. Two forms of LS detection may be used to measure the two latter occurrences:

(a) ***Nephelometry*:** This is defined as the measurement of light scattered by a particulate solution. This method enables the detection of the portion of light scattered at a multitude of angles. The sensitivity depends on the absence of background light or scatter since the detection occurs at a black or null background.

(b) ***Turbidimetry*:** This is defined as the measure of the reduction of light transmitted due to particles in solution. It measures the light scatter as a decrease in the light that is transmitted through the particulate solution. Therefore, is quantifies the residual light transmitted. Sensitivity of this method depends on the sensitivity of the machine employed, which can range from a simple spectrophotometer to a sophisticated discrete analyzer. Thus, the measurement of a decrease in transmitted light from a large signal of transmitted light is limited to the photometric accuracy and limitations of the instrument employed.

Laser Based Scattering Detectors

***Near-Infrared Detectors*:** Operates by scanning compounds in a spectrum from 700 to 1100 mm. Stretching and bending vibrations of particular chemical bonds in each molecule are detected at certain wavelength. This is a fast growing method which offers several advantages: speed (sometimes less than 1 second), simplicity of preparation of sample, multiple analysis from single spectrum, and nonconsumption of the sample (McClure, 1994).

CHAPTER 10

UV & VISIBLE SPECTROSCOPY

Introduction

Spectroscopy is the measurement of Electro magnetic radiation (EMR) absorbed or emitted when molecules or atoms or ions of a sample move from one energy state to another energy state.

Electromagnetic radiation is made up of discrete particles called 'photons'.

Regions of Electromagnetic Spectrum

When a narrow beam of light is allowed to pass through a prism it is dispersed into seven colours from red to violet and a set of colours or band produced is called spectrum.

The arrangement obtained by arranging various types of electromagnetic waves (or) radiations in order of their increasing wave-lengths or decreasing frequencies is called electromagnetic spectrum. The spectrum obtained by white light is called continuous spectrum.

Visible light is a form of electromagnetic radiation which lies in the wavelength range of 3800 $\mathring{A}$ -7600 $\mathring{A}$.

The region of 3800 $\mathring{A}$ wavelength corresponds to violet colour and the region of 7600 $\mathring{A}$ wavelength corresponds to red colour.

If the wave length is less than 380^0 A the radiation is called 'ultra violet light'.

If the wave length is greater than 7600 $\mathring{A}$ the radiation is called 'Infrared light'.

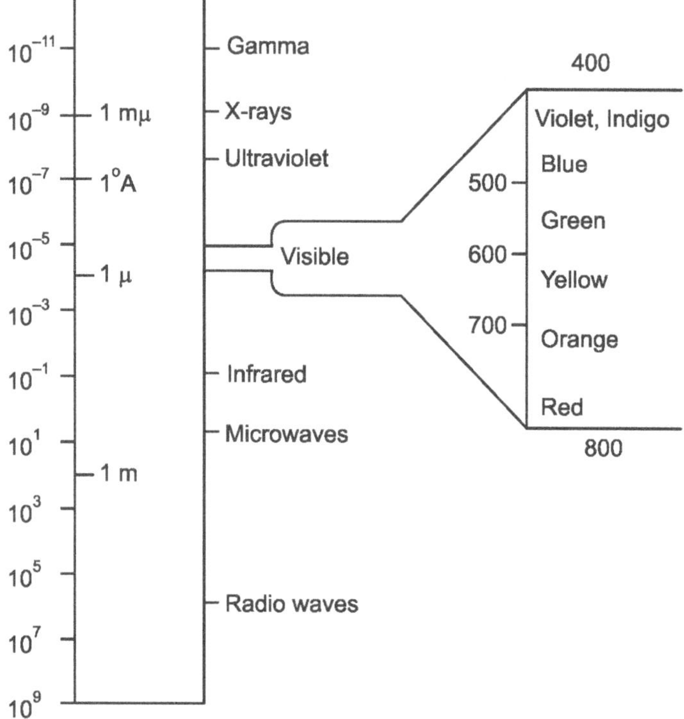

Fig. 10.1 The Electromagnetic spectrum.

The different types of Electro magnetic Radiation are : Visible radiation, UV radiation, IR Radiation, Microwaves, Radio waves, X-rays, Cosmic rays (or) γ -rays.

Entire range over which electro magnetic radiation exists is known as electromagnetic spectrum. The diagrammatic representation of the electromagnetic spectrum is given below :-

(a) ***γ -ray Region*:** This lies between 0.02 to 1 Å. The g-rays are shortest waves emitted by atomic nuclei. Involving energy changes of 10o to 1011 joules/gram atom.

(b) ***X-ray Region*:** This lies between 1 to 10 Å. X-rays are emitted (or) absorbed by movement of electrons close to nuclei of relatively heavy atom, involve energy changes of the order or 10,000 kilo joules.

(c) ***Visible and ultraviolet region*:** These are further made up of following regions.

Vacuum ultraviolet - 1 to 180 nm.

Ultra violet - 180 to 400 nm

Visible - 400 to 750 nm

The distinction between 'vacuum ultraviolet' and 'ultraviolet'is made because air starts absorbing below 180 nano meters.

Colours of visible light

Colour	Wavelength-nm
Violet	400-435
Blue	435-480
Green-blue	480-490
Blue-green	490-500
Green	500-560
Yellow-Green	560-580
Yellow	580-595
Orange	595-610
Red	610-750

(d) ***Infrared Region*****:** This region has been further divided into the following sub-regions.

Infrared (near) - 0.7 to 2.5 m

Infrared - 2.5 to 15 m

Far infrared - 15 to 200m

All the three sub-regions of infrared part of the electromagnetic spectrum are associated with changes in the vibration of molecules.

(e) ***Microwave Region*****:** (0.1 mm to 1 cm wave length) This region corresponds to changes in the rotation of molecules.

(f) ***Radio frequency Region*****:** (10 m-1 cm wavelength)

The energy change involved in this region arises due to the reversal of a spin of nucleus or electron.

Properties of Electromagnetic Radiation

An electromagnetic radiation is said to have a dual nature, exhibiting both wave and particle characteristics.

Wave Properties of Electromagnetic Radiation

An electromagnetic radiation is an alternating electrical and associated magnetic force field in space. Thus, an electromagnetic wave has an electric component and a magnetic component. The two components oscillate in planes perpendicular to each other and perpendicular to the direction of propagation of the radiation.

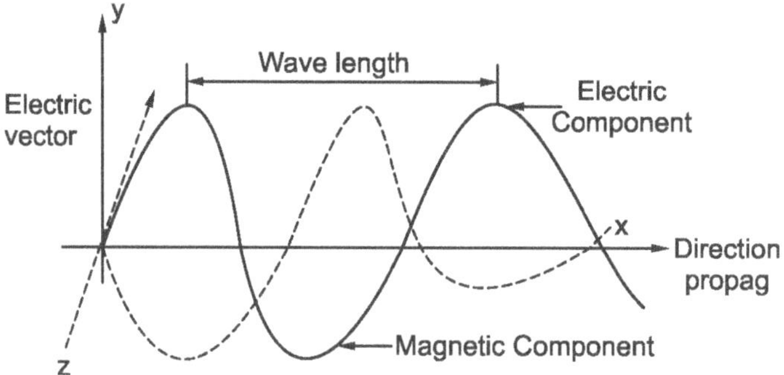

Fig. 10.2 Representation of an electromagnetic wave.

An electromagnetic wave is characterised by the following parameters :

(a) ***Wave length*** **λ :** It is the distance between two successive maxima on an electromagnetic wave. The units are meters, centimetres, millimetres, micrometers, nanometers.

$$1\ \mu m = 10^{-6}\ mm = 10^{-7}\ cm = 10^{-9}\ m = 10^{0} A$$

$$1\ \mathring{A} = 10^{-8}\ cm = 0.1\ nm = 10^{-10}\ m.$$

(b) ***Frequency*:** The number of wave length units passing through a given point in unit time is called the frequency of radiation. It is denoted by n. It is expressed in cycles per seconds or in Hertz (Hz)_.

$$1\ Hz = 1\ cycle\ s^{-1}.$$

(c) ***Wave number*** **$\bar{v}$:** It is defined as the number of waves per centimetre in vacuum. It is denoted by $\bar{v}$.

$$\bar{v} = \frac{1}{\lambda}$$

(d) ***Velocity*:** It is the product of wave length and frequency and is equal to the velocity of the wave in the medium.

Wave length × frequency = velocity

$$\lambda \times n = V$$

Particle Properties of Electromagnetic Radiation

Electromagnetic radiation consists of a stream of discrete packets (particles) of pure energy called photons or quanta. These have definite energy and travel in the direction of propagation of the radiation beam with the velocity equal to that of the light. The energy of the photon is proportional to the frequency of radiation and is given by

$$E = hv$$

Where E = is the energy of photons in ergs

V = frequency of the electromagnetic radiation in cycles/second

h = Planck's constant and has the value of 6.624 × 10–27 erg-sec.

The ultraviolet region extends from 1000 to 4000 Å. The wavelength in the ultra region are usually expressed in Angstrom (Å).

The ultra violet region is subdivided into two spectral regions :

1. The region between 2000 Å - 4000 Å is known as near ultra violet.
2. The region below 2000 Å is called the far or vacuum ultra violet region.

Origin of ultraviolet absorption spectra

Ultra violet absorption spectra arise from transition of electron or electrons with in a molecule or an ion from a lower to a higher electronic energy level. Both organic and inorganic species exhibit electronic translations in which outermost of bonding electrons are promoted to higher energy levels. A compound appears coloured if it absorbs light in the visible region and reflects the light of wavelengths in the rest of the visible region. The main function of the absorbed energy is to raise the molecule from the ground state energy E_0 to the higher excited state (energy E_1)

The difference $E_1 - E_0 = \Delta E$ is given by

$$\Delta E = E_1 - E_0 = h\nu = h\frac{c}{\lambda} \quad (\nu = c/\lambda)$$

where h = Planck's constant

C = Velocity of light

λ = wave length of the absorbed radiation.

Δ E depends upon how tightly the electrons are bound in the bonds and accordingly the absorption will occur in UV or particular region of visible range.

The electrons occupy definite orbits, the energy Δ E and the frequency of light absorbed must have definite values. The frequency of the absorbed light is associated with a particular line in the spectrum. The spectrum of the compound will consist of a large number of lines corresponding to a large number of excited states of the large number of molecules constituting the compound. The values of Δ E are vert close to each other, the lines appear as a band. The existence of the bands in definite parts of the spectrum produces the colour.

The total energy of the molecule is the sum of its electronic energy, its vibrational energy and its notational energy. This is due to the fact that there may be three changes in the molecule as a result of absorption of radiation.

(a) There may be rotation of molecule.

(b) There may be vibration of combining atoms, within the molecule.

(c) There may be electronic transition from one orbit to another.

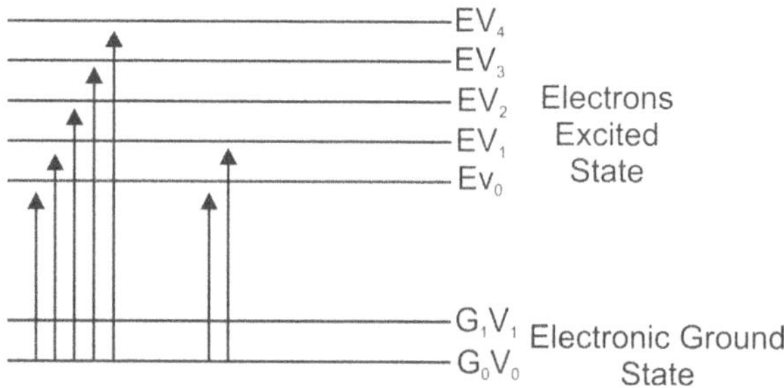

The types of electrons present in organic molecules may be classified as :

(a) ***α-Electrons*:** These electrons are involved in saturated bonds such as those between carbon & hydrogen in paraffins. As the amount of energy required to excite electrons in s bands is much more than that produced by UV light, compounds containing s bands do not absorb UV radiation. For this reason, paraffin compounds are frequently very useful as solvents.

(b) ***π-electrons*:** These electrons are involved in unsaturated hydrocarbons, the compounds with double or triple bonds and aromatic compounds.

(C) **n-*electrons*:** These are the electrons which are not involved in any of the bonding between atoms in molecules. Examples are organic compounds containing nitrogen, oxygen or halogens. As n electrons can be excited by UV radiation, any compound that contain atoms like nitrogen, oxygen, sulphur, halogen compounds or unsaturated hydrocarbons may absorb UV radiation.

Electronic transitions and excitation process

The α, n, π electrons present in a molecule can be excited from the ground state by the absorption of UV radiation.

The various transition are

$$n \rightarrow \pi^* \quad ; \qquad \pi \rightarrow \pi^*$$

$$n \rightarrow \sigma^* \quad ; \qquad \sigma \rightarrow \sigma^*$$

The different energy states associated with such transitions can be given by the diagram –

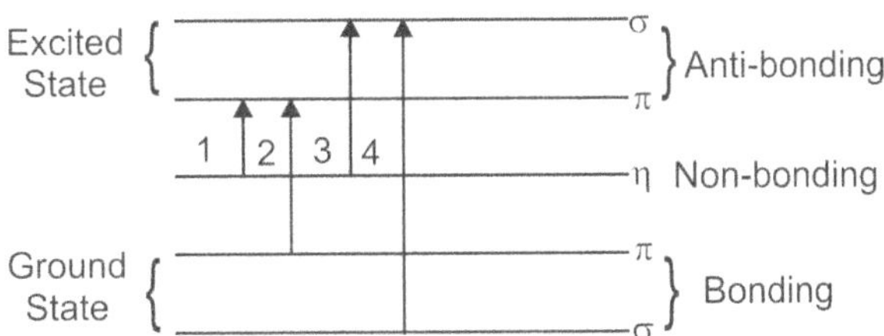

Energy levels of Electronic transitions

The energy required for excitation for different transitions are

$$n \rightarrow \pi^* < \pi \rightarrow \pi^* < n \rightarrow \sigma^* < \sigma \rightarrow \sigma^*$$

Of these transitions n $\rightarrow$ π^* requires the lowest energy and $\sigma \rightarrow \sigma^*$ requires the highest energy, for excitation in the UV region.

After absorption of UV radiations these electronic structures have greater or lesser polar character than in ground state. Some of them exists as biradicals as activated structures.

$$\text{e.g.} > C = O \rightarrow C^+ - O^- \rightarrow C^{\sigma+} - O^{\sigma-}$$

Polar solvents shift n p* & n $\rightarrow$ π^* & n $\rightarrow$ σ^* to shorter wavelengths and $\pi \rightarrow \pi^*$ to longer wavelengths.

Types of Transitions

Transitions	Region	Wave length
$\sigma \rightarrow \sigma^*$	For ultra violet	< 200 nm
$\pi \rightarrow \pi^*$		
$n \rightarrow \sigma^*$	Ultra violet	= 200 nm
$n \rightarrow \sigma^*$	Near UV and visibe	300-600 m

1. ***n → π****

Of all the types of transitions, n → π transition requires the lowest energy (longer wave length). The peaks due to this transition is also called R-bands. This type of peak can be seen in compounds where 'n' electrons (Present in S, O, N or halogens) is present in a compound containing double bond or triple bond e.g. :- aldeydes or ketones, nitro compounds etc.*

Peak occurs between without double or 270-300nm triple bonds

Without double or 300-350 nm

Triple bonds separated by 2 or more single bonds

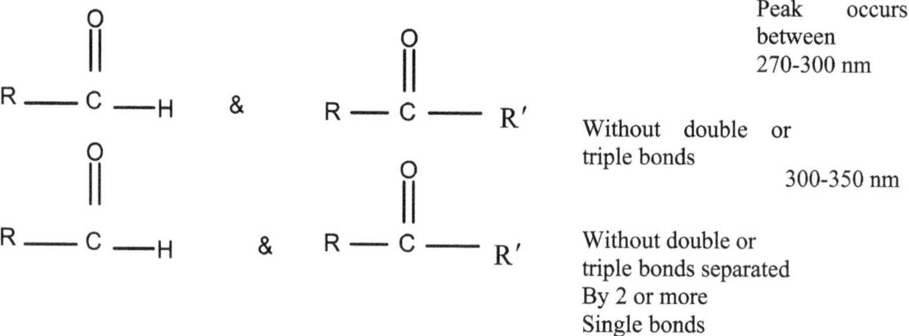

The presence of n $\rightarrow \pi^*$ transition can be identified easily by comparing the UV spectrum of the substance with the spectrum recorded in the acid solution of the same substance. In an acid solution, the band disappears if n $\rightarrow \pi^*$ has been present.

The presence of other hetero atoms can be identified by comparison with a similar compound without hetero atom.

2. p $\rightarrow \pi^*$

This type of transition gives to B, E & K bands.

Type	*Due to*
B-bands (benznoid bands)	*Aromatic & hetero aromatic systems*
E-bands (Ethylenic bands)	*Aromatic systems*
K-bands ($\pi \rightarrow \pi^*$)	*Conjugated systems*

The energy requirement of this transition is between n $\rightarrow \sigma^*$ & n $\rightarrow \pi^*$. But extended conjugation (addition of more double/ triple bonds) and alkyl substituents shifts the λ_{max} towards longer λ (Bathochromic shift). Also trans *isomer of olefin absorbs at longer λ with more intensity than cis isomer. (Bathochormic shift and hyperchromic effect). Extended conjugation (and alkyl substitution) shifts λ_{max} to such an extent that the λ_{max} falls in the colorimetric region.*

e.g., plant pigments like, β-Carotene etc.

The λ_{max} of some chromophores and other systems are given below :-

Chromophore	λ_{max}
$>C=C<$	*174 nm*
$-C\equiv C-$	*178 nm*

3. $n \rightarrow \sigma^*$

This transition occurs in saturated compound with hetero atoms like s, O, N or halogens. It requires lesser energy when compared to $\sigma \rightarrow \sigma^*$ transition. The peaks due to this transition occur from 180nm – 250nm.

These peaks are observed at the lower end of the UV spectrum, it can be called as end absorption. Some compounds with $n \rightarrow \sigma^*$ transitions are :-

Compound	λ_{max}
Methylene chloride	173 nm
Water	191 nm
Methanol	203 nm
Ethanol	204 nm
Ether	215 nm
Trimethylamine	227 nm
Chloroform	237 nm
Carbon tetrachloride	257 nm
Methyl iodide	258 nm

4. $S \rightarrow \sigma^*$

Of all the electronic transition, this type of transition requires the highest energy. This is observed with saturated compounds. The peaks do not appear in UV region, but occur in vaccum UV or for UV region i.e. 125-135nm. Some of the compounds with such transitions are :

Methane	-	*122 nm*
Ethane	-	*135 nm*
Propane	-	*135 nm*
Cyclopropane	-	*190 nm*

UV spectrophotometers are operated above 200nm and these compounds do not absorb above 200nm, they can be used as non polar solvents as they do not give rise to solvent peak.

Choice of Solvent

It should be cheap, a good solvent & transparent down to about 2100^0A. The less polar solvents like cyclohexane and other hydrocarbons can be used for getting fine structure with hydrocarbons.

Solvent	***Wavelength***
Water	*191 nm (910^0 A)*
Methanol	*203 nm (2030^0 A)*
Ethanol	*204 nm (2040^0 A)*
Ether	*215 nm (2150^0 A)*
Chloroform	*237 nm (2370^0 A)*

Instrumentation

Beer-Lambert's law

Beer-Lambert's law is applicable to UV radiation.

Beer's law: *Beers law states that 'The intensity of a beam of monochromatic light decreases exponentially with increase in the concentration of absorbing species arithmetically.*

Accordingly, $$\frac{-dI}{dc} \alpha I$$

The decrease in the intensity of light (I) with concentration (c) is proportional to intensity of incident light (I)

$$\frac{-dI}{dc} = Kdc$$ *(removing and introducing the constant of proportionality 'K')*

$$\frac{-dI}{I} = Kdc$$ *(rearranging terms)*

$$-I_n I = kc + b \qquad ....(1)$$

(On integration b is constant of integration).

When concentration = 0 there is no absorbance. Hence $I = I_0$

∴ *Substituting in equation (1)*

$$-I_n I_0 = K \times o + b$$

$$-I_n I_0 = b$$

Substituting the value of b, in equation (1)

$$-I_n I = K_c - I_n I_0$$

$$I_n I_0 - I_n I = K_c$$

$$I_n \frac{I_0}{I} = K_c \qquad \text{(Since } \log A - \log B = \log \frac{A}{B}\text{)}$$

$$\frac{I_0}{I} = e^{kc} \qquad \text{(removing natural logarithm)}$$

$$\frac{I_0}{I} = e^{-kc} \qquad \text{(making inverse on both sides)}$$

$$I = I_0 e^{-kc} \qquad \text{(Equation for Beer's law)} \qquad .....(2)$$

Lambert's law

The rate of decrease of intensity (monochromatic light) with the thickness of the medium is directly proportional to the intensity of incident light.

i.e. $$\frac{-dI}{dt} \propto I$$

This equation can be simplified by replacing 'c' with 't'

$$I = I_0 e^{-kt} \qquad ......(3)$$

Equation (2) & (3) can be combined to get

$$I = I_0 e^{-kct}$$

$$I = I_0 10^{-kct} \quad \text{(Converting natural logarithm to base 10 \& } K = K \times K \times 0.4343\text{)}$$

$$\frac{I}{I_0} = 10^{-kct} \qquad \text{(rearranging terms)}$$

$$\frac{I}{I_0} = 10^{-kct} \qquad \text{(inverse on both sides)}$$

$$\log \frac{I}{I_0} = kct \qquad \text{(taking log on both sides)} \qquad .....(4)$$

It can be learnt that Transmittance (T) $= \frac{I}{I_0}$ *and absorbance (A)* $= \log \frac{1}{T}$

Hence $A = log \frac{I}{I/I_0}$

$$A = log \frac{I_0}{I} \qquad .....(5)$$

Using equation (4) & (5) since $A = log \frac{I_0}{I}$ *and* $log \frac{I_0}{I} = kct$ *we can say that*

$A = kct$ *(instead of k we can use ε)*

$A = \varepsilon ct$

This is Mathematical equation for Beer's-Lambert's law

where A = Absorbance or optical density or extinction co-efficient.

ε = Molecular extinction coefficient.

C = Concentration of drug (mmol/lit).

t = Path length (normally 10 mm or 1 cm)

ε can be expressed as follows :

$$\varepsilon = E_{1cm}^{1\%} \times \frac{\text{Molecular weight}}{10}$$

where $E_{1cm}^{1\%}$ *means the absorbance of 1% w/v solution using a path-length of 1cm. This value is useful in determining the concentration of drugs in sample formulations or in solutions.*

Instrumentation

The various components of a UV spectrometer are :

Source of light

The best source of light is the one which is more stable, more intense & which gives range of spectrum from 180-360 nm.

The most commonly used sources are hydrogen or deuterium amps, the xenon discharge lamps & mercury arcs. In all the sources, collisions between electrons and gas molecules may result in electronic, vibrational & rotational excitation in the gas molecules. When the pressure of the gas is low only line spectra are emitted and if pressure is high, band spectra & continuous spectra will be obtained.

Various types of radiation sources are :

(a) **Hydrogen discharge lamps:** *In these lamps, hydrogen gas is stored under relatively high pressure. When an electric discharge is passed through the* *lamp, excited hydrogen molecules will be produced which emit UV radiations. The high pressure in the hydrogen lamps causes the hydrogen to emit a continuous spectrum. Hydrogen lamps cover the range 3500 – 1200^0A. These lamps are stable, robust & widely used.*

(b) **Deuterium lamp:** *It is similar to hydrogen discharge lamp, but filled with deuterium in the place of hydrogen. It offers 3-5 times more intensity than other types. This is most widely used but expensive.*

(C) **Xenon discharge:** *In this lamp, xenon at 10-30 atmospheric pressure is filled in and has two tungsten electrodes. The intensity is greater than hydrogen discharge lamp.*

(d) ***Mercury arc:*** *This contains mercury vapour and offers bands which are sharp. The spectrum is not continuous. Hence it is not widely used.*

The following are the requirements of radiation source:

1. Source of light

1. *It must be stable.*
2. *It must be of sufficient intensity for the transmitted energy to be detected at the end of the optical path.*
3. *It must supply continuous radiation over the entire wave length region in which it is used.*

2. Monochromators

The monochromator is used to disperse the radiation according to the wave length. The essential elements of monochromators are :

- *an entrance slit*
- *dispersing element &*
- *exit slit*

The entrance slit sharply defines the incoming beam of heterochromatic radiation.

The dispersing element disperses the heterochromatic radiation into its component wavelengths.

Exit slit allows the nominal wavelength together with a band of wavelengths on either side of it.

The dispersing element may be a prism or grating. The prisms are generally made of glass, quartz or fused silica. Quartz & fused silica prisms which are transparent throughout the entire UV range are widely used in UV spectro photometers.

Mirrors are front surfaced to prevent absorption of radiation.

3. ***Detectors***

There are three common types of detectors which are widely used in UV spectrophotometers. These are :

(a) **Barrier layer cell:** *This cell is also known as photovoltaic cell. The barrier cell consists of a semi conductor such as selenium which is deposited on a stron metal base such as iron. Then a very thin layer of silver or gold is sputtered over the surface of the semiconductor to act as a second collector electrode.*

The rotation falling on the surface produces electrons at the selenium silver interface. A barrier exists between selenium and iron which prevents the electrons from flowing into iron. The electrons are accumulated on the silver surface, produce an electrical voltage difference between the silver surface and the base of cell.

Photovoltaic cell is simple in design & does not require any external power supply.

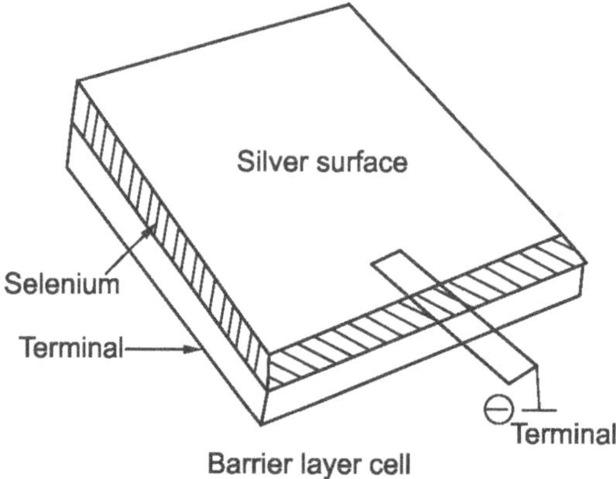

Barrier layer cell

(b) **Photo cell:** *It consists of a light sensitive cathode in the form of half cylinder of a metal which is contained in an evacuated tube. The inside surface of the photocell is coated with a light sensitive layer. When the light is incident upon a photo cell, the surface coating emits electrons. These are attracted and collected by an anode. The current which is created between the cathode and anode is regarded as a measure of radiation falling on the detector.*

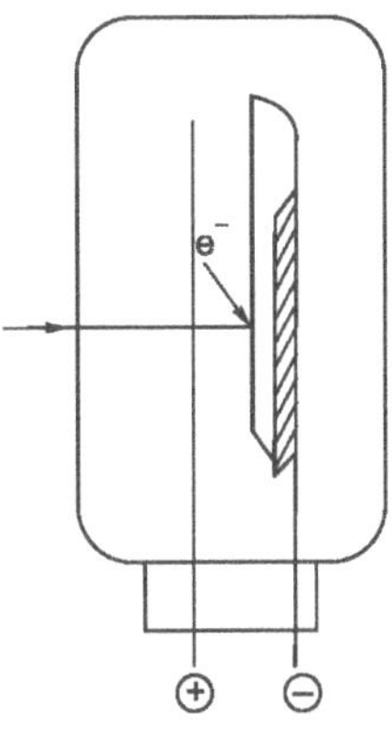

Photocells

(c) **Photo multiplier tube:** *A photo multiplier tube is a combination of a photo diode and an electron-multiplying amplifier. A photo multiplier tube consists of an evacuated tube which contains one photo-cathode and 9-16 electrodes known as dynodes. When radiation falls on a metal surface of a photo cathode, it emits electrons. The electrons are attracted towards the first dynode which is kept at a +ve voltage. When the electrons strike the first dynode, more electrons are then attracted by a second dynode where similar type of electron emission takes place. The process is repeated all over the dynodes present in the photo multiplier tube until a shower of electrons reaches the collector. The number of electrons reaching the collector is the measure of the intensity of light falling on the detector. The dynodes are operated at an optimum voltage that gives a steady signal.*

The transit time between absorption of the photo and the arrival of the shower of electrons is in the range of 10-100 μ sec. For every quantum of light approximately 10^6 electrons are produced.

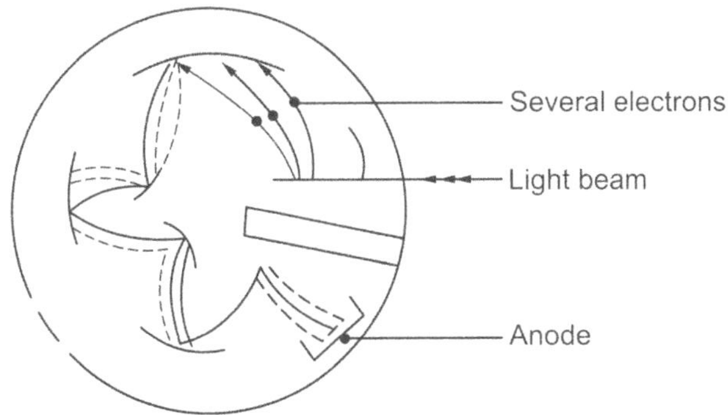

Photomultiplier tube

(d) **Recording system:** *The signal from the photo multiplier tube is finally received by the recording system. The recording is done by recorder pen.*

(e) **Sample Cells:** *The cells that contain samples for analysis should fulfil three conditions :*

1. *They must be uniform in construction; the thickness must be constant and surfaces facing the incident light must be optically flat.*
2. *The materials of construction should be inert to solvents.*
3. *They must transmit light of the wavelength used.*

The most commonly used cells are made up of quartz or fused silica.

(f) **Power Supply:** *The power supply serves a triple function :*

1. *It decreases the line voltage to the instruments ; upto an operating level with a transformer.*
2. *It converts A.C to D.C with a rectifier if direct current is required by the instrument.*
3. *It smooths out any ripple which may occur in the line voltage in order to deliver a constant voltage to the source lamp and instrument.*

Solvents: *Solvent plays an important role in UV spectrum. The solvent for a sample is selected in such a way that the solvent neither absorbs in the region of measurement nor affects the absorption of the sample. Some commonly used solvents & their absorption regions are :-*

Water	-	*191 nm*
Cyclohexane	-	*195 nm*
Methanol	-	*203 nm*
Ethanol	-	*204 nm*
Ether	-	*215 nm*

Single beam and double beam UV spectrophotometer

Source of light - *Hydrogen discharge or deuterium lamp in the place of tungsten lamp.*

Monochromators - *Grating monochromator made up of quartz in the place of filters and prism monochromators*

Sample cells	-	Quartz sample cell in the place of glass or polystyrene cell.
Detector	-	Photo multiplier tubes instead of photo voltaic cell (or) photo tubes.

Single beam ultraviolet spectrophotometers

This consists of a tungsten lamp as source of light. The light radiation is focussed on to a slit by using a concave mirror. This light passes through a simple absorption filter where only the required wavelength of light passes through it and falls on the sample cell where the solution to be analysed is present. The sample or standard solution absorbs a part of the radiation and the rest is transmitted. The intensity of the transmitted or the unabsorbed radiation is determined using a photo voltaic cell using a digital display.

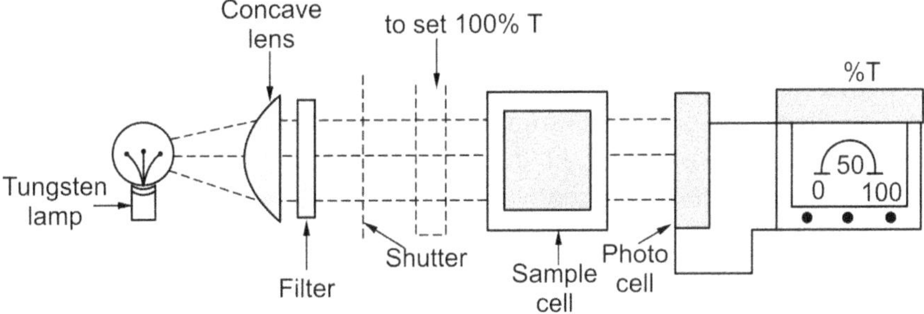

Single beam UV Spectrophotometer

Merits

1. Simple in construction
2. Inexpensive
3. Easy to operate

Demerits

1. The readings are affected by fluctuations in the intensity of source.
2. Recorder cannot be used with single beam type.

Double Beam UV Spectrophotometer

It is similar to that of single beam instrument. Here the light beam after passing through a filter of monochromatic is split into sample beam and reference beam by using a beam splitter. These beams pass through sample and reference solutions and fall on two detectors separately. The final read out is in absorbance or transmittance obtained after electronic manipulation of the two detectors.

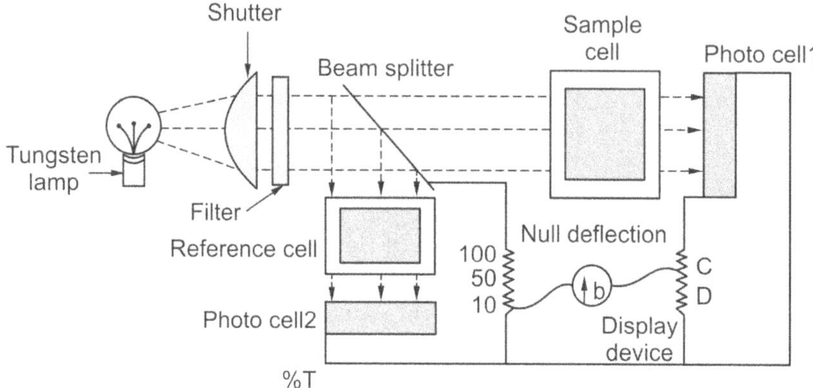

Deviations from Beer's Law

A system is said to obey Beer's law when a plot of concentration vs absorbance gives a straight line. The straight line is obtained by using method of least squares, or by joining the maximum no. of points. The regression line can also be used for determining concentration of a solution whose absorbance is obtained using spectrophotometer. When a straight line is not obtained i.e. a non-linear curve is obtained in a plot of concentration vs absorbance, the system is said to undergo deviation from Beer's law. Such deviation can be positive or negative deviation. Positive deviation results when a small change in concentration produces a greater change in absorbance. Negative deviation results when a large change in concentration produces smaller change in absorbance.

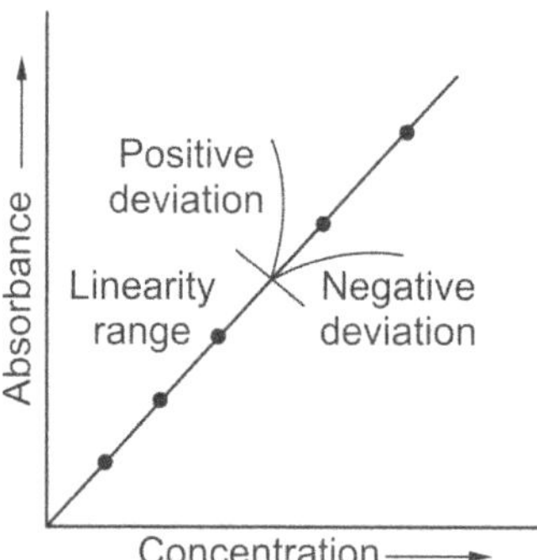

Several reasons for the deviations from Beer's law are:

(a) **Instrumental deviations:** Factors like stray radiation, improper slit width, fluctuations in single beam & when monochromatic light is not used influence the deviation.

(b) **Physico-chemical changes in solution:** *Factors like association, dissociation, ionisation, faulty development of colour, refractive index at high concentrations can influence such deviations.*

Applications in Pharmacy

1. Qualitative analysis

(a) **Detection of Impurities:** *Additional peaks can be due to impurities in the sample and can be compared with that of standard raw material. The impurities can be detected by absorbance measurements at specific wavelengths.*

(b) **Structure elucidation of organic compounds:** *The presence or absence of unsaturation, the presence of hetero atoms like S, O, N or halogens can be determined.*

(c) **Structural analysis of organic compounds:** *Identification of* $n \rightarrow \pi^*$ *transition, effect of conjugation are already discussed under electronic transition. Others like alkyl substitution, effect of cross conjugation, effect of geometric isomerism will be described briefly.*

1. ***Effect of conjugation*** – *Extended conjugation shifts* λ_{max} *to longer* λ *(Bathochromatic shift).*

   Reduction of the compound or saturation of double bonds leads to the opposite effect i.e. hypsochromic shift.

2. ***Effect of geometric isomerism*** – *Of the cis & trans isomers, trans isomer absorbs at long wavelength than cis isomer.*

   e.g. Calciferol (cis isomer) λ_{max} *– 265 nm.*

   Isovit – D_2 *(all trans)* λ_{max}*-287nm*

   Conversion from cis to trans isomer results in bathochromic shift & hyper chromic effect. Conversion from trans to cis isomer results in hypsochromic shift & hypochromic effect.

3. ***Effect of cross conjugation:*** *Cross conjugation has no effect on* λ_{max}.

4. ***Effect of alkyl substitution:*** *Alkyl substitution shifts the* λ_{max} *to longer wave length (Bathochromic shift).*

5. ***Number of rings:*** *The addition of rings causes bathochromic shift.*

2. Quantitative analysis

1. *Using* $E^{1\%}_{1cm}$ *values.*
2. $E^{1\%}_{1cm}$ *not available, but raw material is available.*
3. *Single standard or direct comparison method.*
4. *Calibration curve method or multiple standard method.*

(a) **Simultaneous multi component method:** If a mixture of two components a & b are present in x% w/v & y% w/v respectively by measuring the absorbance of mixture at two wavelengths λ_1 & λ_2 the concentration or amount of components a & b can be estimated. A1 & a_2 & b_1 & b_2 and $E^{1\%}_{1cm}$ values are determined at λ_1 & λ_2 for component a & b respectively.

x% w/v of component a.	λ_1	λ_2
y% w/v of component b.	a_1	a_1
Mixture	b_1	b_2
	S_1	S_2

$$x\ \%\ w/v = 100\left[\frac{b_1s_2 - b_2s_1}{b_1a_2 - b_2a_1}\right] \text{ since } 100\ s_1 = a_1x + b_1y$$

$$100\ s_2 = a_2x + b_2y$$

$$y\%\ w/v = 100\left[\frac{a_1s_2 - a_2s_1}{a_1b_2 - a_2b_1}\right]$$

(b) **Derivative spectrophotometric method:** In this method, spectral isolation is achieved rather than chromatographic isolation. In a derivative spectrum the change in absorbance with respect to wave length (vs) wavelength is recorded. Ist and 2nd derivative spectrum is recorded and the characteristic peak for the individual component can be identified and quantified by using a calibration curve of pure substance.

(c) **Chemical kinetics:** kinetics of a reaction can be studied by using UV spectroscopy. The UV radiation is passed through the reaction cell and the absorbance changes can be followed.

Keto-enol tautomerism: Using this, the percentage of keto & etnol form in a mixture, the presence of enol in ether or alcohols can be calculated.

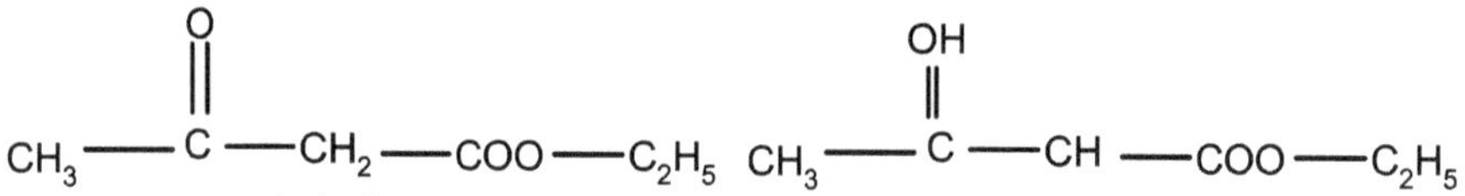

$$CH_3—\overset{\overset{\displaystyle O}{||}}{C}—CH_2—COO—C_2H_5 \qquad CH_3—\overset{\overset{\displaystyle OH}{||}}{C}—CH—COO—C_2H_5$$

keto form λmax = 275 nm — Enol form λmax = 244 nm

(d) **Quantitative analysis of pharmaceutical substances**

Assay of medicinal substances: Many drugs either in the form of raw materials or in the form of formulation can be assayed by making a suitable solution of the drug in a solvent and by measuring the absorbance at specific wavelength.

CHAPTER 11

FLOURIMETRY

Introduction

In nature, any compound can be analysed by using an appropriate analytical technique which basically depends on the nature and properties of the target compound. If the target compounds exhibit phenomenon called as Luminescence where the emission of electromagnetic radiation of a longer wavelength to that of absorbed radiation can be seen, are analysed by using the modern spectroscopic technique called as "FLOURIMETRY".

Flourimetry characterises the relationship between absorbed and excited photons at specified wavelengths. There are two important manifestations of photoluminescence which may constitute possible mechanisms whereby electronically excited molecules can lose energy. They are as follows:

1. Flourescence
2. Phosphorescence

All chemical compounds absorb energy which causes excitation of electrons bound in the molecule, such as increased collisional energy or transitions between discrete electronic energy states. For a transition to occur, the absorbed energy must be equivalent to the difference between the initial electronic state and a high-energy state. This value is constant and characteristic of the molecular structure.

Flourescence occurs when a molecule absorbs photons from the U.V-vis. Light spectrum (200 – 900 nm) causing transition to a high energy electronic state and then emits photons as it returns to its initial state in less than 10^{-9} sec. Some energy within the molecule, is lost through heat or collisions so that excited energy is less than the incident energy i.e. the emission wavelength is always longer than the excitation wavelength.

Flourescence

- When a beam of light is incident on certain substances, they emit visible light/radiations of longer wavelength than incident light.
- The energy of emitted radiations is lesser than that of incident or absorbed radiation because a part of energy is lost due to vibrational transitions.
- In fluorescence the emitted wavelength radiation is higher than absorbed radiation.
- Substances which show the fluorescence are referred to as fluorescent substances.

Phosphorescence

The Phenomenon where the emission of light is continuous by some compounds even when the incident light source is cut off is referred to as phosphorescence.

In short, the delayed fluorescence is called as phosphorescence and substances which exhibit this phenomenon are called as phosphorescent substances.

- Flourescence is more widely used in analysis than the phosphorescence. The measured fluorescent intensity permits the quantitative determination of traces of many inorganic and organic species.
- From earlier days onwards this technique has undergone many modifications in principle levels, instrumental levels, and so as to achieve the superior accuracy, sensitivity and reproductivity in Qualitative and Quantitative analysis of some peculiar compounds (fluorescent & phosphorescent compounds).
- Flourimetry will cover molecular, emission and electronic levels of spectroscopy so as to fulfil the objectives of analysis of fluorescent compounds by controlling some factors.
- Before knowing the flourimetry and its detailed monograph in several aspects we have to know the primary differences between the fluorescence and phosphorescence.

Defination of Flourimetry

Flourimetry is a one of the spectral analytical technique, where the study or measurement of emitted radiation is carried out when electrons undergo transition from singlet excited state to singlet ground state.

Fluorescence	Phosphorescence
1. Emission of radiation is instantaneous	1. Emission of radiation is delayed.
2. In fluorescence, materials remit excess radiation within 10^{-6} to 10^{-4} second of absorption.	2. In phosphorescence, materials remit excess radiation within 10–4 to 20 seconds.
3. Lasts for shorter period	3. Lasts for longer period.
4. This occurs when there is transition from singlet excited state to singlet ground state.	4. This occurs when there is transition from triplet state to singlet ground state.

Flourimetry is

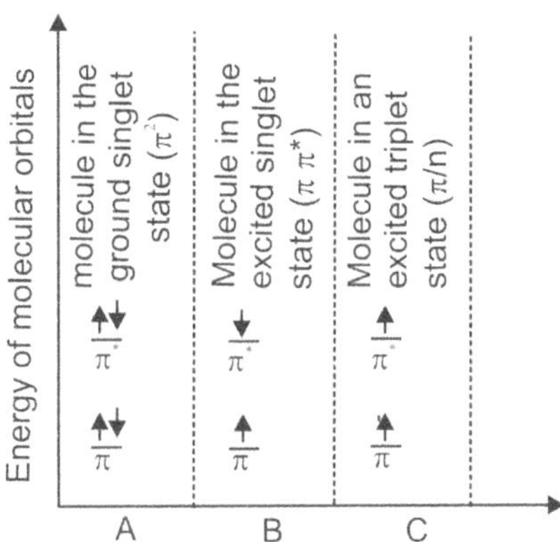

A → Excited singlet state is unstable.

B → Excited singlet state may emit an UV radiation vis. light photon (Flourescence)

C → Stable excited singlet state may undergo transition to a metastable triplet state. (Phosphorescence)

→ Molecular spectroscopy – Where the molecular absorption, emission or collisions are studied.

→ Emission Spectroscopy – Where emission of radiation is studied.

→ Electronic spectroscopy – Where study is done using electromagnetic radiation only.

Flourimetry Principle

To understand principle involved in flourimetry we have to know following basic electronic states as mentioned below.

***Singlet ground state*:** A state in which all the electrons in a molecule are paired (↑ ↓).

Double state : A state in which an unpaired electron is present. e.g. Free radical (↑ or ↓).

***Triplet state*:** A state in which unpaired electrons of same spin are present. (unpaired and same spin) (↑ ↑).

***Singlet excited state*:** A state in which electrons are unpaired but of opposite spin (unpaired and opposite spin) (↑ ↓).

Absorption of UV/visible radiation causes transition from singlet ground state to singlet excited state. As this excited state is not stable, it emits the excess energy and returns to ground state.

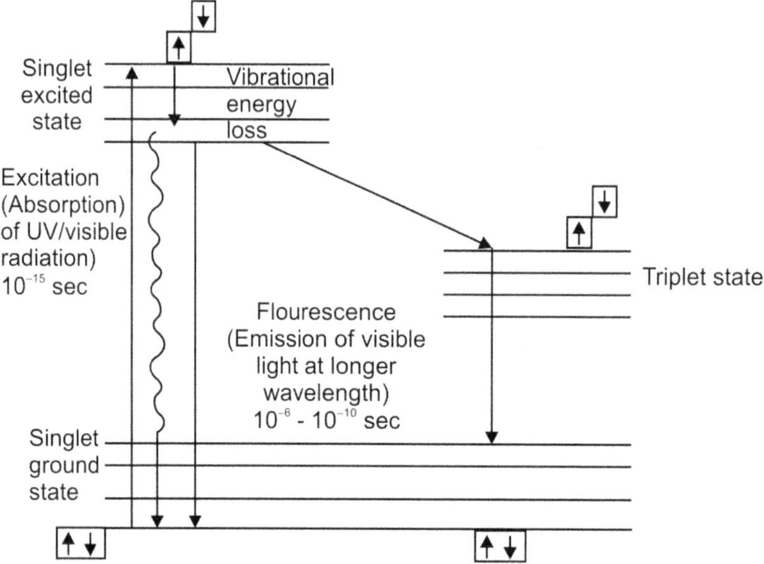

"Flourescence is the phenomena of emission of radiation when there is transition from singlet excited state to singlet ground state".

Excitation wavelength → Wavelength of absorbed radiation.

Emission wavelength → Wavelength of emitted radiation.

These two wavelengths are specific (or) characteristic for a given substance under ideal conditions.

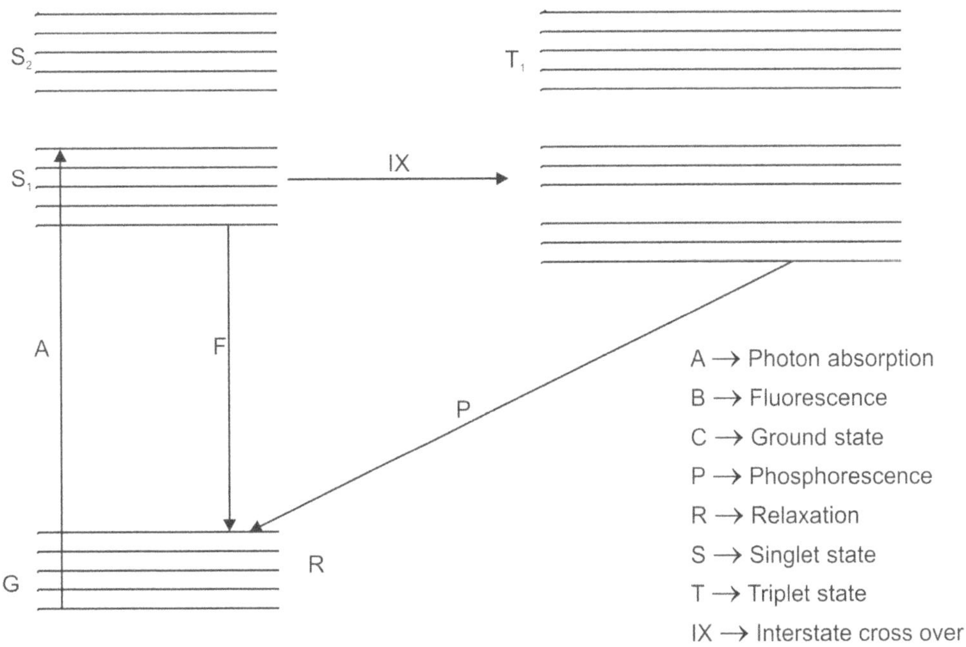

When molecules are irradiated by light of the suitable wavelength, it will be absorbed and the molecules move from ground state to first excited singlet electronic state, as a result of absorption.

From the excited singlet state, the following phenomenon will probably takes place depending on the molecule and the conditions.

(i) Due to unstability of excited singlet state, the excited molecules will return to the ground state by collisional deactivation without emitting any radiations.

(ii) The molecule in excited singlet state may emit radiation as uv or visible light photon (Flourescence).

(iii) The molecules with relatively stable excited state may undergo transition to a metastable triplet state and after some time return to ground state by emission of an ultraviolet or visible photon. (Phosphorescence).

The process of crossing from a singlet state (no unpaired electrons) to a triplet state (2 unpaired electrons) is called as intersystem crossing.

Resonance Flourescence

In fluorescence, the absorbed radiation which is re-emitted at the same wavelength is called as resonance fluorescence.

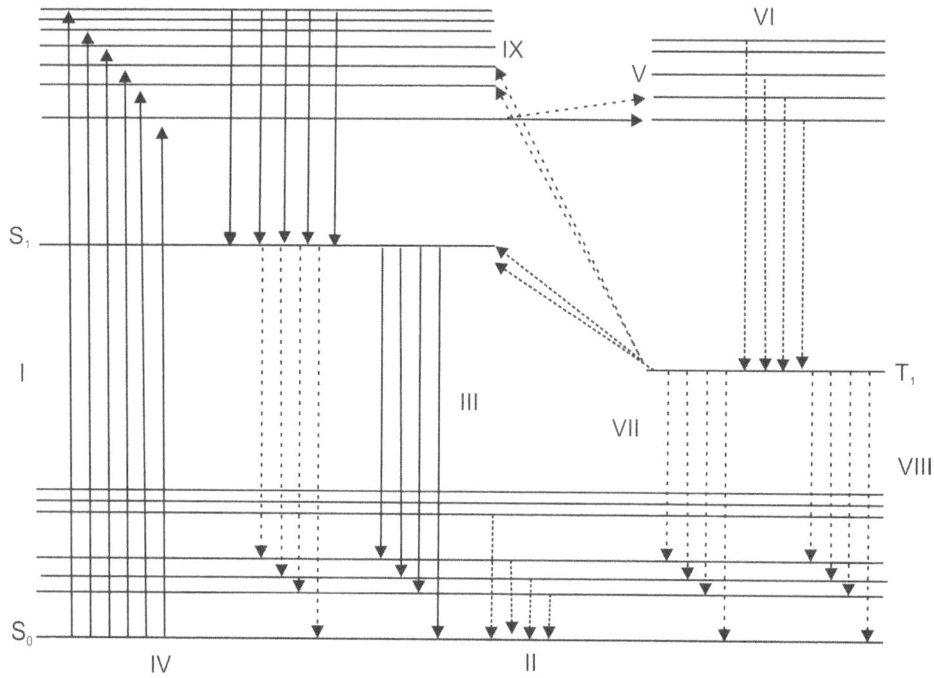

I → Absorption

II Vibrational deviation

III → Flourescence

IV → Quenching of excited singlet state

V → Intersystem crossing to triplet system

VI → Vibrational deactivation in the triplet state.

VII → Quenching of triplet state.

VIII → Phosphorescence

IX → Intersystem crossing to excited singlet state.

The following table gives a summary of transitions and the resultant effect produced by the same :-

Electronic Transition	Effect Produced
$\pi \rightarrow \pi^*$	Only absorption, no fluorescence
$\pi \rightarrow \pi^*$ (+ singlet transition)	Fluorescence
$\pi \rightarrow \pi^*$ (+ triplet transition)	Phosphorescence

Types of Flourescence

Luminescence is the phenomenon of emission of light radiation by substances, when excitation occurs in any form.

1. *Chemiluminescence*: Excitation by chemicals
2. *Electrochemiluminiscence*: Excitation by electrochemical reaction.
3. *Photo Luminescence*: Excitation by electromagnetic radiation.

Examples for photolumonescence : Flourescence

Phosphorescence

Based on wavelength of Emitted Radiation when compared to Absorbed Radiation

***Stocke's Flourscence*:** The wavelength of the emitted radiation is longer than the absorbed radiation.

e.g. Conventional flourimetric experiments.

***Anti Stocke's Flourscence*:** The wavelength of emitted radiation is shorter than the absorbed radiation.

e.g. Thermally assisted fluorescence.

***Resonance Flourescence*:** When the wavelength of the emitted radiation is equal to the absorbed radiation

e.g. Mercury vapour at 254 nm.

Based upon the Phenomenon

***Sensitized Flourescence*:** When elements like zinc, cadmium or an alkali metal are added to mercury vapour, the elements are sensitized and thus give fluorescence.

***Direct Line Flourescence*:** Where, even after the emission of radiation, the molecules remain in metastable state and finally come to ground state after loss of energy by vibrational transition.

***Stepwise Flourescence*:** This is nothing but the conventional type of fluorescence where a part of energy is lost by vibrational transition before the emission of fluorescent radiation.

***Thermally Assisted Flourescence*:** The excitation is partly by electromagnetic radiation and partly by thermal energy.

Factors Influencing Flourescence Intensity

Several factors will influence the fluorescence intensity which are as follows :-

- Conjugation
- Nature of substituent groups
- Rigidity of structures
- Effect of temperature
- Viscosity
- Oxygen
- Effect of pH
- Photochemical decomposition

Conjugation

Conjugation → Molecules will have π (pie) electrons i.e. unsaturation.

So conjugated molecules absorb UB/visible radiation which predominantly leads to fluorescence.

Nature of Substituent Groups

- Element donating groups → Enhance fluorescence intensity (NH_2, OH).
- Electron withdrawing groups → Reduce fluorescence intensity.
- SO_3H, NH_4 + and alkyl groups →No effect.

The given table gives clear picture of substituent group's effect on fluorescent intensity.

S.No.	Substituent	Effect on λ	Effect on Intensity
1.	Alkyl	No effect	Slight increase (or) ↓
2.	COOH, CHO, COOR, CRO	Increase	Decrease
3.	OH, Dme, OEt	Increase	Increase
4.	CN	No effect	Increase
5.	NH_2, NHR, NR_2	Increase	Increase
6.	NO2, NO	Increase	Large increase (or) quenching
7.	SH	Increase	Decrease
8.	SO_3H	No effect	No effect
9.	NH4+	No effect	No effect
10.	F, Cl, Br, I	Increase	Decrease

Rigidity of Structures

Rigid structures → More fluorescence intensity

Flexible structures → Less fluorescence intensity

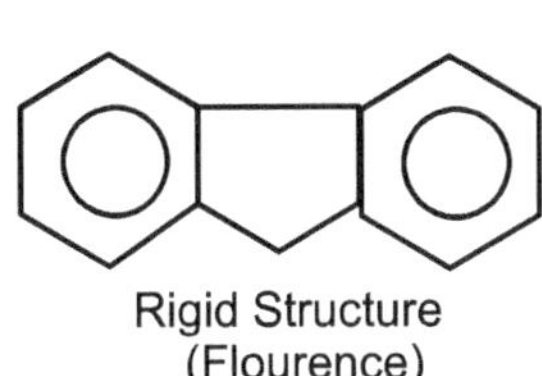

Rigid Structure
(Flourence)

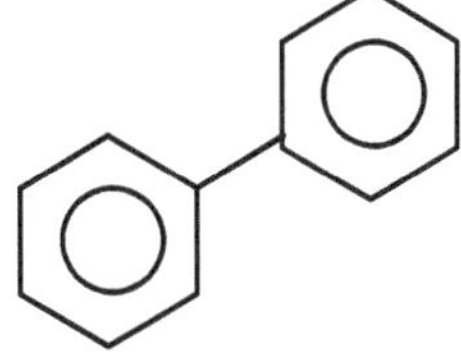

Flexible Structure
(Biphenyl)

Effect of Temperature

Temperature α 1/Flourescence intensity

↑ Temperature ⇒↑collisions of molecules ⇒↓ Flourescence.

Viscosity

Viscosity α Flourescence intensity.

↑ Viscosity ↑⇒ collisions of molecules ⇒↑ Flourescence intensity.

Oxygen

It decreases fluorescence intensity in two ways.

1. It oxidizes fluorescent substance to non-flourescent substance.
2. It quenches (decreases) fluorescence, because of the paramagnetic properties of molecular energy, as it has triplet ground state.

Effect of pH

Effect of pH depends on the chemical structures of the molecule.

1. Aniline + Neutral/Alkaline pH → visible flourescence

   Aniline + Acidic pH → Flourescence in UV region
2. Phenols + Acidic pH → Undissociated → No fluorescence

   Phenols + Alkaline pH → dissociated → good fluorescent

Photochemical Decomposition

UV or visible absorption sometimes leads to photochemical reaction. In such cases, fluorescence cannot be seen. Hence a wavelength which is not strongly absorbed should be chosen to avoid such a reaction. Otherwise errors up to 20% are possible.

When high atomic number molecule is incorporated in the sample, the fluorescence decreases.

Relation Between Concentration and Flourescence Intensity

For quantitative analysis, these should be definite relationship (preferably linear) between concentration and intensity of fluorescence.

From Lambert-Beer law, the intensity of high absorbed by a solution is

$$(I_o - I)$$

where $I = I_0.e^{-acl}$

$\Rightarrow$ Intensity of light absorbed $= I_0 - I_0.e^{-acl}$

$$= I_0 (1 - e^{-acl})$$

where I_0 = Intensity of incident light

I = Intensity of transmitted light

a = Absorptivity (extinction coil) multiplied by 2.303.

c = Concentration

l = Length of optical path

The intensity of fluorescence (F) emitted can be obtained by multiplying the amount of light absorbed by quantum yield (ϕ).

$$\phi = \frac{\text{Light emitted}}{\text{Light absorbed}}$$

$\therefore$ $F = \phi \; I_0 (I - e^{-acl})$

Absorption and emission occur only due to single molecular species and degree of dissociation does not vary with the concentration.

Now e^{-acl} can be exponentially expressed as,

$$e^{-acl} = I - acl + \frac{(acl)^2}{2} - \frac{(acl)^3}{6} + \ldots + \frac{(acl)^n}{n!}$$

If the magnitude of acl is small, all terms after first two can be neglected.

$\therefore$ $e^{-acl} = I - acl$

Putting in equation (2), we get

$$F = \phi \times I_0 (I - I + acl)$$

$$= \phi \times I_0 . acl$$

From given fluorescent compound, solvent and temperature and in a cell of definite dimensions, all factors are constant, then

$$F = K_C$$

where K = proportionality constant

- Flourescent intensity is directly proportional to concentrations of the substance.
- This rule can only be obeyed at low concentrations (mg or ng/ml). But at higher concentration (mg/ml) it does not obey linearity as shown in figures below.

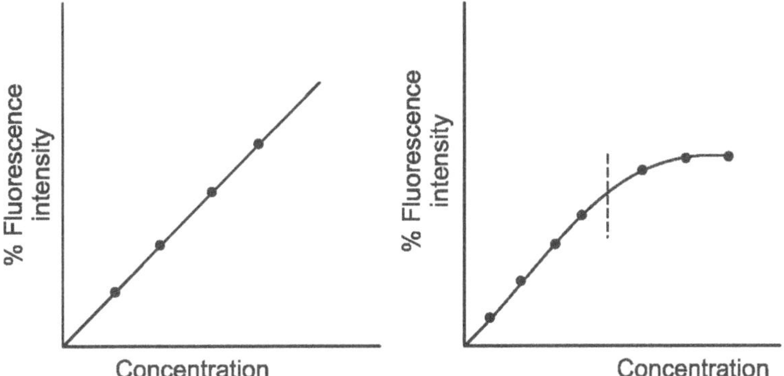

- At higher concentrations, even though concentration increases, fluorescence intensity does not increase proportionately, because of phenomenon called **self quenching** (or) **concentration quenching.**

Reason for Self Quenching

The emitted radiation before falling on detector, is being absorbed and re-emitted by adjacent molecules, leads to internal circulation of radiation (energy). Hence deviation from linearity can be observed.

***Note*:** In quenching, two different concentrations of the same substance shown identical fluorescence intensity. This leads to wrong interpretation of results.

So the concentration range in which a substance undergoes self or concentration quenching and the concentration range in which it obeys Beer's law (linearity) should be determined experimentally. So there must be linearity range.

Calculation of Results

- In flourimetric determination we have a blank and two standards of known composition which cover the range of concentration expected.

- The blanks must be kept relatively low and blank reading should be subtracted from all the readings. In concentration is linear with the fluorescence, then it is evident from equation.

  F standard = K C standard

  F unknown = K C unknown

Note: Standard used should be very close to unknown in composition.

By dividing above equations

$$\text{C unknown} = \frac{C\text{ standard} \times \text{F unknown}}{F\ s\tan dard}$$

Note: Flourescent intensity is measured as percent transmission. F intensity α % transmission. (α = directly proportional)

For 100% transmission level, it requires standardisation.

Standardization may be carried out by either of following:

1. An aqueous H_2SO_4 solution of quinine (quantum yield about 1) or a piece of glass containing uranyl ion (UO_2^{2+}) is inserted into the sample chamber and the instrument set at 100% T.
2. The most concentration standard of the sample being determined is used to set 100%.

After the standardization of the flourimeter (0-100% T) the calibration curve is prepared by measuring % T for series of standards.

Plotting calibration curve

X axis → Concentration ($\mu\ gm^{-1}$).

Y axis → Flourescence intensity.

Quenching of Flourescence and Types

Quenching: It is the decrease in fluorescence intensity due to specific effects of the constituents of the solution itself.

Factors Affecting Quenching

1. Concentration
2. pH
3. Presence of specific chemical substances
4. Temperatures
5. Viscosity

Self Quenching (or) Concentration Quenching

At low concentrations (μg or μg/ml), linearity was observed. At high concentrations (μg/ml) of the same substance, proportionate increase in fluorescence intensity does not occur. This is called as self quenching.

Chemical quenching

pH : Aniline at pH = 5 – 13 → Blue fluorescence 290 nm

Aniline at pH < 5 (exists as cation) → No Flourescence

Aniline at pH > 13 (exists as anion)

Oxygen

Presence of oxygen → Paramagnetic property
↓
Triplet ground state
↓
Quenching

Halides and electron withdrawing groups

Halides → Cl, Br, I

Electron withdrawing groups → Nitro (NO_2)
Carboxylic (COOH)

They lead to quenching because of the paramagnetic property and decrease influorescent intensity.

***Heavy Metals*:** They lead to quenching because of collisions and triplet ground state.

Static Quenching

This occurs because of complex formation. For example, caffeine reduces Riboflavin fluorescence intensity by complex formation.

Collisional Quenching

It results from several factors like presence of halides, heavy metals, increased temperature, decrease in viscosity, results in increase in collisions forming quenching.

M + hv	→	M* (Absorption)
M*	→	M + hv (Flourescence)
M* + Q	→	Q* + M (Quenching)
Q*	→	Q + Energy
M	→	Sample in ground state

M* → Sample in excited state
Q → Quenching agent
hv → Photon of radiant energy

During quenching there is no permanent reaction between the fluorescent substance and the quencher. There is usually a reversible oxidation – reduction reaction involved between the quencher and the excited molecule and then the regeneration of the original substance.

Quenchers → Iodide, Thiocyanate
Polyhydroxy phenols
Amines

Instrumentation

1. Source of light
   (a) Mercury vapour lamp
   (b) Xenon are lamp
   (c) Tungsten lamp
2. Filters and monochromators
   (a) Primary filter
   (b) secondary filter
   (c) Excitation monochromator
   (d) Emission monochromator
3. Sample cells
4. Detectors

Source of Light

(a) ***Mercury Vapour lamp*****:** It gives intense lines on a continuous background above 350 nm under high pressure (8 atmospheres).

- Lines are seen at 365, 398, 436, 546, 579, 690 amd 734 nm.
- Low pressure mercury vapour gives an additional line at 54 nm. It is used as source in filter type of flourimeters.

(b) ***Xenon arc lamp*****:** It gives a more intense radiation when compared to mercury vapour lamp. It is used as the source of light in spectroflourimeters.

(c) ***Tungsten lamp*****:** If excitation has to be done in visible region, this can be used. It doesn't require UV radiation, moreover the intensity of this lamp is too low.

Filters and Monochromators

In flourimetry two thirds are important:

1. Excitation wavelength
2. Emission wavelength

Whenever these two wavelengths are different, in most cases, a filter or monochromator is used for the purpose.

Filter flourimeter → Primary filter
Secondary filter

Filters are of two types :

1. Absorption filters
2. Interference filters

Absorption Filters

- Filters are made up of glass, coated with pigments or made up of gelatin.
- Filters are selected according to opposite colour present as described below.

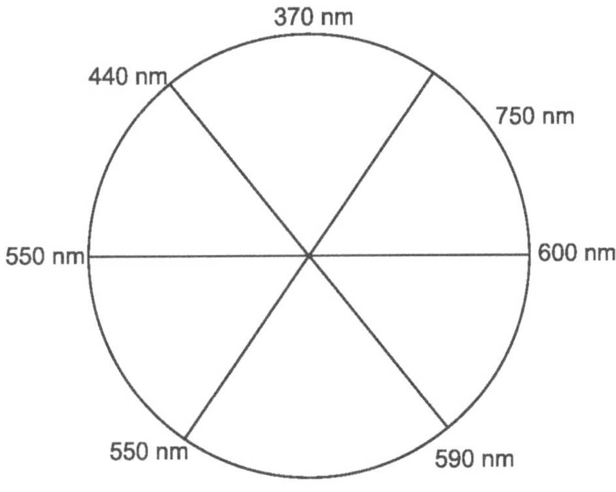

Absorption filter

Merits

- Simple in construction
- Not expensive
- Selection or filter is easy

Demerits

- Less accurate

- Band base is more $\pm$ 20 to 30 nm. (If we have to measure at 400 nm, we get radiation from 370 nm to 430 nm.) Hence less accurate results are obtained.
- Intensity of radiation becomes lessened due to absorption by filters.

Interference Filters: (Faby-Perot Filter)

- It has dielectric spacer filter made up of CaF_2 or SiO between two parallel reflecting silver films.
- The thickness of dielectric spacer film can be ½ λ (1st order), 2λ/2 (2nd order). 3λ / 2 (3rd order) etc.
- The mechanism is the radiation reflected by the 2nd film and the incoming radiation undergoes constructive interference to give a monochromatic radiation which is governed by

$$\lambda = 2\,\eta\,b/m$$

$\lambda \rightarrow$ Wave length of light obtained

$\eta \rightarrow$ Dielectric constant of layer material

$b \rightarrow$ Layer thickness

$m \rightarrow$ Order No (0, 1, 2, 3, ……)

- Band pass is 10-15 nm.
- Maximum transmission is 40%

Merits

- Inexpensive
- Lower band pass when compared to absorption filters and hence more accurate.
- Use of additional filter cuts off undesired wavelengths.

Demerits

- Peak transmission is low, and becomes so when additional filters are used to cut off undesired wavelength.
- The band pass is only 10-15 nm and hence higher resolution like monochromators or gratings can't be achieved.

In Flourimetry

1° Filter	→	Absorbs visible radiation
(Primary)	→	Transmits UV radiation
Placed	→	Between sample and radiation source.

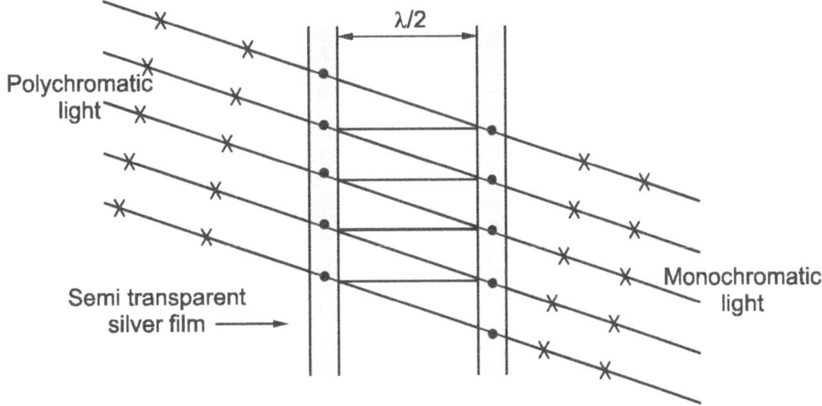

2° Filter	→	Absorbs UV radiation
(Secondary)	→	Transmits visible radiation
Placed	→	Between sample and detector

Monochromators

- Better and more significant and more efficient than filters.
- They convert a polychromatic light or heterochromatic light into monochromatic light.
- Monochromator has the following units.
  1. Entrance slit (to get narrow source).
  2. Collimator (to render light parallel).
  3. Grating or prism (to disperse radiation)
  4. Collimator (to reform the images of entrance slit).
  5. Exit slit (to fall on sample cell).

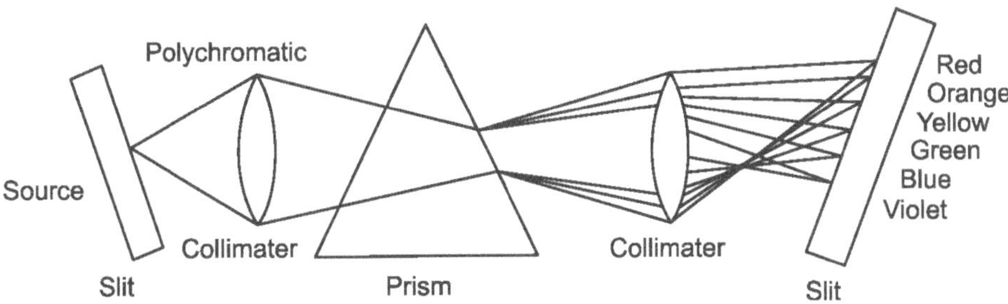

In spectro flourimeters, excitation monochromators and emission monochromators are present which have gratings.

Excitation monochromator → Provides a suitable radiation for excitation of molecule (Radiation which is absorbed by molecule).

Emission monochromator → Isolates only the radiation emitted by the fluorescent molecule.

Gratings

- They are the most efficient in converting a polychromatic to monochromatic light in the real sense.
- By using these, resolution of $\pm$ 0.1 nm could also be achieved.
- As the gratings are expensive, they are used in spectrophotometer.

  Types will be

  1. Diffraction grating.
  2. Transmission grating

Diffraction grating

Gratings → Rulings made on some material like glass, quartz or alkyl halides depending on instrument whether it is visible UV/IR Spectrophotometer.

Spectrophotometer		**Rulings/mm**
IR	→	20 grooves/mm
UV/visible	→	3600 grooves/mm

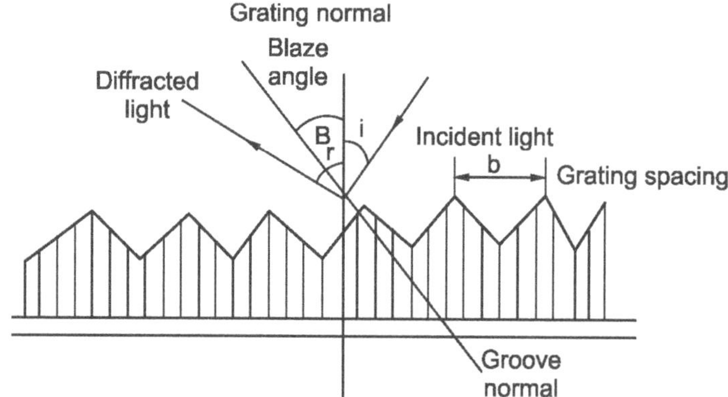

- Gratings are made from master grating, by coating the original master with epoxy resin and are removed after setting.
- To make surface refractive, a deposit of 'Aluminium' is made.

Mechanism

Diffraction produces reinforcement. The ray which is incident upon the grating gets reinforced with the reflected ray and hence resulting radiation has wavelength which is governed by equation.

$$m\lambda = b(\sin i \pm \sin r)$$

λ → Wavelength of light produced

B → Grating spacing, I → Angle of incidence

r → Angle of reflection (Angle of diffraction)

m → order (0, 1, 2, 3 ....)

Transmission Grating:

→ Similar to diffraction grating

→ But refraction takes place instead of reflection

→ Refraction produces reinforcement.

The wavelength of radiation produced by transmission grating can be expressed by the following equation.

$$\lambda = \frac{\partial \sin\theta}{m}$$

λ → Wavelength of radiation produced

d → 1/lines per cm m → Order no. (0, 1, 2, 3 etc.)

θ → Angle at deflection / diffraction.

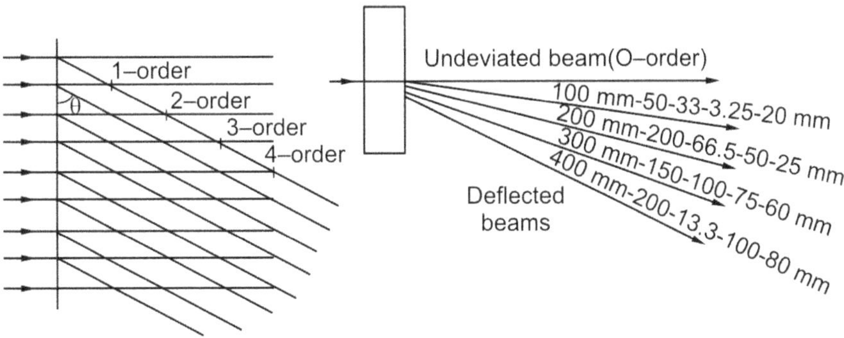

Note **:** Light radiation at any angle (θ) or any order can be collected and used in the instrument by either moving the grating and fixing the slit or moving the slit and keeping the grating constant.

Sample Cells

- Sample cells or cuvettes are used to hold a sample solution.

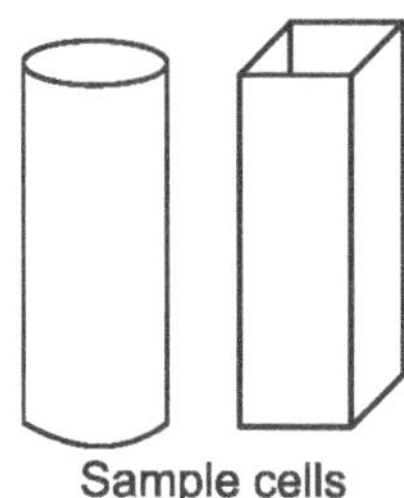

Sample cells

Shape of cell	→	Cylindrical
		Rectangular
Sample volume	→	Smaller (0.5 ml)
		Larger (5 – 10 ml)
Path length	→	1 cm (or) 10 mm (Internal distance)
Material	→	glass for visible region .
		Quartz for UV radiation

Note

- In quadrangular cells, two are polished surfaces (through which light is transmitted) and two are ground surfaces (for handling the cells.)
- All the surfaces are polished in flourimetry because emission measurements are made at 90° angle.

Detectors

- Detectors used in UV/visible spectrophotometers can be called as photometric detectors.
- When a radiation is passed through a sample cell, part of it gets absorbed by the sample solution and the rest is transmitted.
- This transmitted radiation falls on the detector and the intensity of absorbed radiation can be determined or displayed.

  Light energy → Electrical signal → Recorded

  Commonly used detectors are :

  1. Barrier layer cell (or) photo voltaic cell
  2. Photo tubes (or) photo emissive cells.
  3. Photo multiplier tubes.

Photo Voltaic Cell

- These cells are the cheapest and used in inexpensive instruments.

Construction

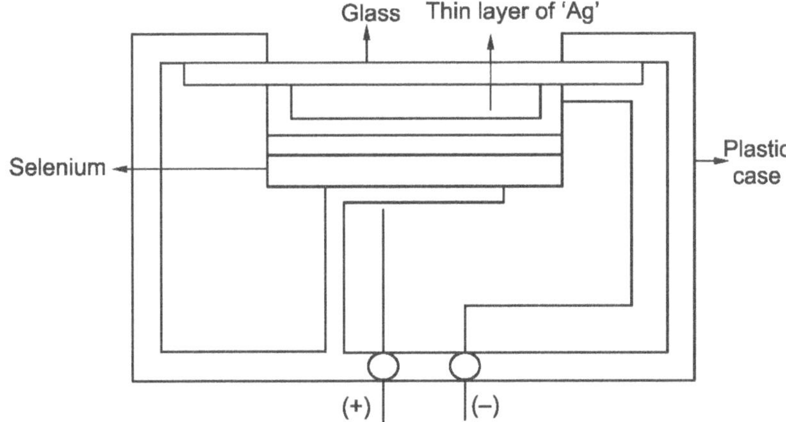

- The detector has transparent metal layer coated with silver or gold and acts as electrode.
- It also has a metal base plate which is the other portion of electrode.
- These two are separated by a semi conductor layer of selenium.

Working

- Light radiation when falls on the silver or gold surface, creates an electric voltage difference between the top surface and base plate.
- A low external resistance is connected in the circuit, which causes the flow of current which depends on the wavelength and intensity of radiation.
- This current signal can be converted to digital read-out or analogue output (panel meter).

Photo tubes (or) Photoemissive cells

- Better sensitivity when compared to photo voltaic cell and most widely used.

Construction

The detector is composed of

1. An evacuated glass tube
2. Photo cathode
3. Collector anode

Photo cathode is made up high atomic volume material (caesium, potassium, Ag_2O)

- which can liberate electrons when light radiation falls on it.

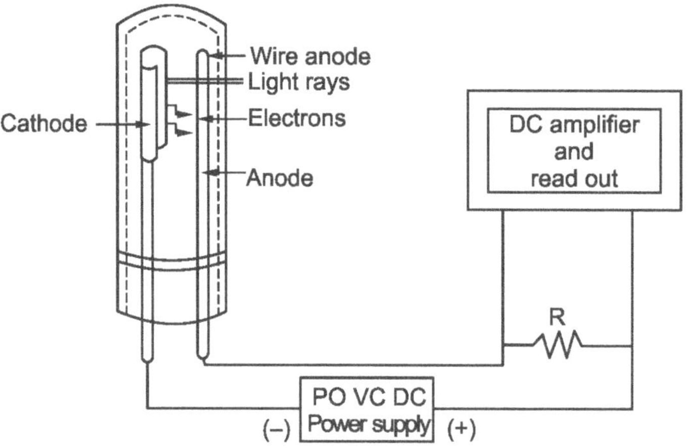

Working

- Cathode liberates electrons.
- These electrons move towards anode, produce a current proportional to the intensity of light radiation.
- Caesium, caesium oxide and silver oxide can increase the sensitivity and range of wave length in which the detector can be used.
- The signal from the detector can also be amplified using an amplifier circuit.

Photomultiplier Tubes

- It is most sensitive to all the detectors.
- Expensive and used in sophisticated instruments.
- It can detect vary weak signals, even 200 times weaker than that could be done using photo evacuated cell.
- Widely used in fluorescence measurements.

Note: It should be shielded from stray light inorder to have accurate results.

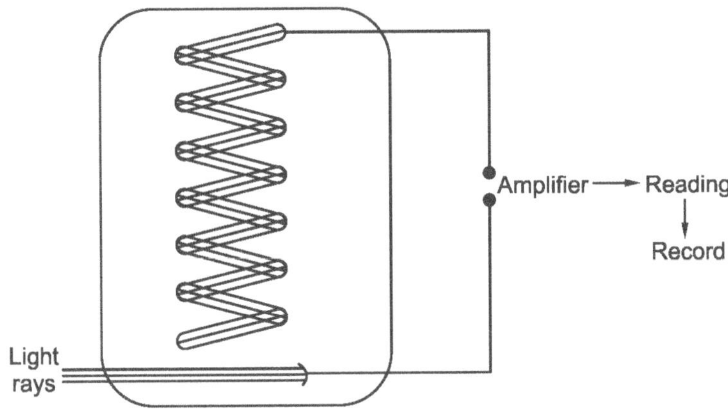

Construction

- Consists of photo cathode and a series of anodes (dyanodes). Upto 10 dyanodes are used. Each dyanode is maintained at 75-100 V higher than the preceding one.

Principle: Multiplication of photoelectrons by secondary emission of electrons. This is achieved by photocathode and anodes.

- At each stage, the electron emission is multiplied by a factor of 4 or 5 due to secondary emission of electrons and hence an overall factor of 10^6 is achieved.

Instruments

The measurement of fluorescence is usually carried out by making use of instruments as follows. They are :

1. Fluorometers
   (a) Single beam (Filter) flourimeter.
   (b) Double beam (Filter) flourimeter.
2. Spectroflourometers
   (a) Those consisting of fluorescence attachment for a spectrophotometer.
   (b) Self contained instruments usually with two monochromators.

Fluorometers

- They are filter instruments and are used for routine measurements of fluorescence from 350-780 mm.
- Analogous to photometers in that filters are employed to restrict the wavelength of the excitation and emission beams.

- Resemble Nephelometers in that the illumination is at right angles to the direction of observation.
- It differs from photometers in that.
- The head of filter between receptor and filter.
- Measurement of light emitted by the sample at right angles to the source to avoid interference from the direct beam of source.
- The choice of appropriate filter depends on
  1. The wavelength of the exciting mercury line.
  2. The wavelength of the emitted light.

Single Beam Filter Flourimeter

- An inexpensive instrument
- Contains tungsten lamp as source of light.
- Has optical system compared of primary filter.

  1° Filter ⇒ Absorbs visible radiation

  ⇒ Transmits UV radiation

  ⇒ Which excites the molecules present in sample.
- The emitted radiation (fluorescence) is measured at 90^{0} by using a secondary filter and a detector.

  2^{0} Filter ⇒ Absorbs UV radiation

  ⇒ Transmits visible radiation.
- Unabsorbed radiation and fluorescent (emitted) radiation will produce detector response and give false results if other than 90^{0} is employed.

Advantages

- Simple in construction.
- Cheaper and easy to operate
- Range of application can be widened by using different combinations of 1^{0} and 2^{0} filters.

Disadvantages

- Not possible to use sample and reference solution at the same time.
- Rapid scanning is not possible.
- At first we have to adjust to zero by using blank.
- We have to standardise at different wave lengths.

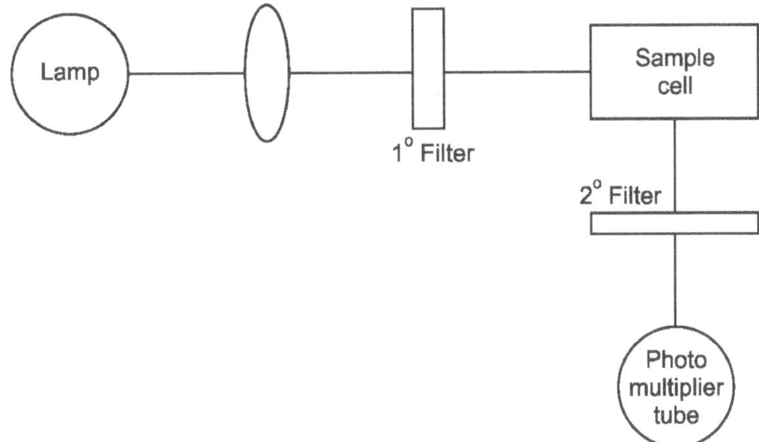

Double Beam Filter Fluorimeter

- It is similar to single beam except that two incident beams from a single light source pass through primary filters separately and fall on the either sample or reference solution.
- The emitted radiation from sample or reference passes separately through secondary filter and produces combined response on a detector.
- The analyses can be completed by means of calibration curve prepared in usual manner.

  e.g. The kleft fluorometer
  The Beckman Radio fluorometer

Beckman's Radio Fluorometer

Advantage

- Sample and standard solution can be analysed simultaneously.

Disadvantages

- Rapid scanning is not possible due to use of filters.
- Expensive one.

Spectro Fluorometers

A fluorometer constructed with two monochromators is called as spectro fluorometer.

- 1^0 filter in double beam filter fluorometer replaced by excitation monochromator.
- 2^0 filter replaced by emission monochromator.

  Excitation source → Mercury core xenon lamp
  Detector → Photo multiplier tube

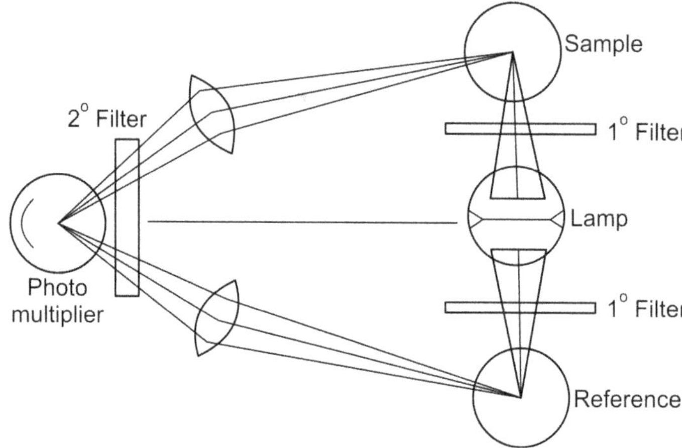

- The source was dispersed by prism or grating placed for high efficiency at shorter wavelengths and other prism or grating placed at some what greater wavelengths to disperse the emitted wavelengths.
- The fluorescent intensity was recorded by detector.
- Using spectro fluorometers we can know

  1. The wavelength of best excitation
  2. Wavelength of strongest emission.

Operation

1. A suitable wavelength for the emission spectrum is chosen by rough preliminary observations.
2. Second monochromator is set at this point.
3. An excitation spectrum is plotted by scanning the first monochromator.
4. An emission spectrum is obtained by scanning the second monochromator with the first set at a suitable value.

Result

For each fluorescent material on recorder two curves are obtained

1. Excitation curve
2. Emission curve

Excitation Spectrum

→ Can be produced by plotting wavelength of the exciting source against the intensity of emission.

→ The exciting wavelength produces a greater intensity of emission.

The data for making such a correlation may be obtained by measuring the intensity of the exciting source, at the sample position with a thermopile or by fluorescent solution.

Advantages

1. Rapid scanning to get excitation and emission spectrum.
2. More sensitivity
3. More accuracy
4. Continuous reading
5. Latest and precise manner results

Selection of an Excitation wavelength for Analysis

The best excitation wavelength to be used for a particular wavelength is governed by several considerations as follows.

1. It should be at a strong absorption band of the compound.
2. It should be easily separated from the emission by a grating prism or filter.
3. It should be at a strong intensity point of the radiation source of the instrument.
4. The wavelength of least decomposition of the sample should be chosen.

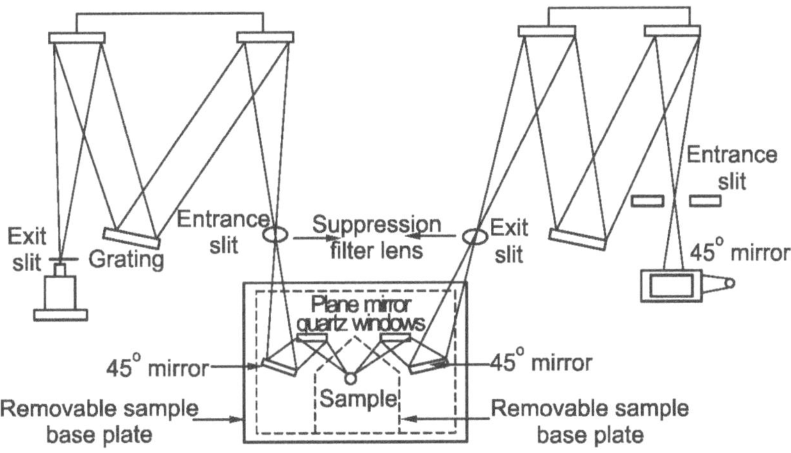

Reporting Flourescence Spectra

1. The spectrum should be corrected or reference should be made to a correction curve of the instrument.
2. The spectrum should be plotted as relative quanta per unit interval on the vertical scale V_{λ} wave numbers in reciprocal microns or reciprocal cms.

3. The spectra should be corrected for background fluorescence of the cuvette, scattered light and Raman emission, or the total background should be recorded on the graph from a measurement on the pure solvent.
4. Following experimental data should be given:
   - The spectrum of exciting light.
   - The light source and the band width.
   - The transmission curves of filters and the nature of light source.
   - The geometrical arrangement and the path lengths of the exciting as well as fluorescent light through the liquid.
   - Estimate the distortion of the spectrum by self absorption.
   - Concentration and purity of solute and the nature of solvent.
   - Temperature of the solution and a statement whether it is aerated or air free.
   - The type of analysing monochromator.

If gratings are used, we have to change wavelength to wave-numbers.

If prisms are used, we have to change wavelength to wave number compulsarilly.

Precautions

1. To eliminate the contaminants of the samples.
2. Common solvents, such as methyl alcohol, ethyl alcohol, dimethyl formamide etc, must be redistilled and used middle fractions only.
3. Rubber and cork stoppers contain fluorescent materials and these are extracted if the solvent touches them. (Same for filter papers also).
4. Grease from stopcocks and other sources are contaminant.
5. The interfering agents to flourometry are:
   - Raman lines from the solvent.
   - Solutions and extractable impurities from containers (Boron from pyrex glass) and from reagents.
   - All glasses contain Al, Ca, SiO_2.
6. Concentration should be expressed in micromolecules so that the ratio of the reagent to metal may be estimated easily.
7. Large temperature change between sample and standard should be avoided.
8. Should not expose the solutions to ultraviolet radiation for long periods.

Advantages of Flourescence

1. ***Sensitivity***: This technique is more sensitive since concentrations as low as μg/ml or even mg/ml can be determined.
2. ***Precision***: Upto 1% can be achieved easily.
3. ***Specificity***: As both emission and absorption wavelength are characteristic, it is more specific than absorption methods, when absorption maxima may be same for two compounds.
4. ***Range of applications***: Even non fluorescent materials can also be converted to fluorescent compounds by chemical reaction.

Limitation of Flourimetry

1. Careful pH buffering is necessary.
2. Dissolved oxygen may cause photochemical destruction (or) quenching.
3. Traces of halides, heavy metals can affect fluorescent intensity.
4. UV absorption sometimes causes chemical changes.
5. All elements and compounds may not be fluorescent, inspite of chemical reaction.
6. This method is not suited for the determination of major constituents of a sample, because the accuracy is very less for large amounts.

Applications of Flourimetry

So many applications are there in several fields as follows :

1. Determination of inorganic substances
2. Determination of organic substances
3. Biological applications.
4. Pharmaceutical applications
5. Special fluorescent applications.

Determination of Inorganic substances

Ion	Reagent	Wavelength (nm)		Seinsitivity μ g/ml
		Excitation	Flourescence	
Al^{3+}	Alizarin garnet	470	500	0.007
Zn^{2+}	Benzoin	-	Green	10.0
Sn^{4+}	Flavonol	400	470	0.1
Li^{+}	8-hydroxy quinoline	370	580	0.2
Be	Naphthoic Acid	380	460	2

Determination of Organic Substances

1. Determination of ruthenium in the presence of other platinum metals.

   pH = 6 ; Ruthenium range = 0.3-2.0 m μ .mh^{-1}.

2. Determination of vanadium with benzoic acid

   pH = 2 (Acetate buffer) ; Range = 0.5-400 ppb

3. Determination of traces of boron in steel by forming complex with Benzoin.

4. Small amount of Aluminium in alloys.

   Reagent → Dye pontachrome blue black F

   pH = 4.8

5. Chromium and Manganese in steel when it is dissolved in acid and the solution is oxidised with persulphate.

6. Determination of Uranium salts.

7. Determination of other organic compounds as follows:

Reagent	Structure	For Ions	Flourescence
2, 21 Dihydroxy - 1, 1[1] – azonapthalene - 4 – Sulphonic acid, Sodium salt	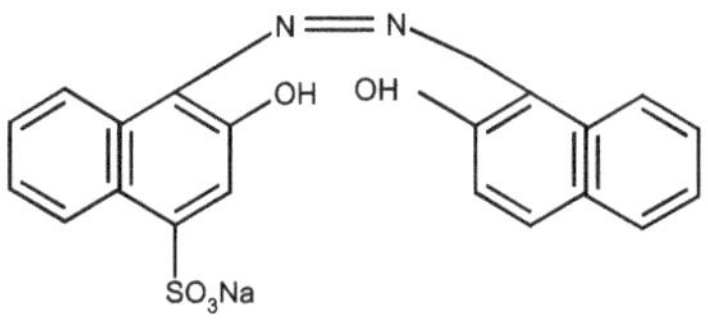 N=N, OH, OH, SO_3Na	Al	Red
2, 2[1] Dihydroxy-1, 11 napthalene-azobenzen - 5sulphonic acid, sodium salt	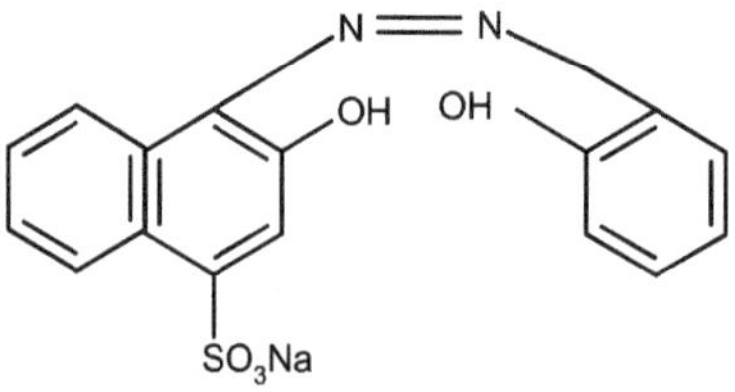 N=N, OH, OH, SO_3Na	Al	Orange
2, 4, 2[1] – trihydroxy azobenzene-5[1]-sulphonic acid, Na salt	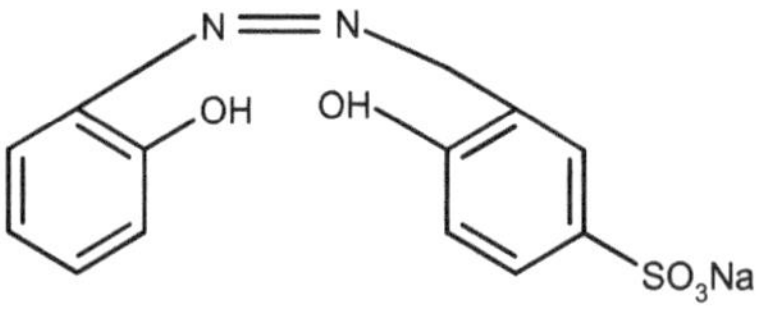 N=N, OH, OH, SO_3Na	Al	Yellow

Contd...

Reagent	Structure	For Ions	Flourescence
Salicylidene-o-aminophenol	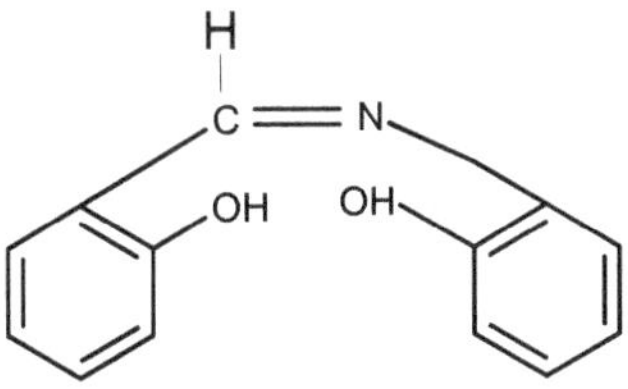	Al, Ga	Green
3-hydroxy favone (Flavonol)	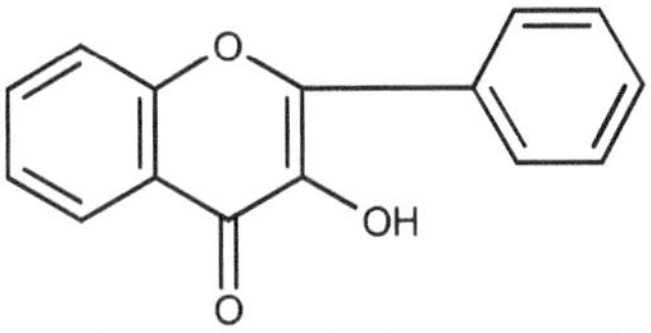	Zn, Sn	Blue
2^1, 3, 4^1, 5, 7-pentahydroxy Flavone (morin)	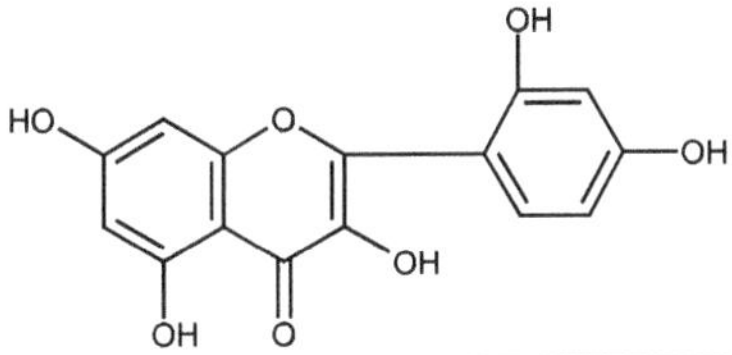	Al, Be	Bluish
3, 3^1, 4^1, 5, 7-pentahydroxy Flavone (Quercetin)	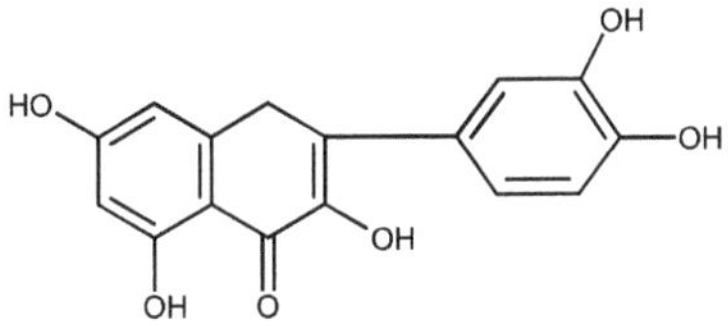	Zn or paper	Blue-White
Benzoin	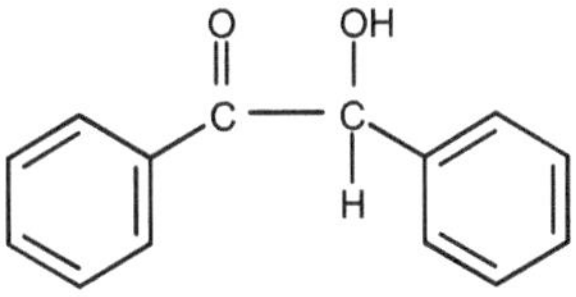	B, Zn, Ge, Si	Blue-White
1-Amino 4-hydroxy Anthraquinone (or) 1, 4-dihydroxy Anthraquinone	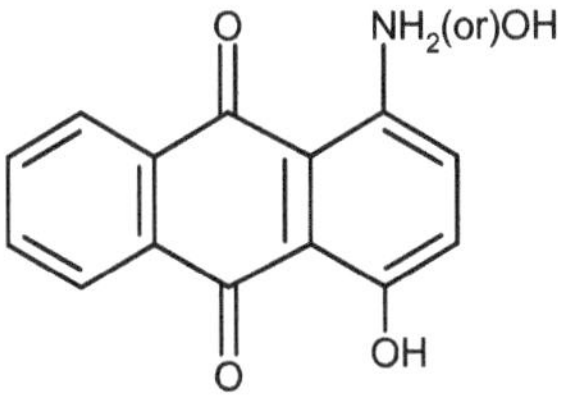	Be, Th	Red
2 hydroxy 3-Napthoic Acid	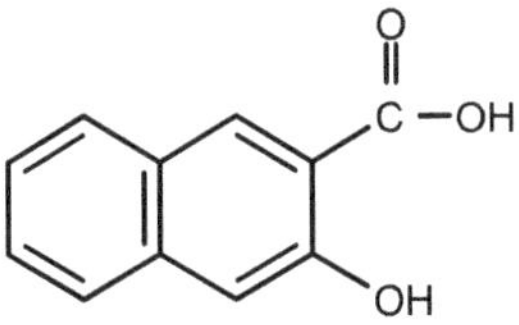	Al, Be	Blue

Contd...

Reagent	Structure	For Ions	Flourescence
8-hydroxy quinoline	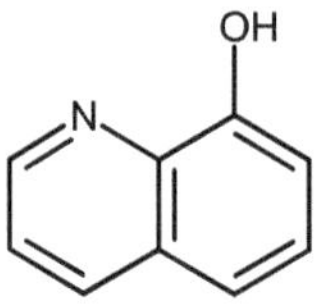 OH, N	Al, Be	
Alizarin garnet Red	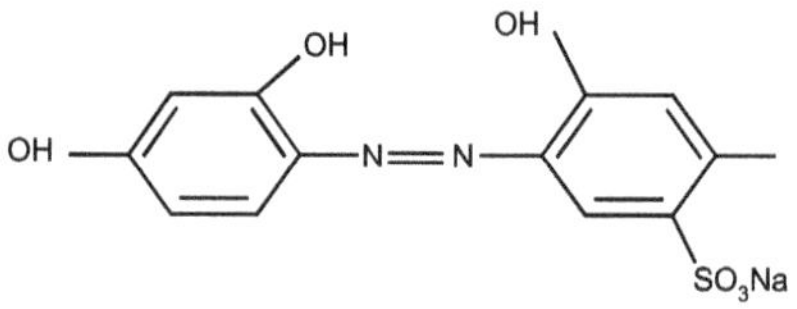 OH, OH, OH, N=N, SO_3Na	Al, F-	

- Anthranalic acid
- Aromatic polycyclic hydrocarbons
- Indole
- Napthols
- Nerve gases
- Proteins
- Salicylic acid
- Uric acid
- Tryptophan
- Skatole

Determination of Plant Products

- Chlorophyll
- Ergot alkaloids
- Flavonoids
- Retinone

Determination of Medicinal Agents

- Tridextran
- 5-Amino salicylic acid
- Amino methyl coumarin
- Staurosporine
- Ciprofloxacin
- Amphetamines
- Adrenalin
- Noradrenalin

- Chloroquin
- Digitalis principles
- Pencillin
- Procaine
- Reserpine
- Aureomycin
- Chlorpromazine
- Cinchonidine
- Cinchonine
- Hydro cortisone
- Pento barbitone
- Procainamide
- Physostigmine
- Quinine
- Terramycin
- Riboflavin
- Vit-A

Various options available are: (Mixture of medicinal substances)

→ A wavelength at which only one drug is excited is chosen.

→ Using separation methods & analyzing the compounds

→ Using chemical reaction

→ Preparation of derivatives.

e.g. EOSIN + ATROPINE → CHLOROFORM SOLUBLE COMPLEX (FLOURESCENT)

Pharmaceutical Applications

Compound	Wave length (nm)		Requirement
	Excitation	Flourescence	
P-amino Salicylate	300	405	pH = 11.0
Desipiramine	295	415	Alkaline pH
Ergometrine	325	465	1% tartaric acid-solvent
Griseofulvin	295	450	pH = 7.0

Contd...

Compound	Wave length (nm)		Requirement
	Excitation	Flourescence	
Indomethacin	300	410	Alkaline pH
Morphine	285	350	pH = 7.0
Quinine	350	450	0.1 N H_2SO_4
Riboflavin	270, 370, 445	520	AQ, butter, pH = 6.0
Vitamin – A	325	470	0.01 mg/ml conc
Amytal	265	410	0.1 mg/ml ; pH = 14
Aureomycin	355	445	0.02 mg/ml ; pH = 14
Chloroquine	335	400	0.05 μg/ml ; pH = 11
Chlorpromazine	350	480	0.1 μg/ml ; pH = 11
Cinchonidine	315	445	0.01 μg/ml ; pH = 1
Cinchonine	320	420	0.01 μg/ml : pH = 1
Epinephrine	295	335	0.07 μg/ml ; pH = 1
Folic acid	365	450	0.01 μg/ml ; pH = 1
Hydrocortisone	460	520	75% WN in H_2SO_4 ; is ethanol
LSD	325	465	0.02 μg/ml ; pH of is CNCL
Nicotinamide	250	430	"
Norepinephrine	295	335	0.06 at pH = 1
Pentorbarbitone	265	440	0.1 μg/ml; pH = 13
Procaine	275	345	0.01 μg/ml ; pH = 11
Procainamide	295	385	0.01 μg/ml ; pH = 11
Physostigmine	300	360	0.04 μg/ml ; pH = 1
Reserpine	300	375	0.008 μg/ml ; pH = 1
Terramycin	390	520	0.05 μg/ml ; pH = 11

Compounds Converted to Flourescent Products by Chemical Reaction

Compound	Method	Wave length (nm)	
		Excitation	Flourescence
Chlordiazepoxide	Formation of lactam	380	480
Chloroquine	Photochemical induction	-	-
Heroin	Heating with strong acid	-	-

Contd...

Compound	Method	Wave length (nm)	
		Excitation	Flourescence
Hydrocortisone	75% w/v of H2SO4 in ethanol	460	520
Isoniazid	Reaction with salicylaldehyde followed by reduction	-	-
Nicotinamide	Cyanogen bromide	250	430
Oxytetracycline	Complexation with Mg^{2+} and EDTA	-	-
Reserpine	Oxidation	-	-
Tetracycline	Conversion to anhydrous tetra cycline	-	-
Thiamine	Complexation with Aluminium	-	-
Imipramine	Reaction with formaldehyde & Acetyl acetone	-	-
Diphenyl hydantoin	Oxidation using $KMnO_4$ in alkaline condition to Benzophenone.	355	485
Methyldopa	Oxidation & alkali rearrangement to dihydroxyindole derivative	400	510

Flourescent Indicators

→ The intensity and colour of the fluorescence of many substances depends on pH of the solution. For this purpose we are using fluorescent indicators.

→ Mainly using in acid base titrations.

Indicator	pH Range	Colour change
Eosin	3.0 - 4.0	Colourless to green
Flourescein	4.0 - 6.0	Colourless to green
Quinine sulphate	3.0 - 5.0	Blue to violet
Acridine	5.2 - 6.6	Green to violet – blue
2-Naptha quinine	4.4 - 6.3	Blue to colourless
2-Hydroxy cinnamic acid	7.2 - 9.0	Colourless to green

Special Fluorimetric Analysis

1. Investigation of chemical structures & processes
    - Hydrogen bonding
    - Cis-trans isomerism
    - Polymerisation
    - Tautomerism
    - Rates of reactions

    e.g.

    Slow rate of reactions → recorder

    Fast rate of reactions → Cathode ray oscilloscope

    Free radicals → Spectrograph
2. Qualitative and Quantitative Chemical Analysis
    - Detection of impurity (Cyclohexane free from benzene bands at 2600 Å)
    - Estimation of single component – vitamin A at 3280 Å
    - Vitamin – A from liver oil
3. Estimation of fluorescent intensity by addition method in which fluorescent intensity is measured before and after the addition of a known amount of the pure substance being estimated.
4. Estimation of Rare Earth Terbium
    - Formation fluorescent complex with EDTA and SSA (sulphosalicylic acid) at λ max = 3200 Å.

CHAPTER 12

NEPHELOMETRY AND TURBIDIMETRY

Introduction

Naturally any compound, irrespective of its origin, can be normally analysed by Qualitative and Quantitative analysis. Qualitative and Quantitative analysis respectively tell us about what species are present and in which concentrations they are present.

For choosing an analytical technique five important concepts we need to appreciate are :

1. Range
2. Sensitivity
3. Accuracy
4. Reproducibility
5. Interference

In order to fulfill the objective of Analysis of any compound, the above concepts should be considered. They will depend on the target compound characteristics and nature. Depending on these characteristics, we have to select and appropriate analytical method to achieve objective.

If we want to analyse suspensions and like compounds, we have to consider the characteristics of suspended particles. These particles are having refractive index different from that of the medium. When light is passed through moderately stable suspensions, a portion of the incident radiant energy is dissipated by virtue of the absorption, refraction, and reflection whereas the remaining portion gets transmitted. When suspension is viewed at 90° (i.e., right angles) to the direction of the incident light, the system appears opalescent on account of the reflections of light from the particle of the suspension. This scattering of light is termed as Tyndall effect.

Depending on the properties of suspended particles, the light may be scattered or unscattered when passed through the turbid solution. Based on either scattered light (or) unscattered light measurement of a turbid solution, two techniques are available.

1. Nephelometry
2. Turbidimetry

Nephelometry

It is defined as the measurement of light scattered by a particulate solution (suspended particles) of concentration less than 100 mg/L.

Turbidimetry

It is defined as the measurement of the reduction of light transmitted due to suspended particles in solution of concentration more than 100 mg/L.

These two methods are dependent either directly or indirectly on the 'turbidity'. So before knowing the above methods, we have to study the theory of turbidity.

Theory of Turbidity

Suspension of particles in water interfering with passage of light is called turbidity.

- Turbidity is caused by wide variety of suspended matter which range in size from colloidal to coarse dispersions depending upon the degree of turbulence and also ranges from pure inorganic substances to those that are highly organic in nature.
- Turbid waters are undesirable from aesthetic point of view in drinking water supplies and may also affect products in industries. Turbidity is measured evaluate the performance of water treatment plant.
- Turbidity can be measured either by its effect on the transmission of light which is termed as "Turbidimetry" or by its effect on the scattering of light, called as "Nephelometry'.

In short turbidimetry is the measurement of the degree of attenuation of a radiant beam incident beam incident on particles suspended in a medium, the measurement being made in the directly transmitted beam.

$$\therefore \quad \text{Turbidity (T)} = \frac{1}{\lambda} . \lambda n \frac{I_0}{t}$$

λ – Length of dispersion through which the light passes

I_0 – Intensity of incident light

I_t – Intensity of transmitted light

n – Refractive index of the dispersion medium

The International pharmacopoeia describes Turbidance (S) as – 'a measure of the light-scattering effect of suspended particles; and turbidity (V) as – 'a measure of the decrease in incident beam intensity per unit length of a given suspension:

Acidic water is normally crystal clear, while basic/neutral water is turbid. The reason is that the oxides, hydroxides and carbonates of heavy metal ions found in basic conditions are insoluble substances, while the nitrates, chlorides and sulphates of the same metal ions present under acidic conditions are soluble.

Further, acidic conditions are toxic to algae and other organisms, which can survive in very basic pH waters creating turbidity.

Environmental Significance of Turbidity in Public Water Supplies

***Aesthetics*:** Turbidity in drinking water is automatically associated with possible waste water pollution and the associated health hazards.

***Filterability*:** Satisfactory operations of rapid sand filters generally depend on effective removal of turbidity by chemical coagulation before the water is admitted on the filters.

***Disinfection*:** Turbidity caused by municipal waste water solids encases the pathogenic organisms in particles and protects from disinfection.

EPA Limit in Public Water Supplies (EPA-Environment Pollution Audit)

Between 0.5-1.0 units (1 mg SiO_2/L = 1 unit) of turbidity, depending upon the treatment process used.

Techniques for Measuring Turbidity

Turbidity and Nephelometry involve the measurement of the amount of radiation that passes through the sample in the forward direction (turbidimetry) or the amount of radiation scattered (Nephelometry).

Principle

Nephelometry

- At low concentrations of a suspension, there is uniform scattering. Hence the intensity of scattered light is proportional to the concentration. The intensity of scattered light is normally measured at 90°, 45°, 60°, 135° etc.
- The intensity of the scattered light can also be measured directly in order to gain sensitivity. The direction of incident light as a function of the concentration of the dispersed phase.
- It is based upon the measurement of the power of scattered light at right angles to a collimated beam.

- It should be noted that in nephelometry, the intensity of the scattered light is measured, usually, but not necessarily, at right angles to the incident light beam.
- The intensity of scattered light can be approximately related to the concentration of suspended particles.
- These methods are applicable to colourless, opaque suspensions that do not show selective absorption.
- In practice, light scattered at right angle s to the incident beam is plotted against concentration. Light scattering intensity units have been used for some nephelometric methods in clinical chemistry laboratories. These units relate to standardised suspensions of polystyrene latex particles which are used to calibrate the instrument.

Tubidimetry

- At high concentrations of a suspension, scattering is not uniform and light is scattered in all directions. Hence the intensity of transmitted light is measured at 180°.
- Here intensity of transmitted light is inversely proportional to concentration.
- In turbidimetry, consideration must be given to the question of colour of the final solution. If the solvent and dispersed particles are both free colour, then a wavelength in the blue or near ultraviolet should be selected for maximum sensitivity. If colour is present, a coloured filter must be used. If a blue filter is used with a red solution, a certain amount of the light will be absorbed resulting in false measurement.

This method is best suited for the determination of relatively high concentrations of suspended particles ranging from 0.05 to 0.5 mg/100 mL. Under favourable conditions, the low end and be extended from 0.02 mg/100 mL and high end upto 2 mg/100mL.

S.No.	Nephelometry	S.No.	Turbidimetry
1.	It is the measurement of scattered light.	1.	It is the measurement of unscattered light.
2.	Requires a special measuring instrument, where the detector is set at an angle to the incident light beam	2.	Requires instruments such as photometers (or) colorimeters.
3.	Sensitivity depends on absence of background light (or) scatter.	3.	Sensitivity depends on sensitivity of machine employed (From simple spectrophotometer to a sophisticated disctete analysis).

Contd...

S.No.	Nephelometry	S.No.	Turbidimetry
4.	Used at low concentrations of a suspension.	4.	Used at high concentrations of a suspension.
5.	Scattering is uniform	5.	Scattering is not uniform
6.	Intensity of scattered light is proportional to the concentration.	6.	Intensity of transmitted light is inversely proportional to the concentration.
7.	Intensity of scattered light is measured at 90°, 45°, 60°, 135° etc.	7.	Intensity of transmitted light is measured at 180°.
8.	Resultant scattered light is measured using a photo detector.	8.	Consideration must be given to the questions of colour of the final solution.
9.	Proportionality constant is related to the concentration of suspended paticles.	9.	Proportionality constant depends upon – Particle size and shape – λ of incident light – Refractive index of both medium and particle
10.	Detection limit is appx. 10 g/mL.	10.	Detection limit is approx. 20-30 μg/mL.
11.	Better detection limit in case of lipeamic sample of purer media like CSF when compared to turbidimetry	11.	Lesser detection capacity than nephelometry in several views.

Comparison between Colorimetry and Turbidimetry

	Colorimetry	Turbidimetry
Similarly	1. Intensity of transmitted light is measured (It) 2. 'It' is measured at 180°.	1. Intensity of transmitted light (It) is measured. 2. 'It' is measured at 180°.
Difference	The decrease in intensity of incident light is due to absorption of radiation.	The decrease in intensity of incident light is due to scattering of radiation.

Comparison between Flourimetry and Nephelometry

	Flourimetry	Nephelometry
Similarly	Intensity of emergent radiation is measured at 90°.	Intensity of emergent radiation is measured at 90°.
Difference	1. Intensity of emergent radiation is measured. 2. Emitted radiation has longer wavelength than incident light.	1. Intensity of scattered radiation is measured. 2. Scattered light has same wavelength as that of incident light.

Choice of Method

Choice of method, viz. Nephelometry or Turbidimetry depends on the concentration of suspension and amount of light scattered.

Nephelometry as the Choice

When the concentration of suspension is less, scattering of light is less and hence can be accurately measured at 90° or any convenient angle. This makes Nephelometry as the choice in low concentrated suspensions.

Turbidimetry as the Choice

When the concentration of suspension is more, since scattering is also more, only transmitted light (unscattered light) can be measured at 180°. This makes Turbidimetry as the choice of method in high concentrated suspensions.

Precautions

To make measurements reproducible it is important that the particle size in maintained constant. Therefore the following items are considered strictly.

1. The relative concentration of ingredients must be controlled.
2. The relative ratios of reactants must be constant.
3. The manner, order of addition and rate of mixing must be constant.
4. The nature of other solutions present must be considered and, if necessary, protective colloids added to avoid protein precipitation.
5. The temperature must be maintained constant.
6. Constant time lapse before reading.
7. Extremely dilute suspensions of bacterial cells may be employed to encounter the problems caused due to biorefrigeration.

Factors Responsible for Producing Uniform Turbidity

For Nephelometric or turbidimetric measurements, it is important to have uniform turbidity of suspension, otherwise accuracy may not be obtained. Hence to produce uniform turbidity, the following factors must be considered.

1. The manner, order and rate of mixing substances.
2. Agitation of suspension.
3. Temperature (affects solubility and viscosity of substance).

4. Presence or absence of inert electrolytes, salts, protective colloids like gelatin, acacia, dextrin etc. which affects flocculation and deflocculation.
5. Concentrations of solutions mixed to get a suspension.

Factors Responsible For Intensity of Scattered Radiation

The following factors affect the intensity of scattered radiations, appearing at any angle.

1. Number of suspended particles (concentration).
2. Size and shape of particles (the size should be equal to or greater than the wavelength of incident light).
3. Wavelength of radiation used; it should be selected in such a way there is no absorption, but only scattering.
4. Difference in the refractive index of particles and the medium.

Effect of Concentration and Wavelength on Scattering

Concentration

The intensity of transmitted light is expressed using an equation similar to that of Beer-Lambert's law, i.e.

$$P = P_0 . e^{-Tb}$$

where $P \rightarrow$ Power of transmitted beam

$P_0 \rightarrow$ Power of incident beam

$T \rightarrow$ Turbidity or turbidity coefficient

$b \rightarrow$ Path length

$$\therefore \qquad Tb = \log \frac{P_0}{P}$$

'T' was found to be proportional to the concentration (c) of suspended particles.

Hence, as $$T = K_c,\ K_{cb} = \log . \frac{P_0}{P}$$

Wavelength

The expression will be as follows

$$T = \frac{S}{\lambda_t}$$

T → Turbidity

S → Constant for a given system

λ → Wavelength

t → Depends on size of particles and is 'u' when particle size is smaller than wavelength

Limitations of Nephelometry and Turbidimetry

1. Their object is mostly towards suspension materials.
2. Choice of method is some what difficult.
3. So many factors will be considered.
4. Calibration of instruments will decide accuracy and sensitivity.

Instrumentation

Nephelometric and Tubidimetric measurements may be made with a fairly reasonable accuracy precision by using either standard instruments available commercially or by improving other similar devices.

For measuring the accurate results of Nephelometry and Turbidimetry there are many instruments available with genuine as well as slight modifications of colorimeter or flourimeter. Whatever be the design of instruments, the following components are used for their construction.

1. Source of light
2. Filters and Monochromators
3. Sample cells
4. Detectors

Source of Light

It is must for any spectroscopic analytical method which gives adequate intensity of radiation. In order to fulfill the objective of a source of light, it should follow some characteristics as follows:

1. It should provide continuous radiation.
2. It should provide adequate intensity.
3. It should be stable and free from fluctuations.

Normally for Nephelometry and Turbidimetry the following types of light sources are used:

(a) Tungsten lamp.

(b) Mercury lamp.

Tungsten Lamp

It is used when a polychromatic light is used. The lamp finds its place in most of colorimeter and spectrophotometer. The lamp consists of a tungsten filament in a vacuum bulb similar to the ones used domestically but it offers sufficient intensity.

Mercury Arc Lamp

Mercury arc lamp is used when a monochromatic light is used. This is used to avoid any light absorption, since we require only scattering of light.

Filters and Monochromators

- When light or polychromatic light is used, filters and monochromators are not required.
- When monochromatic light is required, then only filters and monochromatrors are used.

Filters

For Turbidimeter → Blue filter or 530 nm.

For Nephelometer→ Visible filter as secondary filter.

Description of various types of filters:

Basically filters are two kinds:

1. Absorption filters
2. Interference filters

1. Absorption filters

These are made up of glass, coated with pigments or by dyed gelatine. They absorb the unwanted radiation and transmit the rest of the radiation which is required.

We can select the required filter in a colorimeter, based upon the colour of the solution.

Merits

1. Simple in construction
2. Cheaper
3. Selection of filter is easy.

Demerits

1. Less accurate since band pass is more ($\pm$ 30 nm)
2. Intensity of radiation becomes less due to absorption by filters.

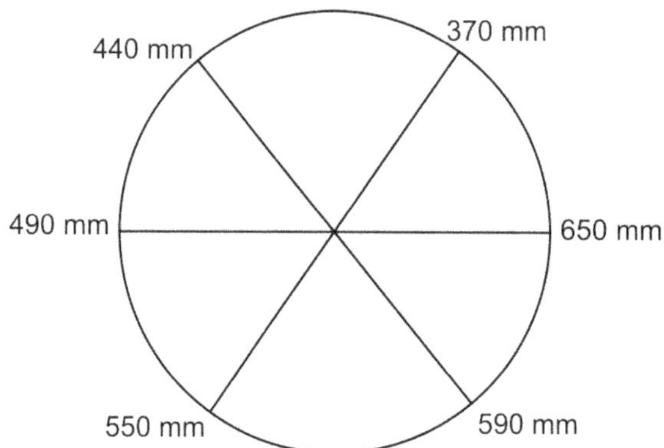

2. Interference Filters : (Fabry-Perot Filter)

- It has dielectric spacer film made up of CaF_2, MgF_2 or SiO between two parallel reflecting silver films.
- The thickness of dielectric spacer film can be ½ λ (1-order), 2λ / 2 (2-order), 3λ / 2 (3-order) etc.
- Band pass is 10-15 nm.
- Maximum transmission is 40%.

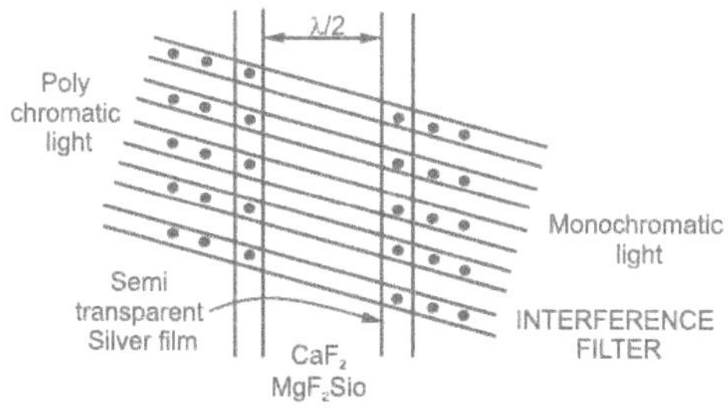

Mechanism: The radiation reflected by the 2nd film and the incoming radiation undergoes constructive interference to give a monochromatic radiation,

which is governed by following equation

$$\lambda = \frac{2\eta b}{m}$$

λ → Wavelength of light obtained

η → Dielectric constant of layer material

b → Layer thickness

m → Order no. (0, 1, 2, 3, etc.)

Merits

1. Inexpensive
2. Lower band pass when compared to absorption filters and hence more accurate.
3. Use of additional filter cuts off undesired wavelengths.

Demerits

1. Peak transmission is low, and becomes so when additional filters are used to cut off undesired wavelength.
2. The band pass is only 10-15 nm and hence greater resolution obtained with monochromators or gratings cannot be achieved.

Monochromators

These are more efficient than filters in converting a polychromatic light or heterochromatic light into monochromatic light.

Naturally monochromator has the following units :

1. Entrance slit → To get narrow source
2. Collimator → To render narrow parallel
3. Granting or prism → To disperse radiation
4. Collimator → To reform the images to entrance slit
5. Exit slit → To fall on sample cell

Types

1. Prisms
   (a) Refractive type
   (b) Reflective type (Littrow type mounting)
2. Gratings
   (a) Diffraction grating
   (b) Transmission grating

Prisms

- They disperse the light radiation into individual colours or wavelengths.
- Used in inexpensive instruments.
- Band pass is lower than that of filters which results better resolution. Resolution depends upon the size and refractive index.
- Material of the prism is normally glass.

(a) Refractive Type Prisms

- Here the source of light, through entrance slit falls on acollimator.

- Parallel radiations from collimator are dispersed into different colours or wavelengths.
- By using another collimator, the images of entrance slit are reformed. The reformed ones will be either violet, indigo, blue, green, yellow, orange or red.
- The required radiations on exit slit can be detected by rotating the prism or by keeping the prism stationary and moving the exit slit.

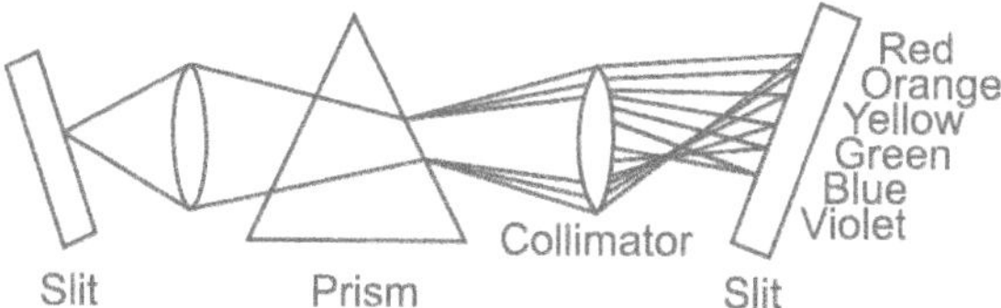

(b) Reflective Type Prism

Principle of working is similar to that of refractive type except that, a reflective surface is present on one side of the prism. Hence the dispersed radiation gets reflected and can be collected on the same side on the source of light.

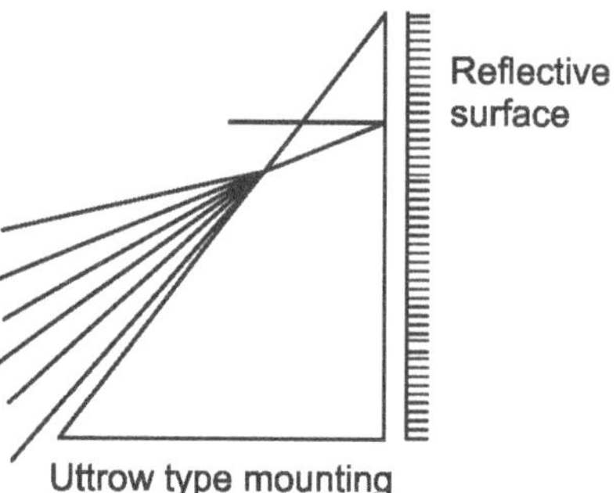

Gratings

- More efficient ones in converting a polychromatic to monochromatic light.
- As a resolution of $\pm$ 0.1 nm could be achieved by using gratings, commonly used in spectrophotometers.

(a) Diffraction Gratings

- Gratings are nothing but ruling made on some material like glass, quartz or alkyl halides depending on the instrument (visible/UV/IR Spectrophotometer)

Instrument		*Ruling*
IR Spectrophotometer	→	20 grooved/mm
UV/visible	→	3600 grooved-more/mm

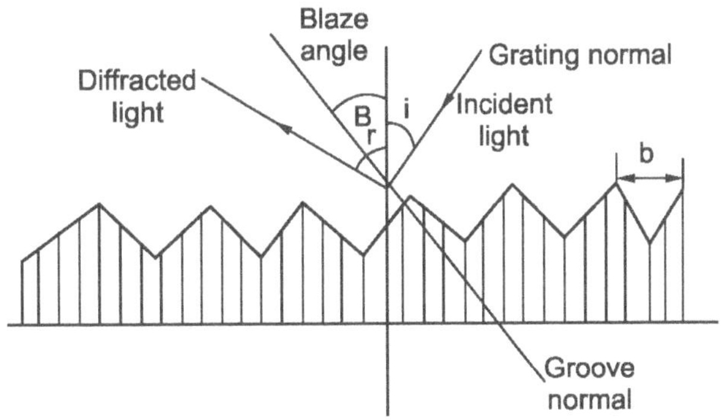

Diffraction Grating

- These gratings are replica made from master grating by coating the original master grating with epoxy resin and are removed after setting.

***Mechanism*:** Diffraction produces reinforcement. The rays which are incident upon the grating gets reinforced with the reflected rays and hence the resulting radiation has wavelength which is governed by the equation.

$$m\lambda = b\,(\sin i \pm \sin r)$$

$\lambda \rightarrow$ Wavelength of light produced

b $\rightarrow$ Grating spacing

i $\rightarrow$ Angle of incidence

r $\rightarrow$ Angle of reflection

m $\rightarrow$ Order (0, 1, 2, 3 etc).

The band pass of these gratings are $\pm$ 0.1 nm, which means they are most efficient and hence gratings are preferred.

(b) Transmission Grating

Here instead of reflection, refraction takes place. Refraction produces reinforcement. This occurs when radiation transmitted through grating reinforces with the partially refracted radiation.

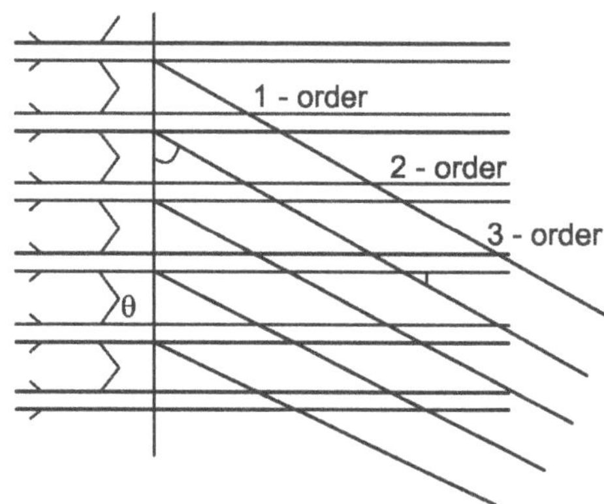

The wavelength of radiation produced by transmission grating can be expressed by following equation.

$$\lambda = \frac{d \sin \theta}{m}$$

λ → Wavelength of radiation produced

d → 1/lines per cm

m → Order (0, 1, 2, 3 etc).

θ → Angle of deflection/diffraction

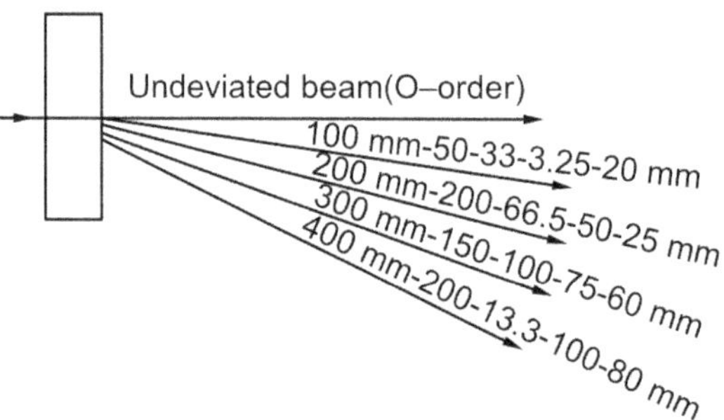

Thus a light radiation at any angle (θ) or any order can be collected and used in the instrument either by moving the grating and fixing the slit or moving the slit and keeping the grating constant.

Sample Cells

Various shapes of sample cells are used in Nephelometry and Turbidimetry.

Cylindrical – like ordinary small test tube with 1 cm path length

Rectangular – cell walls may be coated with black to avoid any reflection that may affect detector response.

Special cells– To measure scattered light at different angles like 15°, 90°, 135° and 180°. These cells are made up of glass.

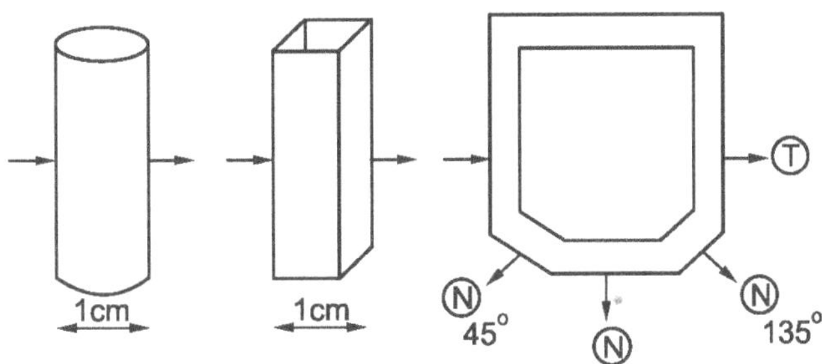

Detectors

Turbidimeters – Photovoltaic cells phototubes

Nephelometer – Photomultiplier tubes (Scattered radiation is weak)

Photovoltaic Cell (Barrier Layer Cell)

Advantages

- Cheaper and used in inexpensive instruments.
- Useful for colorimeters, flourimeters and Nepheloturbidimeters.

Disadvantages

- Amplification of the signal is not possible.
- The resistance of the external circuit has to below,
- Fatigue effects and the lesser response of the detector with light other than blue and red.

***Construction*:** The detector has a thin metallic layer coated with silver or gold and acts as electrode. It also has a metal base plate which acts as another electrode. These two layers are separated by a semiconductor layer is selenium. Selenium has an extremely low electrical conductivity and hence the electrons are not mobile.

***Working*:** When light radiation falls on the selenium layer, these electrons become mobile and are taken by the transparent metal layer. This creates a potential difference between the two electrodes and causes flow of current causes deflection of the galvanometer needle, which depends on the wavelength and intensity of radiation. The sensitivity of the instrument is similar to that of human eye.

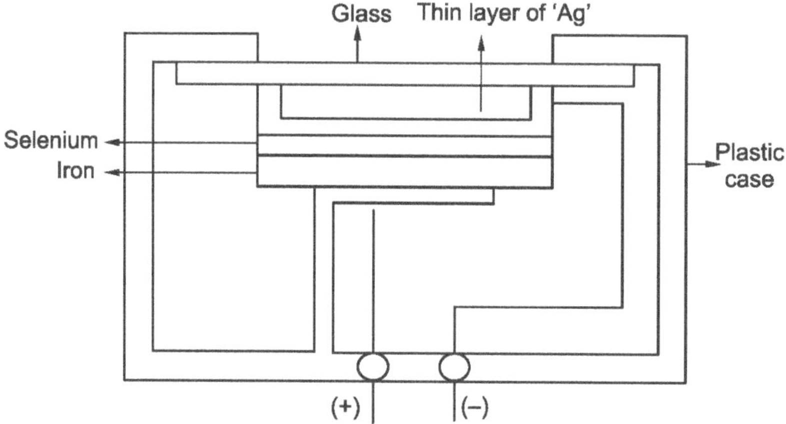

Photo Tubes (Photo Emissive Cells)

- They have better sensitivity when compared to photo voltaic cell and hence more widely used.

Construction: This detector is composed of an evacuated glass tube, which consists of a photocathode and a collector anode. The photocathode is coated with elements of high atomic volume like caesium, potassium or silver oxide.

Working

- Photocathode can liberate electrons, which flow towards anode producing a current proportional to the intensity of light radiation.
- Composite coatings like caesium / caesium oxide / silver oxide can also be used, which increase the sensitivity and range of wavelength in which the detector can be used.
- Signal from the detector can also be amplified using an amplifier circuit.

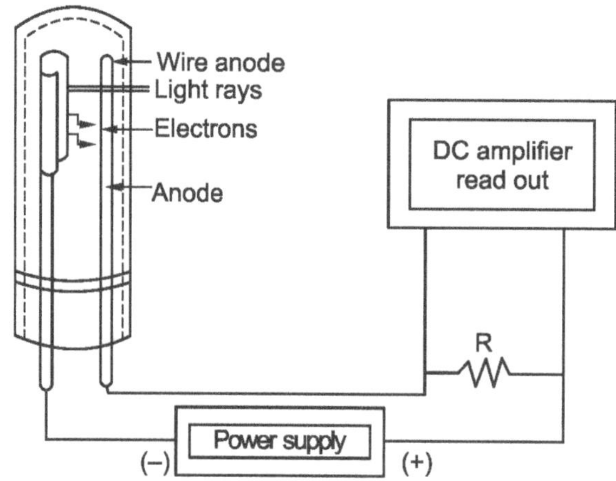

Photo Multiplier Tubes (PMT)

Advantages

- Most sensitive of all the detectors.
- Used in sophisticates instruments.

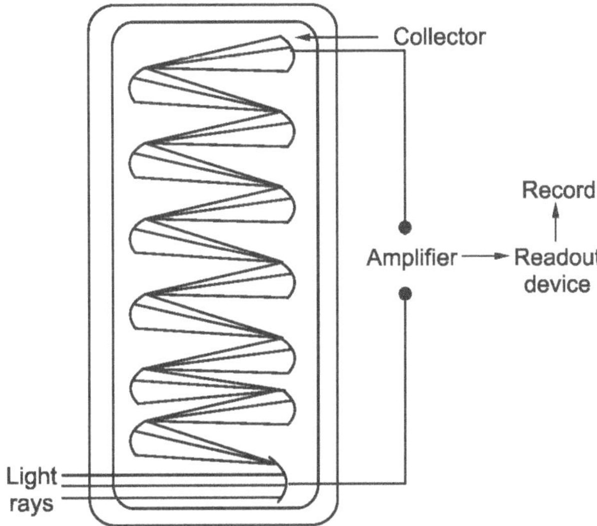

- It can detect very weak signals (200 times weaker are also detected when compared to photovoltaic cell).
- Useful in flourescence measurements.

Working: The principle employed in this detector is the multiplication of photoelectrons by secondary emission of electrons.

This is achieved by using a photo cathode and a series of anodes (Dyanodes). Upto 10 dyanodes are used.

Each dyanode is maintained at 75-100V higher than the preceding one. At each stage, the electrons' emission is multiplied by a factor of 4 or 5 due to secondary emission of electrons and hence an overall factor of 10^6 is achieved. PMT should be shielded from stray light in order to have accurate results.

Instruments: Several instruments have been designed for turbidimetry and Nephelometry and many Colorimeters and Spectrophotometers may also be used this purpose.

1. Nephelometers
2. Turbidimeters
3. Nephlotubidimeters

Nephlometers

These instruments are used for the nephelometry measurements. The advantages of these type are as follows.

Advantages

- Simple
- Inexpensive
- Easy to operate
- Has reasonable precision and accuracy

The most important characteristic feature of a Nepholometer is the 'reflector' that has been specifically designed so as to collect the light which has undergone scattering by the particles present in a turbid or cloudy solution.

Construction: It consists of a tungsten lamp as source of light and the sample cell (flat bottom) is placed on top of source. Light passing through filter falls on suspended particles. These particles scatter the light. The light scattered by the particles are collected by curved mirror and reflected to the photovoltaic cell, kept at bottom of the instrument. These instruments have provisions for setting the illumination at right angles to the direction of observation.

Working: The test solution is placed in a test tube (F) that has been duly nested on a light source as exhibited in figure.

The scattered light caused by the particles in a turbid or cloudy solution is immediately directed by the reflector (E) on to an annular photo cell.

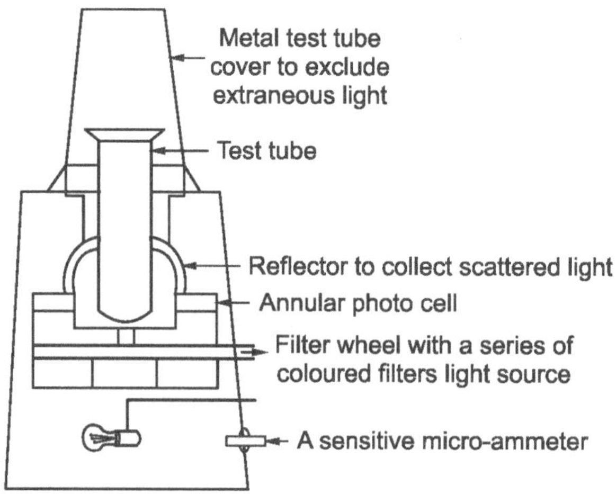

A series of standard colour filters are usually provided in the form of a filter where so as to facilitate analysis of coloured solutions; taking care that the filter chosen must be similar in colour to that of the solution.

The current passed through the photocell (i.e. light energy is being converted to electrical energy) is recorded by a sensitive micro ammeter.

The test tube is provided with a metallic cover to get rid of any extraneous light. Usually a Nephlometer is provided with zero-setting controls sensitivity adjusting device and a set previously matched test tubes.

Duboscq Colorimeter

A Duboscq colorimeter with a slight modification may be used as nephelometer: For instance:

1. The path of light should be arranged in such a fashion that the light enters the side of the cups at right angles to the plungers rather than through bottom.
2. Clear glass tube with opaque bottoms are to be used instead of the normal cups.
3. The glass plungers are precisely filted with opaque sleeves.
4. The light that enters at right angles to the clear glass tubes should be monitored carefully so as to achieve an equal-illumination on either sides.

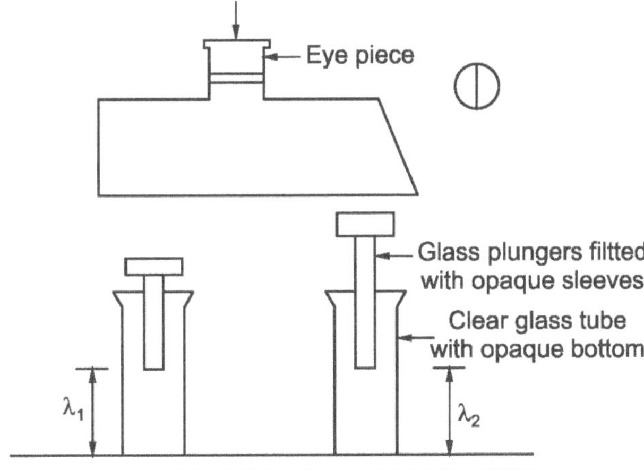

Working: A standard suspension is placed in one clear glass-tube and the unknown solution is treated exactly in an identical fashion and placed in the other clear galss-tube. Finally the dividing line existing between two folds in the eye-piece must be distinct and sharp, and it must disappear when the two folds are matched properly.

Subsequently, set the unknown solution at a scale reading of 10.0 mm and simultaneously adjust the standard until the fields are matched equally. Perform at least five similar adjustments with the celar-glass-tube containing the standard solution, and calculate the mean value.

***Principle*:** Assuming Beer's law holds good, the concentration of the solution in question (unknown) may be determined by following expression:

$$\underset{\text{(known)}}{C_1\lambda_1} = \underset{\text{(unknown)}}{C_2\lambda_2}$$

C_1 = Concentration of known solution

C_2 = Concentration of unknown solution

λ_1 = Average readings for the clear glass-tube having the solution of known calculations.

λ_2 = Average readings for the clear glass-tube having the solution of unknown calculations.

It may, however, be observed that if $\lambda_2 = 10$, the standard scale when multiplied by 10 shall give the percentage concentration of the sample in terms of the standard.

Precautions

- To ensure that the readings are zero when the plungers just touch the bottoms of the clear glass-tubes.
- Equal volume of known and unknown solutions are placed in clear glass-tubes; bearing in mind the fact that the clear glass-tubes should never be filled above their respective shoulders.
- Care must be taken that the plungers always remain below the surface of the liquid, it is advised to visualise the match-point from above and below.

Flourimeter

A flourimeter can also be converted to a Nephelometer by using a visible filter as secondary filter as given in the diagram

1. Fisher Neflurophotometer
2. Coleman Universal Spectrophotometer

These may be used for measurement of scattered radiation in nephelometry.

One may use white light in photometer, but it is desirable to use monochromatic radiation. Similarly, monochromatic radiation is used in turbidimeters to reduce absorption.

A mercury arc or a laser with appropriate filter concentration for isolating one of its emission lines is the most convenient source of radiation.

A polychromatic source, such as tungsten lamp is useful, if one has to determine the concentration of a particular material.

In Nephelometer, photomultiplier tube should be used as a detector, because of the fact that the intensity of scattered radiation is usually very small.

For sampling, cylindrical cells are used but rectangular cells are usually preferred.

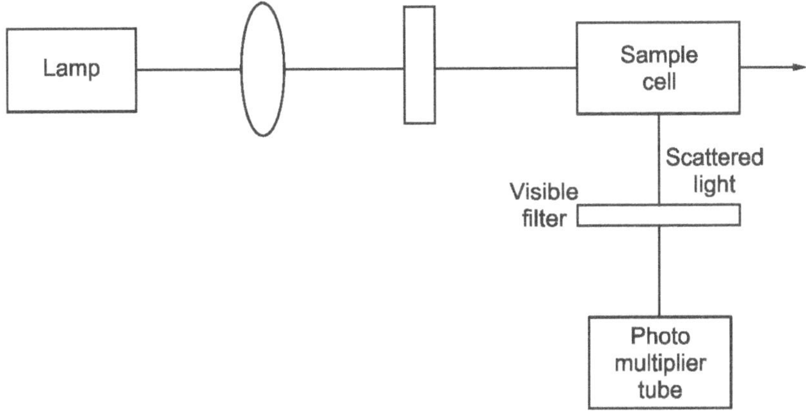

Flourimeter Converted to Nephelometer by using Secondary Filter as Visible Filter

Photo Electric Nephelometer

Optical and electrical system on a photoelectric Nephelometer are same as in photoelectric colorimeters except that the photo cell in photo electric nephelometer is situated on one side of the cuvette.

Turbidimeters

***Simple Turbidimeter*:** The viewing tube is adjusted in the suspension until the special S-shaped lamp filament just disappears.

Measurement is then made of the length of the turbid solution necessary to extinguish the image of the lamp filament. The length of the solution is then related to the concentration by calibration. This turbidimeter gives accurate results for the analysis of sulphate at low concentration. Here $BaSO_4$ suspension is formed by the addition of $BaCl_2$.

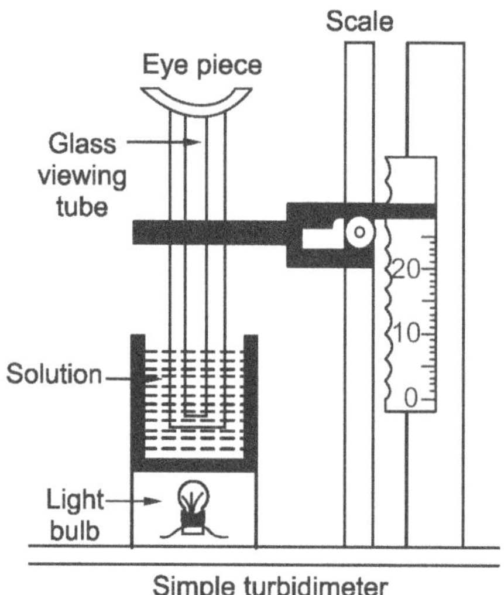

Simple turbidimeter

Parr Turbidimeter: The parr turbidimeter is a special type of instrument which consists of a cylinder to contain the turbid suspension, a lamp filament of fixed intensity of the base and an adjustable plunger through which visual observation is made. The depth of the turbid solution necessary to extinguish the image of the lamp filter filament is measured. A calibration curve is prepared using standard suspension. The curve is a plot of depth versus concentration.

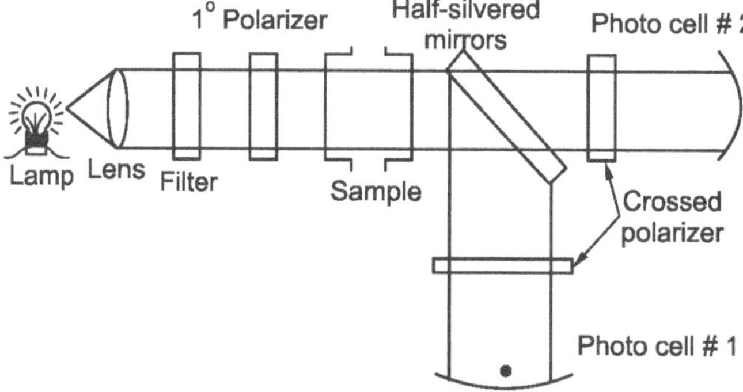

Simple Diagram of Dupont Model 430 Turbidimeter

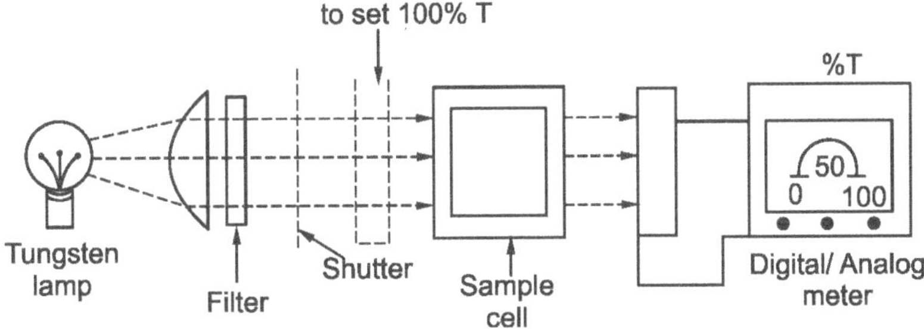

Turbidimeter (Use Blue Filter to Set at 530 nm in a Single Beam Colorimeter)

Colorimeter: A colorimeter can be used as Turbidimeter by selecting 530nm or by using blue filter. Here the filter is monochromatic and photoelectric detector may be used both for the nephelometric and tubidimetric analysis. This instrument may be used for viewing either at right angles to or in direct line with the incident light.

Nepheloturbidimeter

If a suspension has to be analysed, it is important to know whether it can be analysed by nephelometry and turbidimetry. But in practice, it is not essential to know this, because recent instruments are a combination of the above two.

These Nephlo-turbidimeters have the design as shown in figure. They have two detectors, one for measuring the scattered light at 90° and the other at 180° for measuring the transmitted light. The ratio of the two detectors is displayed as Nepheloturbidimetric units (NTU) which is proportional to the turbidity of the suspension.

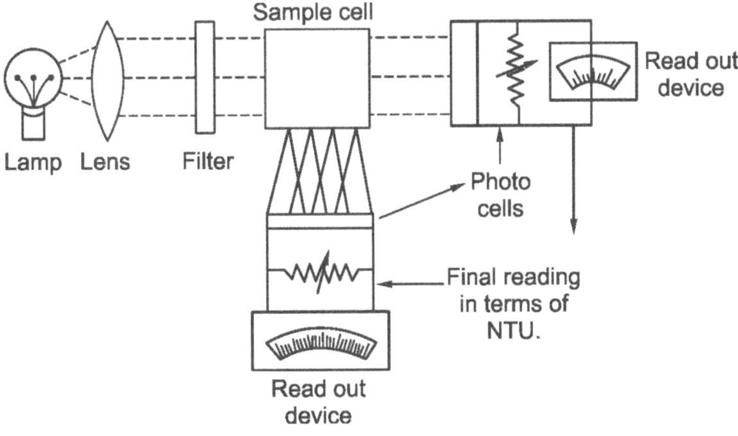

Nepheloturbidimeter

Nepheloturbidimetric Analysis

To know the correct method of Nephelotubidimetric analysis, the following concepts should be considered.

1. Why Analysis is conducted
2. Analysis-correct sampling
3. Analysis of metal finishing baths
4. Planning our Analysis strategy
5. Principal stages
6. Representing our data

Analysis-Why?

Metal finishing process baths, including electroplating solutions, electrolysis plating baths, conversion coating solutions, anodising baths, cleaners and degreasing solutions, not forgetting rinse baths-all perform optimally only when their chemical composition lies within set limits. So to determine whether they are within limits or not by using specific methods, Analysis of compounds is done.

For choosing an Analytical Technique, important concepts we need to appreciate, are;

1. Range
2. Sensitivity
3. Accuracy
4. Reproducibility
5. Interference

1. ***Range***: An analytical method will only give good results within a certain concentration range. If the sample is too concentrated, we can easily dilute by known amount. If the sample is too dilute, it can be concentrated.
2. ***Sensitivity***: The lowest concentration at which the analytical method gives satisfactory results. Thus the lower end of the range limit.
3. ***Accuracy***: Also referred as resolution. Is the answer 33 × 33.4 × 33.47 × grams/litre? Could the method distinguish between two solutions of concentration 33.4 and 33.5 gm/litre? Don't be deceived by an instrument with lots of numbers digitally displayed. The digital display has to show something but the last digits could be quite meaningless.
4. ***Reproducibility***: If we try to analyse, the same solution at different period, will be method give us the same answer? This takes into questions concerning calibrations and standards which we won't discuss.

5. ***Interferences*:** You might wish, for example, to analyse cadmium. But may be there can also be zinc present in the same solution, the method would not distinguish between them. So rather than giving the cadmium concentration, it would give you (cadmium) and (zinc) which is a wrong answer. Sometimes we will be told that a method is vulnerable in this way. At times, we'll have to use our instinct and judgement, over a few tests to see if there is a problem.

Analysis-Correct Sampling

We need to know the chemical composition of our process solutions. How? We need to take a sample from the solution in the bath, and analyse it, using, usually, a chemical analysis method, but some times a physical method too.

1. Sampling is not a clinch.
2. Look after your sample.

***Sampling is not a Clinch*:** We have to think carefully about how to take a meaningful sample. The composition of a bath may differ from top to bottom of a tank, or as between inlet and outlet. The concentration may differ when the bath works and when it is idle. They may be zoned in the baths especially if it is not thoroughly stirred, which are more or less dilute than the rest of the baths. Chemical and electrochemical reactions take place at or around the anodes and the cathode sampling too close to these could give the wrong answer.

***Look after your Sample*:** Try and carryout your analysis as soon as possible after sampling. Don't let your sample become heated or be exposed to direct sunlight, before analysis. In some cases (Hydroflouric acid) don't forget that the solution can react with the container (when this is made of glass) and this will certainly result in a false result. Don't forget to label each sample like when and where it was taken, may be who took it. Use a label which won't wash off by mistake.

Analysis of Metal Finishing Baths

This permits the compound lies within set limits. The performance of a plating plant is to be optimised; some parameters which have to be maintained are:

- Too concentrated
- Too dilute
- Incorrect pH
- Too high a concentration of impurities
- Surrounding environment

***Bath too Concentrated*:** If the bath contains excessive concentrations of acids, alkalies, buffers, the main reagents (metal ions, cations), organic or inorganic additives, the consequences could be as follows:

1. Defective work
2. Too many rejects increase production costs.
3. Chemical costs
4. Greater will be the rate at which organic compounds will break down, in solution or at the anode (cathode).
5. Additional load on the effluent treatment plant.

Bath too Dilute

1. Defective work
2. Wasted energy
3. If the electrical conductivity is too low, cell voltage will be high.
4. Waste of electrical energy
5. Problems with excessive bath heating.

Planning Our Analysis Strategy

First of all, we have to decide what we are going to look for. Our first task will be to determine the concentrations of all known bath constituents, as set out by the supplier. Looking for impurities contaminating species is more difficult because in many cases, we have to take a guess at what the contaminant might be. So one approach is to start using qualitative analysis. If our plates or other components have an obvious defect, we could try another approach. In many cases, the defective nature of the finished surface can give you a clue to the type of impurity present.

Principal Stages

1. Sampling
2. Sample preparation
3. Evaluation of results
4. Calibration curves.

***Sampling*:** During initial step of Analysis, the sample portion should be chosen so that it is representative of the bulk material. Statistics is used to determine the sample size and the number of samples.

The Analyst should consider

- Detailed description of the information required.
- An estimate of the accuracy to be achieved.

- Estimate the amount of time and money that can be spent on sampling
- Samples must be multipled at varying locations with in the basic materials.

***Sample Preparation*:** After the sample has been collected; it may be necessary to chemically or physically treat at the sampling site. The nature of treatments is dependent on the sample and the substance for which it is being analysed.

- Sealing the sample containers.
- Trace element samples, metallic pollutants are precipitated
- Metallic adsorption can be minimised by adding HNO_3.

***Evaluation of Results*:** After completion of assays, quantitative results are mathematically manipulated and both quantitative and quantitative results are presented in a meaningful manner.

Two values are reported for quantitative analysis.

I Value – Estimates the correct value for anlysis.

II Value – Estimates amount of random error in analysis.

Mean of the values (average) – Report.

Median – Central value when the results are arranged in order of size.

Mode – The value obtained most often.

Accuracy – Degree of agreement between experiment result and the true value.

Precision – Degree of agreement among a series of measurements of same quantity.

- Errors may be systematic (determinant) or random (indeterminant). The errors can be minimised but not eliminated.
- Statistics is used to estimate the random error that occurs during each step.
- The variance (V) is the source of the standard deviation and is useful in many cases.

Calibration Curves

- Signal depends on particle size and concentration, calibration curves are usually empirical.
- In turbidimetry, Beer's law is sometimes followed over only a limited range, but the addition of protective colloid (gum anlabic, gelatine) often stabilises the suspension and extends linear range.
- The reference suspension is one containing weighed 5g of hydrogen (2^+) sulphate and 50g of hexamethyl-enetetramine dissolved in IL of distilled water which is described 4000 nephelometric turbidity (NTU).

- After standing for 48 hrs, the insoluble polymer formatin formed from condensation polymerisation polymetric reaction, develops a white turbidity. The turbidity can be prepared repeatedly with accuracy $\pm$ 1%.
- Analytical standards can be prepared from the solution.

Applications

Applications of Nephelometry and turbidimetry are widely varied in analysis. They find numerous applications in water treatment in plant, in sewage work, in power and steam generating plant, in beverage bottling industry, in pulp and paper manufacturing, in petroleum refineries and in pharmaceutical industry.

1. ***Analysis of Water*:** For determination of clarity and for determining the concentration of various ions by adding selective precipitants, Nepheloturbidimetry is applied.
2. Light scattering methods are applicable to continuous on-stream analysis, including aerosol systems and solids suspended in liquids.
3. The growth of test bacteria in a liquid nutrient can be measured turbidimetrically.
4. ***Determination of CO_2*:** The sample of gas is passed through alkaline solution of Barium salt and then analysed for barium carbonate suspension with Nepheloturbidimetry.
5. Turbidimetry can be used for analysis of sugar products and clarity of citrus juices. Benzene in alcohol can also be determined by dilution with water to make an immiscible suspension.
6. They are applied for determining the end point in precipitation reactions by using chemical indicators.
7. Gaseous, liquid or even transparent solid samples especially when samples contain precipitates that are difficult to filter either because of small particle size or the particles that are gelatinous in nature.
8. Light scattering measurements are used to establish the concentration of smog, fog, smoke, and aerosols by using EPA method.
   - Test water is added to a tube until light from a standard could be at the bottom is extinguished.
   - The Nephelometers measure scattered light at 90o to incident light with a photodetector.
   - The readings are in Nephelometric Turbidity units (NTU's)
   - Samples are quantified versus standard of freshly prepared polymer (Hydrazine + hexamethylene, tetramine, 1:10 w/w in water, 25°C, 24 hrs.) or standard styrene divinyl benzene copolymer beads.

9. ***Quantitative Analysis of Ions (Even at ppm levels)***: This can be done by using calibration curve of standard substance. In this method, a series of standard solutions is prepared, treated with reagent to produce turbidity and NTO is measured using Nepheloturbidimeter. The sample solution is treated in the same ways as standard and from the calibration curve, the concentration of ion in the unknown solution can be determined.

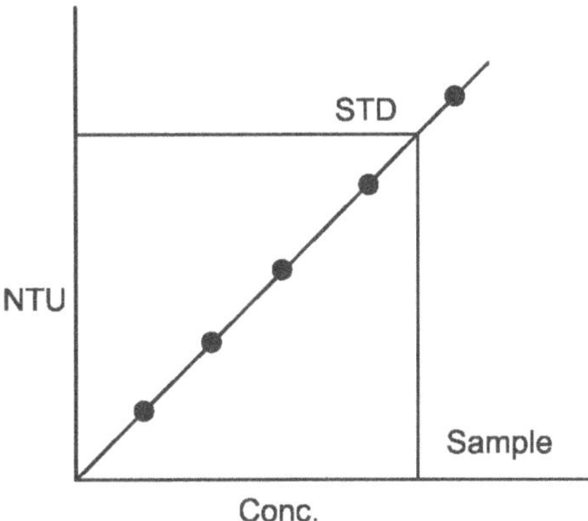

10. **Use of Nephelometry in Clinical Immunology**

A. Serum Immunoglobulins

- IgG, IgA, IgM, are widely available.
- Kappa and lambda light chains are also used.
- IgD, IgE concentration are too low for nephelometric detection.
- Abnormal immunoglobulins (myeloma)

B. Complement Components

C_3, C_4, C_3d, Factor B complement factors are detected as antigens, not functionally.

C. Acute Phase Reactant Protein

- C-reactive protein
- Haptoglobin
- Transtennin
- Ceruloplasmin

D. Cerebrospinal Fluid

Daily determinations of CSF IgG in multiple screlosis IgG index is often used.

E. **Rheumatoid Factor**

Immuno nepheloturbidimetric assay for the in vitro quantitative determination of rheumatoid factors in human serum and plasma.

11. ***Turbidimetric Titrations***: It is similar to spectro-photometric titrations. In this, NTU is monitored against the volume of titrant added. The titrant and titrate gives a product which is turbid. The end point of the titration can be known from the point of inflection on the graph.

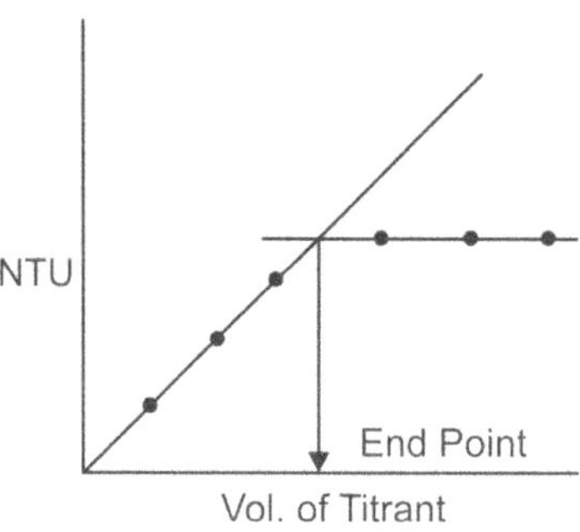

12. Determination of Inorganic Substances

Element	Method	Suspensions	Reagent	Interference
Ag	T, N	AgCl	NaCl	–
As	T	As	KH_2PO_2	Se, Te
Au	T	Au	$SnCl_2$	Ag, Hg, Pd, Pt, Ru, Se, Te
Ca	T	CaC_2O_4	$H_2C_2O_4$	Mg, Na, SO_4^{2-}
Cl^-	T, N	AgCl	$AgNO_3$	Br^-, I^-
K	T	$K_2NaCO(NO_2)_6$	$Na_3CO(NO_2)_6$	SO_4^{2-}
Na	T, N	$Na_2N(VO_2)_3(OCH_3COO)_9$	$Zn(OCH_3COO_2)_2$ $UO_2(OCH_3COO)_2$	Li
SO_4^{2-}	T, N	$BaSO_4$	$BaCl_2$	Pb
Se	T	Se	$SnCl_2$	Te
Te	T	Te	NaH_2PO_2	Se

N → Nephelometry, T → Turbidimetry

Others
- Carbonate as $BaCO_3$
- Chloride as AgCl

- Flouride as CaF_2
- Cyanide as AgCN
- Zinc as Ferrocyanide

Miscellaneous

- Biological oxygen demand
- Temperature
- Total dissolved solids (TDS)
- Chromium
- Manganese
- Copper
- Selenium
- Arsenic
- Mercury Ambient Air Analysis.
- Confirm hardness
- Conductivity
- Boron
- Nitrate
- Iron
- Aluminium
- Cyanide

Assay of Pharmaceutical Substances

(a) Turbidimetric Assay

No.	Antibiotic	Micro Organism	Medium pH	Phosphate Buffer pH	Potency of Solution v/ml	Incubation Temp (°C)
1.	Doxycycline	S. aureus	7.0	4.5	0.003-0.010	35-37
2.	Gentamycin	–do–	7.0	8.0	0.6-1.25	35-37
3.	Neomycin	Klebsiella	7.6	8.0	1.5-4	35-37
4.	Streptomycin	–do–	7.0	8.0	2.4-3.8	35-37
5.	Tobramycin	S. aureus	7.0	7.0	0.75-1.87	35-37

(b) Nephlometric Assay

- Assay sulphate Ion (SO_4^{2-})
- Assay of phosphate Ion (PO_4^{3-}) ……etc.

CHAPTER 13

ATOMIC ABSORPTION SPECTROSCOPY

Introduction

The characteristics of atomic particles are described using the Theorems of quantum mechanics.

Quantum mechanics–or quantum chemistry–describes the geometry of atoms and molecules in terms of complex mathematical models. It also describes the relative states of atomic matter. The atomic absorption spectrometer uses the principles of quantum chemistry to detect the presence of certain metals (i.e. iron, aluminium, copper etc.) and determines the concentration of these metals in samples.

It was introduced first time by a scientist called Walsh in 1950. It is one of the most powerful analytical tools for the qualitative determination of trace metals in liquids.

The technique provides the total metal content of the sample and is almost independent of the molecular from of the metal in the liquid.

The versatility (universal application) of this spectroscopy is form the fact that 60-70 elements including most of the common rare earth metals have been determined by this technique in concentration ranging from trace to micro quantities. By then these techniques, the determination can be made in the presence of bivalance elements. It means that it becomes unnecessary to separate the test elements from the other elements present in the sample and then taking time and in the process eliminates several forces of error. The technique is not restricted only to aqueous solution, but can be applied to nonaqeous solution as well.

The technique does not demand sample precipitate. Hence it is an ideal too for non-chemist (clinician) who is interested only in the significance of results.

Energy Transitions

All atoms and their components have energy. The energy level at which an atom exists is referred to as its state. Under normal conditions, atoms exist in their most stable states. We refer to that most stable level as the ground state. Although we cannot measure the precise energy state for an atom, we can usually measure changes to its energy relative to its ground states.

Certain processes can change the energy state for an atom. For example, adding Thermal energy (heat) can cause an atom to raise to a higher energy state. This change in energy is written as E. We refer to energy states which are higher than the ground state is excited states. In theory, there are infinite excited states, however there are decreasing numbers of atoms from a population that reach higher excited states.

The laws of quantum mechanics tell us that atoms do not increase their energy levels gradually. An atom goes directly from one state to another without going through intermediates. We refer to these "quantum leaps" as transitions. The transition from the ground state (E_o) to the first excited state (E_1) requires some from of energy input. This energy is adsorbed by the atom. That energy absorption is equal to $\Delta E_0 \rightarrow 1$. When this energy absorption takes place in the presence of ultraviolet light, some of that light will be absorbed. This UV absorption occurs at a specific wavelength.

Each element in the periodic table will have a specific ΔE that will absorb a specific wavelength of UV light. The relationship between the energy transition and the wavelength (λ) can be described by

$$\Delta E = \frac{h}{\lambda}$$

Where h is plank's constant. Atomic absorption uses this relationship to determine the presence of a specific element based on absorption at a specific wavelength. For example, calcium absorbs light with a wavelength of 422.7nm. Iron absorbs light at 248.3nm.

Principle

When a solution of metallic salt is sprayed on to a flame, fine droplests are formed. Due to the thermal energy of the flame, the solvent in the droplets evaporate, leaving behind fine residue, which are converted to neutral atoms. These neutral atoms are converted to excited state atoms by the thermal energy of the flame. As the excited state is not stable, these excited atoms return to ground state, with the emission of radiation of specific wavelength. The wavelength of the radiation emitted is characteristic of the element and is used to identify the element (Qualitative analysis).

The intensity of the radiation emitted depends upon the concentration of the element analysed (quantitative analysis).

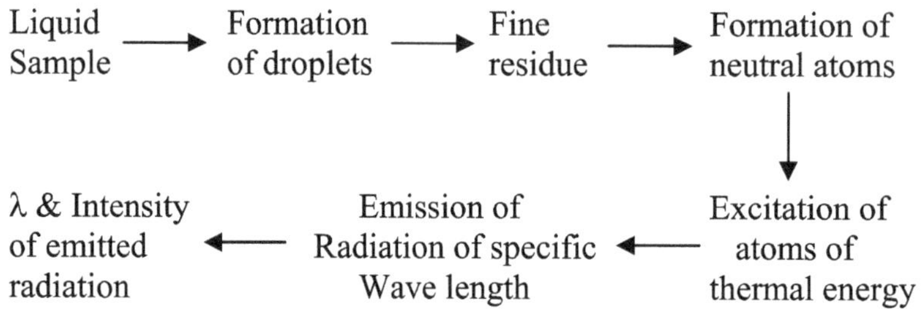

Liquid Sample → Formation of droplets → Fine residue → Formation of neutral atoms
↓
Excitation of atoms of thermal energy → Emission of Radiation of specific Wave length → λ & Intensity of emitted radiation

Although it is theoretically possible to analyse all the elements by flame photometry, the availability of burner, fuel and oxidant combinations and technical reasons make it practically possible to analyse group IA elements (Li, Na, K) and group IIA elements (Ca, Mg). The intensity of the radiation emitted depends up on the proportion of thermally excited atoms, which in turn depends up on the temperature of the flame.

$$\text{Fraction of free atoms thermally excited} = \frac{N^*}{N_0} = A_e^{-\Delta E/KT}$$

where N^* = no. of atoms in excited state

N_0 = no. of atoms in ground state

A = constant for element

ΔE = difference in energy levels of excited and ground state

K = Boltzmann constant

T = Frame temperature

The wavelength of the light emitted depends up on the difference in the energy levels of atoms in the excited and ground state.

Since atoms of each element has specific excited and ground state energy level, the wavelength of radiation emitted is different for different elements. For example, Sodium emits yellow radiation (589 nm), Potassium emits orange (767 nm), Calcium emits brick red colour (422, 554 and 626 nm) and Lithium emits blue at 670 nm.

Some of the elements emit at a single wavelength (primary emission), whereas other elements emit secondary emissions at different wavelengths.

The wavelength of the radiation emitted is given by the following equation:

$$\text{Wavelength of light emitted } (\lambda) = \frac{hc}{E_2 - E_1}$$

where h = Planck's constant

c = velocity of light

E_2, E_1 = Energy levels of excited and ground state respectively.

The intensity of the radiation emitted depends upon the concentration of the elements present in the solution. Higher the concentration, more is the flame intensity and lower the concentration, lesser is the flame intensity. The intensity of the spectral emission line is given by the following equation.

$$\text{Intensity of spectral emission line } (I_V) = \frac{V_{AT} h y_0 N_0 g_a}{B(T)} e^{\frac{-E}{KT}}$$

where
E = Energy of excited state
T = absolute temperature
Y_0 = freq. of radiation
AT = no. of transitions each excited atom undergoes per second
N_0 = no. of free metal atoms in ground state per unit volume
g_a = statistical weight of excited atomic state
B(T) = partial function of the atom overall states
K = Boltzman constant
h = Plank's constant
V = Flame volume (aperture ratio)

Components of Atomic Absorption Spectrophotometer

Hollow Cathode Lamp

The lamp or the source of light in AAS is a hollow cathode lamp. The cathode, is made up of specific element or alloys of elements or coating of elements on cathode.

When current is applied between anode and cathode, metal-atoms emerge from hollow cup and collide with filter gas, which is normally argon or neon. Due to these collisions, number of metal atoms are excited and emit their characteristic radiation. This characteristic radiation is absorbed by neutral atoms of the same element in ground state, which occur in the flame, when sample solution is sprayed.

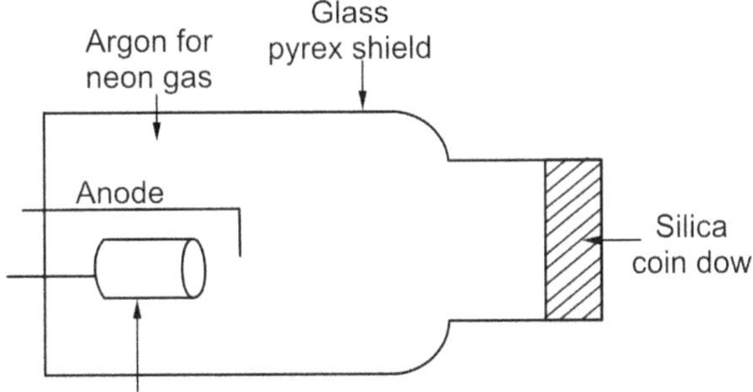

It is not possible to use a source of light with a monochromator because this arrangement gives a radiation with a band width of 1 nm, whereas the hollow cathode lamp gives a band width of 0.001 to 0.01 nm, which is highly desirable to achieve specificity. Moreover, the light source should provide a line width less than the absorption line width of the element to be determined.

The demerit in AAS is that, for determination of every element, separate hollow cathode lamp has to be used. This can be overcome by using multi element lamps e.g. Two element lamps like Na/K, Ca/Mg; Cu/Zn and three element lamps like Ca/Mg/Zn are available.

Burner (With Fuel and Oxidant)

The temperature of the flame is not critical, but atomization of sample solution like in flame photometry is required.

Burners, with fuel and oxidant as specified in flame photometry are used.

There are different burners available, which are used to spray the sample solution in to fine droplets, mix with fuel and oxidant, so that a homogenous flame of stable intensity is obtained. The most common ones are Mecker Burner, Total Consumption burner and laminar flow (premix) burner.

Total Consumption Burner: The construction of a total consumption Burner is simple and in this, the sample solution is aspirated through a capillary by the high pressure of fuel and oxidant and burnt at the tip of the burner. The advantage is that, the design is simple and the entire sample is consumed.

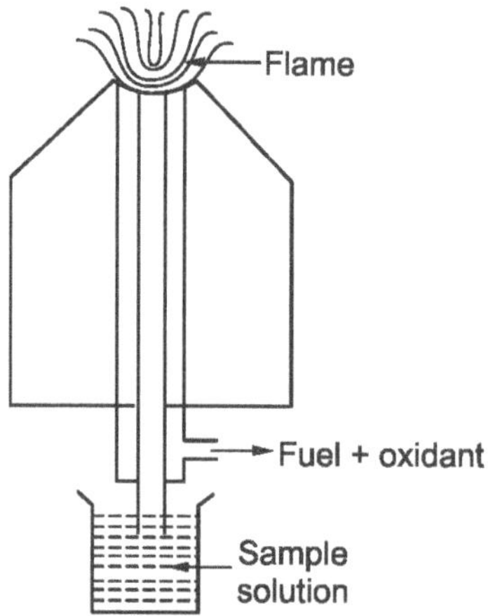

But the demerit is that, a uniform and homogenous flame is not obtained, since droplet sizes vary. This leads to fluctuations in the flame intensity.

***Laminar Flow (premix) Burner*:** This burner is the most widely used, because of its merits like uniformity in the flame intensity. In this type, the sample solution, fuel and oxidant are mixed before they reach the burner tip.

Only few droplets of uniform size reaches the flame and the remaining are drained through an outlet at the bottom.

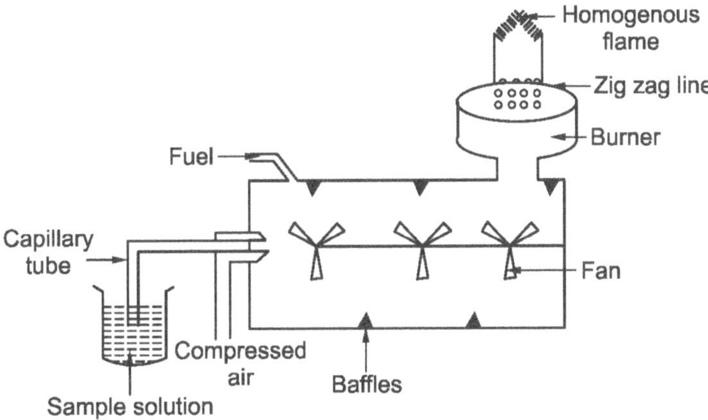

***Fuel and Oxidants*:** If the temperature of the flame is too low, it may not cause excitation of neutral atoms. If the temperature is too high, it may cause ionisation of atoms and thus sufficient population of atoms in excited state may not occur. Hence the temperature of the flame is critical. This makes it necessary to select ideal combination of oxidant and fuel which gives the desired temperature in flame photometry.

The different combinations of fuel and oxidant are used to get desired flame temperature. In most cases, a conventional flame photometer uses compressed air as oxidant and liquified petroleum gas (LPG) as fuel.

Fuel	Flame Temperature	
	Oxidant	
	Air	Oxygen
Propane	2100 °C	2800 °C
Hydrogen	1900 °C	2800 °C
Acetylene	2200 °C	3000 °C

Chopper

In the earlier instruments, choppers, which rotate like a fan, allow alternatively, radiation from flame alone or the radiation from hollow cathode lamp and flame. This produces a pulsating current (signal), which is used to measure the intensity of light absorbed by elements, without interference by radiation from the flame itself.

In modern instruments, where flameless techniques (electrothermal technique) are used, the lamp itself is modulated at a frequency. The amplifier is switched in synchronisation with the lamp and hence acts as a phase sensitive detector. This eliminates all errors in signals (other than hollow cathode lamp), hence only the intensity of the absorption by the element is measured.

Monochromator

Some elements have a single absorption line (principal line). But several elements have more than one absorption line (secondary lines). Hence it is necessary to select the spectral line for absorption measurements. Moreover, it is necessary to isolate the line spectrum of element from that of the emission by the gas in the lamp, or from the back ground signal of the flame. Hence a monochromator which can provide good resolution of 1 nm or less, is required.

Monochromators are better and more efficient than filters in converting a polychromatic light or heterochromatic light into a monochromatic light. A monochromator has the following units.

1. Entrance slit (to get narrow source).
2. Collimator (to render light parallel).
3. Grating or prism (to disperse radiation)
4. Collimator (to reform the images of entrance slit).
5. Exit slit (to fall on sample cell).

1. Prisms

The prisms disperse the light radiation into individual colours or wavelength. These are found in inexpensive instruments. The Band pass is lower than that of filters and hence it has better resolution.

The resolution depends upon the size and refractive index of the prism. The material of the prism is normally glass.

The two types of prisms available are:

(i) ***Refractive Type***

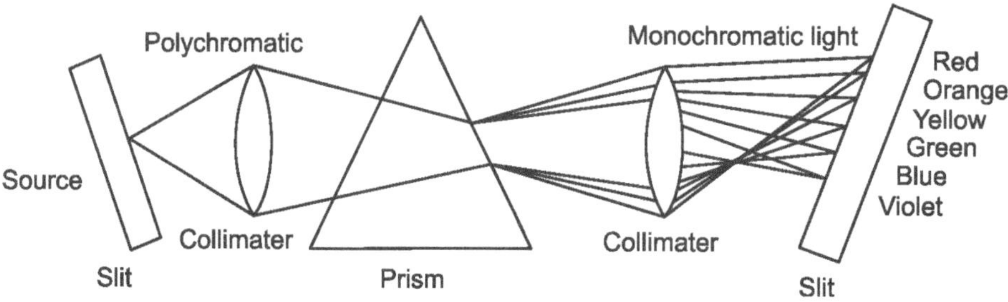

The above figure shows a prism, where the source of light, through entrance slit falls on a collimator. The parallel radiations from collimator are dispersed into different colours or wavelengths, and by using another collimator, the images of entrance slit are reformed. The reformed ones will be either Violet, Indigo, Blue, Green, Yellow, Orange or Red. The required radiation on exit slit can be selected by rotating the prism or by keeping the prism stationary and moving the exit slit.

(ii) ***Refractive Type (Littrow Type Mounting)***: The principle of working is similar to the refractive type except that, a reflective source is present on one side of the prism. Hence the dispersed radiation gets reflected and can be collected on the same side as the source of light.

2. Grantings

Gratings are the most efficient ones in converting a polychromatic to monochromatic light in the real sense. As a resolution of ± 0.1 nm could be achieved by using gratings, they are commonly used in spectrophotometers.

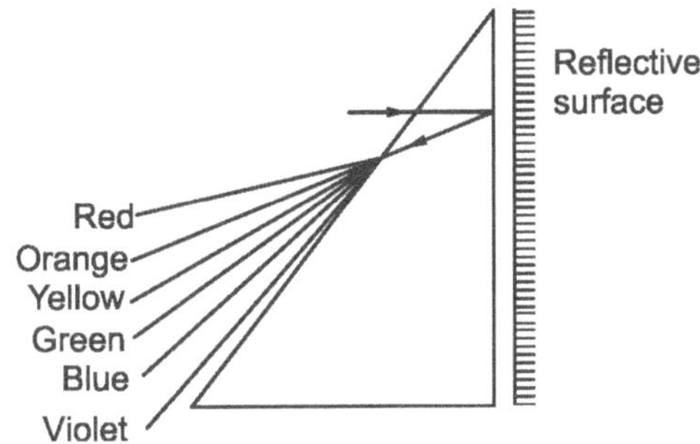

Gratings are of two types:

(i) Diffraction grating (ii) Transmission grating

(i) **Diffraction Grating**

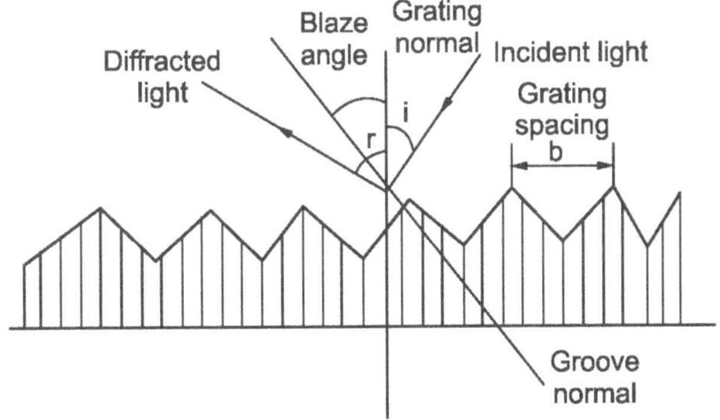

Gratings are nothing but rulings made on some material like glass, quartz or alkyl halides, depending upon the instruments, whether it is visible/UV/IR spectrophotometer. The number of rulings per nm also ranges from 20 grooves or lines per nm for IR spectrophotometer to 3600 grooves or more per nm for UV/visible spectrophotometer.

These gratings are replica made from master grating, by coating the original master grating with epoxy resin and are removed after setting. To make the surface reflective, a deposit of aluminium is made on the surface.

The mechanism is that diffraction produces reinforcement. The rays which are incident upon the grating get reinforced with the reflected rays and hence the resulting radiation has wavelength which is governed by the equation.

$$m\lambda = b\,(\sin i \pm \sin r)$$

where λ = wavelength of light produced

b = grating spacing

i = angle of incidence

r = angle of reflection

m = order (0, 1, 2, 3, etc).

The band pass of these gratings is 0.1nm which means they are the most efficient and hence gratings are preferred.

(ii) ***Transmission Grating*****:** Transmission grating is similar to diffraction grating, but refraction takes place instead of reflection. Refraction produces reinforcement. This occurs when radiation transmitted through grating reinforces with the partially refracted radiation.

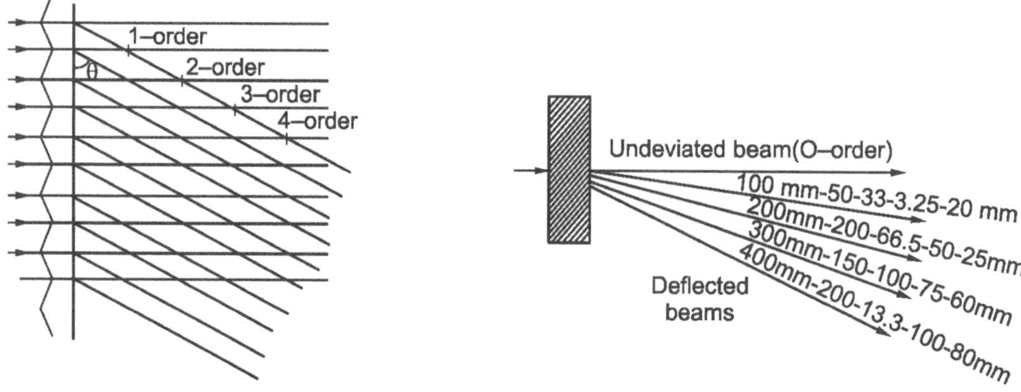

Transmission grating

The wavelength of radiation produced by transmission grating can be expressed by the following equation.

$$\lambda = \frac{d \sin \theta}{m}$$

where λ = wavelength of radiation produced

d = 1/lines per cm

m = order no. (1, 2, 3, etc.)

θ = angle of deflection/diffraction

Detector

The radiation emitted by the elements is mostly in the visible region. Hence conventional detectors like photo voltaic cell or photo tubes can be used. In a flame spectrometer, photomultiplier tube is used as detector.

Detector used in UV/Visible spectrophotometers can be called as photometric detectors. When a radiation is passed through a sample cell, part of it is being absorbed by the sample solution and the rest is being transmitted. This transmitted radiation falls on the detector and the intensity of absorbed radiation can be displayed. In these detectors, the light energy is converted to electrical signal which can be read or recorded. The most commonly used detectors are:

1. Barrier layer cell or photo voltaic cell
2. Photo tubes or photo emissive cells and
3. Photo multiplier tubes

1. Barrier Layer Cell or Photo Voltaic Cell

These cells are the cheapest and are used in inexpensive instruments, like filter type colorimeters, fluorimeters and nepheloturbidimeters.

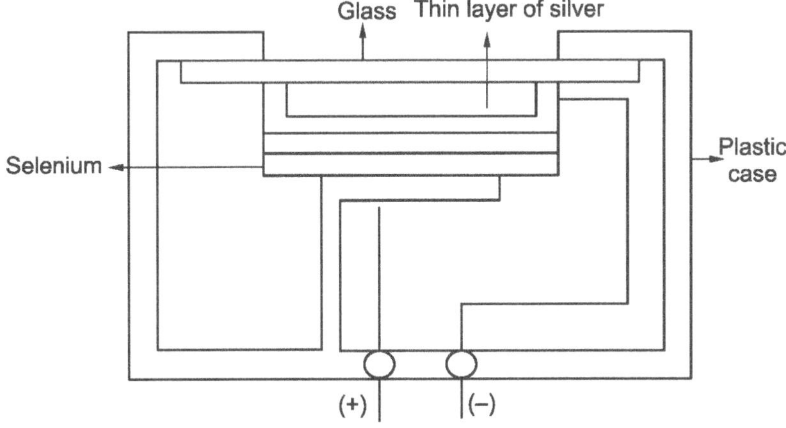

Photo Voltaic Cell

The detector has a thin metallic layer coated with silver or gold and acts as an electrode. It also has a metal base plate which acts as a another electrode.

These two layers are separated by a semiconductor layer of selenium. Selenium has extremely low electrical conductivity and hence the electrons are not mobile. When light radiation falls on the Selenium layer, these electrons become mobile and are taken up by the transparent metal layer. This creates a potential difference between the two electrodes and causes the flow of current, when the resistance in the external circuits is small. This flow of current causes deflection of the galvanometer needle, which depends on the wavelength and intensity of the radiation. The sensitivity of the instrument is similar to that of human eye.

The disadvantages of this detector are:

The amplification of signals is not possible, because the resistance of the external circuit has to be low, fatigue effects and the lesser response of the detector with light other than blue and red light.

2. Photo Tubes (or) Photo Emissive Cells

This detector is composed of an evacuated glass tube, which consist of photo cathode coated with elements of high atomic volume like caesium, potassium or silver oxide, which can liberate electrons, when light radiation falls on it.

This flow of electrons towards anode produce a current proportional the intensity of light radiation. Composite coatings like caesium/caesium oxide/silver oxide are also be used, which increase the sensitivity and range of wavelength in which the detector can be used (UV/Visible region). The signal from the detector can also be amplified using an amplifier circuit. Photo tubes have better sensitivity when compared to photo voltaic cell and hence are more widely used.

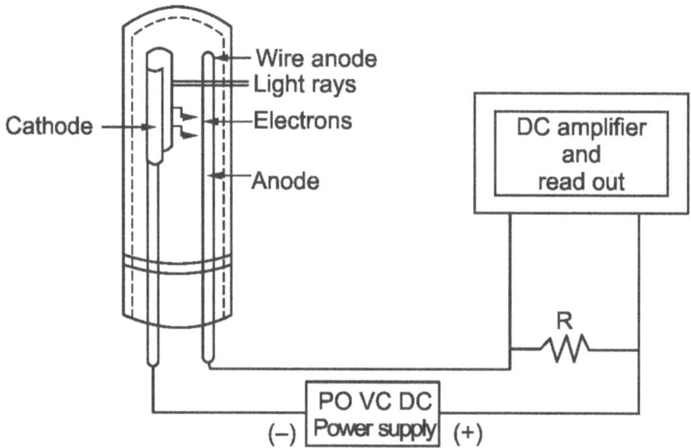

3. Photo Multiplier Tubes (PMT)

This type of detector is the most sensitive of all the detectors, expensive and used is sophisticated instruments.

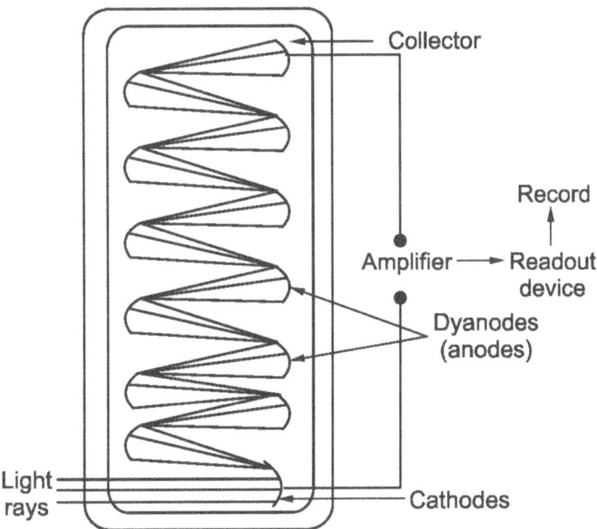

The principle employed in this detector is that, multiplication of photo electrons by secondary emission of electrons. This is achieved by using a photo cathode and a series of anode (dyanodes), upto 10 dyanodes are used. Each dyanode is maintained at 75-100V higher than the preceding one. At each stage, the electron emission is multiplied by a factor of 4 to 5 due to secondary emission of electrons and hence an overall factor of 10^6 is achieved.

PMT can detect very weak signals, even 200 times weaker than that could be done using photo voltaic cell. Hence it is useful in fluorescence measurements. PMT should be shielded from stray light in order to have accurate results.

Read Out Device

The readout device is capable of displaying the absorption spectrum as well as the absorbance at a specified wavelength (similar to UV spectroscopy). Beer's law is obeyed over a wide concentration range.

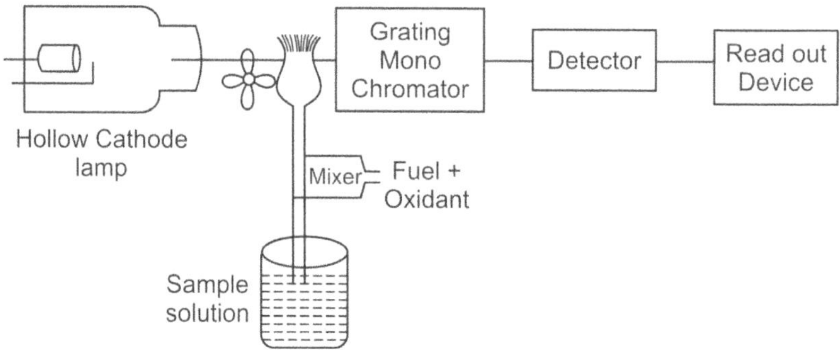

Schematic diagram of atomic absorption spectrophotometer

A single beam AAS consists of the components which are described below:

The sample solution is sprayed into a flame with the use of a fuel and oxidant, using an efficient mixer/burner (as used in a flame photometer). The neutral atoms present is the flame absorb light radiation emitted by the hollow cathode lamp (of same element to be analysed) and passes on through a monochromator. (To isolate the required radiation) and the intensity of radiation absorbed is measured by using a photometric detector. Thus the intensity of radiation absorbed by neutral atoms is measured and displayed by readout device. To eliminate the detector response due to radiation, choppers were used in olden days. In modern instruments, electronic devices are used which eliminate such background signal from the flame.

Double Beam AAS (Two Channel)

The two channel double beam AAS consists of two hollow cathode lamps for the determination of two elements. This type of instrument has the advantages like measurement of concentration of two different elements simultaneously and use of internal standard in one of the channels. This double beam design eliminates the errors

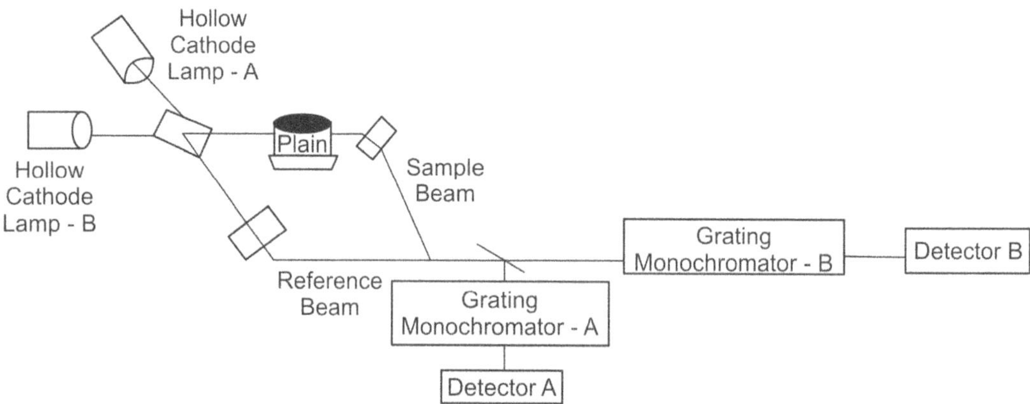

Schematic Diagram of Double beam AAS

due to fluctuations in the conditions of the flame, like viscosity of sample, temperature of sample solution, spraying rate etc. This double beam AAS offers the above advantages, when compared to single beam AAS.

Applications of AAS-Quantitative Analysis

AAS is mainly used for quantitative analysis of various elements present in different samples. It is not used for quantitative analysis since useless separate lamps are used and it is not possible to identify various elements present in the given sample.

Calibration curve method is used in quantitative analysis, where various standard solutions of the element to be determined are prepared and the absorbance of each solution is determined. A calibration curve of concentration of elements VS absorbance is made, from which the concentration of the element in the sample solution is determined. Beer's law is obeyed over a wide range of concentration. Low levels of detection such as 0.001ppm of elements are possible in quantitative analysis by AAS.

The following are some of the applications of AAS:

1. Estimation of trace elements in biological fluids (*e.g.* blood, urine, etc).
2. Estimation of elements like Copper, Nickel and Zinc in food products.
3. Estimation of Magnesium, Zinc, etc. in blood.
4. Estimation of Zinc in Zinc insulin injection.
5. Estimation of Mercury in Thiomersal solution.
6. Estimation of lead in Calcium Carbonate, petrol, etc.
7. Estimation of elements in Soil samples, water supply, effluents, ceramics, etc.

The following table shows some of the elements estimated by AAS along with the wavelength of principal absorption line and the lower detection limit.

Element	λ (nm)	ppm		Element	I (nm)	ppm
Lead	217	0.01		Copper	324.7	0.1
Bismuth	223	0.1		Calcium	442.7	0.05
Nickel	232	0.1		Barium	553.5	0.2
Cobalt	240.7	0.1		Sodium	589	0.01
Iron	248.3	0.1		Potassium	766.5	0.01
Mercury	253.7	1.0				

Comparison of Atomic Absorption Spectroscopy (AAS) with Flame Photometry (FP)

Parameter/Characteristics	Fp	AAS
Concentration of element depends on	Radiation emitted by exited atoms	Radiation absorbed by ground state atoms
Temperature dependency	Excited atoms are obtained by thermal energy of flame. Hence it is temperature dependent.	The thermal energy of flame is just enough to get neutral atoms. Hence it does not depend on temperature.
Linearity: Concentration vs parameters measured	Nearly linear over a narrow range of concentration.	Beer's law is obeyed and is linear over a wide range of concentration.
The number of elements that can be analysed by the technique	Very few elements especially group IA and IIA only can be analysed.	Wide range of elements can be analysed.

Differences between flame emission spectroscopy (EFS) and atomic absorption spectroscopy (AAS)

S.No.	EFS	S.No.	AAS
1.	The atoms when put in a flame become excited. The excited atoms which are unstable quickly emit a photon of light and return to a lower energy state eventually reaching to the unexcited (or) ground state. The determination of this emitted radiation forms the basis of flame emission spectroscopy. Analytical signal in flame emission is the sum of all energies emitted as excited atoms drop to the ground state. The signal comes directly and entirely from the emitted atoms.	1.	In A.A.S. the signal obtained from difference between the intensity of the source in the absence of metallic elements present in the liquid and decreased intensity obtained, when metallic elements are present in the optical path.
2	The emission intensity is dependent up on the number of excited atoms and therefore greatly influenced by temperature variations	2.	Atomic absorption depends up on the number of unexcited atoms and the absorption intensity does not depend up on the temperature of flame directly.

Contd...

S.No.	EFS	S.No.	AAS
3.	The relation between the absorption and concentration is not true in case of F.E.S.	3.	The relation between the absorption and the concentration is linear, that is the Beer's law obeyed over a wide concentration range.

Advantages of A.A.S. over F.E.S.

1. The atomic absorption technique is specific because the atom of a particular elements can only absorb radiation of their own characteristic wavelength i.e. the light of a particular frequency can easily be absorbed by the specific element to which it is characteristic. Spectral interferences which occur in F.E.S. are not seen.
2. Because of the much larger number of metal atoms that contribute to an A.A.S signal variation in flame temperature shows relatively less effect in A.A.S. than F.E.S. In other words A.A.S. is independent of flame temperature.

Disadvantages of A.A.S.

1. A separate lamp (radiation source) for each element is required. This difficulty is overcome by using a continuous source with a very high source with high mono chromator.
2. This technique is unsuccessful for estimation of elements like Al, Mo, vanadium because, these elements give rise to red metallic oxidises in the flame. However the estimation can be carried out under modified condition.

Interferences

AAS is less liable to be affected by interferences, when compared to flame photometry. The technique of AAS is especially free from cationic interferences. This is because of the absorption of sharp resonance lines from hollow cathode lamp. However, AAS the following interferences.

(a) ***Physical Interferences*: as described in flame photometry**

1. ***Back Ground Absorption*:** This occurs due to the sample matrix, flame itself, scattering, absorption by similar alkali halides, etc.

   ***Remedy*:** Use of gratings will avoid or minimise these interferences.
2. ***Spectral Interference*:** Atomic line interference, occurs due to the presence of other cations, which can emit radiation in the same region of emission by that of the element under analysis.

This is also called as cation-cation interference or molecular spectral interference for *e.g.*:

(a) Orange band of Ca – 543 – 622 nm interference with Na doublet 588 and 589.6 nm and Ba line at 553.6 nm

(b) Iron 324.7 nm interferences with copper 324.8 nm

Iron 285.2 nm interferences with Mg 285.2 nm

(c) Aluminium interferences with emission lines of Ca and Mg.

(d) Na and K mixture interfere with each other.

Remedy

1. Extraction of the ions interfering with each other.
2. Calibration curve of interfering material
3. Use of gratings instead of prisms/filters

(b) ***Anionic Interference***: The methods to overcome this type of interference is also given in flame photometry.

(c) ***Vapourisation Interference***: Chemical type, which occurs due to presence of some acids, by affecting the dissociation with other metals.

Physical type, due to high viscosity dextrose, sucrose overcome by the following techniques:

1. **Choice of flames, burners, atomisers and Additives**

   e.g.: Use of Acetylcholine/Nitrous oxide flame for thermally stable phosphates, sulphates, silicates, aluminates, etc.

2. **Additives**

   Releasing agents: Add few PPM of Lanthalum/strontium as ionisation suppressant to overcome interference due to PO_4. chelation/masking: Add EDTA to mask Ca in the presence of PO_4 (Cation-anion-interference).

(d) ***Scattering Effects***: This occurs due to the presence of high concentration of interfering element. This can be eliminated by using a continuous light source (deuterium lamp), in addition to hollow cathode lamp.

(e) ***Ionic Interferences***: Such interferences are seen in hot flames, when the thermal energy of the flame is sufficient for ionisation. This decreases the proportion of neutral atoms in the ground state. Hence easily ionizable elements like potassium (2000 μg/ml) are added to the sample solution, which is preferentially ionized than the elements of interest.

(f) ***Ionisation Interference***: More ionisation depopulates neutral atom both in ground state and excited state. Hence it decreases the sensitivity of the method.

Remedy: Add excess of easily ionisable ions like K, Cs, strontium. Hence it decreases the sensitivity of the method.

Experiment: Atomic spectrometry determination of calcium and magnesium in pharmaceuticals with statistical treatment of the measurement

Purpose

The analysis of field sample requires three operations

1. Acquiring the raw sample employing representative sampling technique.
2. Preparing the raw samples to convert them to an analysable form.
3. Analysing the prepared samples to determine the analyte(s) of interest. The result of the analysis will be affected not only by the raw sample composition but also by the three operations performed to collect the results. Two types of atomic spectrometry will be used to perform the measurements. Analysis of variance (ANOVA) will be used to quantify the effects of the three analytical operations on the data obtained.

Introduction and Theory

Atomic spectrometry is an analytical measurement method relying on the spectroscopic processes of excitation and emission. Atoms are capable of under going electronic transitions due to absorption of light or through excitation and emission of light. Since atoms have no rotational or vibrational energy, these transitions are a function of the quantized energy levels available for the atom.

These will be unique to each element and produce a narrow, sharp, spectral bands when measured. Since the bands are narrow, multiple elements are often resolved without interference, as might occur, in molecular spectroscopy.

The first type of atomic spectrometry used in this experiment is atomic absorption (AA).

Electromagnetic radiation from a suitable source passes through the atomic aerosol, resulting in absorption, due to excitation of electrons to higher energy levels. The radiation transmitted by the sample then passes through the monochromator and is quantified by a detector. For AA, the signal strength reaching the detector is small when a large concentration of the anlayte atoms is in the atomic aerosol.

The atomic aerosol for the instrument utilized in this experiment is provided by a combination of a concentric tube nebulizer and an air acetylene flame. Pressurized air is passed through an outertube causing the sample solution to be drawn into a concentric inner tube. The velocity of the rushing air then breaks the sample solution stream in to a fine mist. This mist is then mixed with acetylene and burned to produce a stable flame. The flame creates the atomic aerosol. Naturally, the sample must be in solution form in order to employ this process.

The very narrow absorption lines of atoms, about 0.02 Å are required. The used of a discrete source, such as the tungsten or deuterium lamps used in molecular spectroscopy cannot be employed. Such a source would swamp the signal. The very narrow absorption band, would appear as only a minute charge against the broad incident radiation, if it could be detected at all. In atomic absorption, a specialized source, a hollow cathode lamp, is generally used. A hollow cathode lamp is constructed such that the cathode contains the elements of interest. The lamp used in this experiment contains both calcium and magnesium. When such a lamp is energized, atoms are vaporized from the cathode and excited by this process. The atoms then relax back to the ground state, emitting light that is used as the source radiation for AA. The hollow cathode lamp will emit an atomic spectrum that matches the spectrum of the analyte.

This emission spectrum provides the source radiation. This should suggest a major drawback of AA. Lamps are required for each element to be measured. Even with multi-element lamps, such as used in this experiment, this can become cumbersome, especially if many elements must be measured. It also makes it impractical to perform quantitative work with AA.

The second atomic spectrometric method employed in this experiment is atomic emission (AE). When atoms are excited by the absorption of thermal energy to a higher electronic state, they will tend to relax to a lower state. This relaxation process is often accompanied by the emission of light. The measurement of the light emission can be used as analytical tool and is the basis for AE.

AE can take on many forms. Both solid and solution sample may be employed, in contrast to AA. This experiment focuses on the solution techniques. Excitation can occur by flame, furnace or noble gas plarma. By far the most popular technique is plarma. The very high temperature available in a plasma provides a stronger signal and makes many more element available as compared to flame and furnace techniques.

The air-acetylene flame used in this experiment provides only a small amount of excitation energy and is, therefore, useful only for easily excited elements like sodium and calcium. It does not provide sufficient excitation energy for magnesium. To summarize, in AE the thermal energy is the atomic aerosol which provides excitation energy to the atoms. The atoms then relax and emit photons that can be detected. These photons, as with the absorbed photons in AA, occur in a narrow band that is essentially unique to the element of interest. Unlike AA, in AE the signal strength reaching the detector will increase as the concentration of atoms in the aerosol increases.

There exists an interesting relationship between AA and AE measurements. Since the air-acetylene used in this experiment provides sufficient energy to cause emission for calcium, this could adversely affect the absorption measurements for calcium. As the calcium concentration in the flame increases, the emission signal as the detector will also increase. This occurs at the same wavelength as is used for absorption. This is in conflict with the absorption measurement where it is expected that the detected signal will decrease.

This error is eliminated by modulating the system. The source is pulsed to produce intermittent light for the absorption measurement. The detector is coupled to the frequency of this pulse. In this way, the detector can correct for the emission signal.

The most serious source of error in atomic spectrometry is chemical interference, Interference occur, when matrix components, cause a variation in the observed absorbance of an analyte compared with that observed for a pure standard of the same concentration. This is alleviated by matrix matching. Wherever possible, standards are prepared in the same matrix as the samples. We will be using a solution of ammonium chloride and strontium chloride to prepare the sample solutions. The standard must use the same solution. Further chemical interferences are also present when analysing sand and soil samples for calcium. Such sample may also contain phosphate, aluminium, silicates and sulphate. These can combine with calcium to form non volatile compounds that are not readily available in the aerosol for AA or AE. This problem can be overcome by the addition of a releasing agent such as strontium. Strontium will also combine with these compounds. It it is added in excess, it will tend to keep the calcium available for AA and AE. The purpose of the ammonium chloride in the preparation of the sample is to extract the calcium and magnesium from the drug through an ion exchange process.

Experimental Procedure

1. Extraction solution (25.9 g/L NH_4Cl and 2.3 g/L SrC_{12} in deionized water)
2. Stock standard solution (10 mg/L Mg and 50 mg/L Ca in the extraction solution)
3. Unknown sample solution (Mg and Ca in the extraction solution)

Part A: Acquisition of Samples

Obtain sample from the sample box. It has been divided into a $5' \times 5'$ grid. Before arriving in the lab to perform the experiment, generate 3 pairs of random numbers corresponding to coordinates (x, y) on the grid. You can use a computer, calculator, random number table, or less preferably, dice or drawing lots. You don't want any bias to result in your selection.

Select three clean dry beakers to collect the samples. Carefully mix the drug in the grid locations selected. Obtain three separate drug samples of about 2 g from each of the selected grid locations.

Part B: Chemical treatment of raw samples to convert them to analyzable form

In order to perform atomic spectrometry on the instrument, a solution is needed. In this experiment the calcium and magnesium will be extracted from the drug. The drug will then be filtered out and the resulting solutions are analysed. Complete extraction of Ca and Mg is assumed.

1. Choose one of the three samples. Using an analytical balance, weigh three 0.5 g portion of this sample into 3 separate 50 ml Erlenmeyer flasks.
2. For the remaining two samples, weigh a single 0.5 g portion each and place each into a 50ml Erlenmeyer flask. You should have a total of 5 flasks containing drug samples.
3. Add approximately 25 ml of the extraction solution to each of the drug samples in the Erlenmeyer flasks. Seal the top of the flasks with paraffin.
4. Place these on a shaker and shake vigorously for 30 minutes.
5. After shaking, filter the solutions using filter paper and glass funnel, with several rinses of extraction solution, into 50 ml volumetric flasks. Be careful to avoid spillage during filtration and rinsing. Be careful not to overfill the volumetric flasks during rinsing. Dilute to the mark with extraction solution. Seal the flask tightly and mix well.

The second analytical operation is now complete. The samples are now in an analyzable form.

Part C: Instrumental Analysis of the Samples

The instrument may now be started and prepared for the analysis. The Perkin Elmer 3100 atomic absorption spectrometer will be used. In order to obtain maximum sensitivity and precision, the instrument operating parameters must be optimized. Start by adjusting the measurement wavelength, lamp alignment, flame height, and gas flows and pressures.

I. Instrument start up and Optimization

1. Turn on the instrument when the message "Perkin-Elmer-Model 3100" appears, press. Enter the lamp current (probably 15 mA-consult the instrument log book for the specific value). Enter the lamp current value selected in the log book.
2. On the top of the instrument are some settings for the monochromator optics. Set the slit width lever to 0.7 nm and the slit height to "High".
3. Press (energy). A bar chart for CTS and EN will appear on the instrument display. This is a relative measure of the strength of the signal reaching the detector. Now locate the wavelength control dial on the left side of the instrument. Set the value of the optimum wavelength setting of Mg, 285.5 nm. The CTS and bar chart display should change as you rotate the dial. Delicately adjust the wavelength control dial so that the maximum value is obtained for CTS and EN. If the bar chart goes off scale during this adjustment, press the (gain) key. The EN value should increases when this is done. By maximizing the CTS and EN values, the wavelength setting is optimized.

4. Locate the vertical and horizontal alignment screws for the lamp on the top right side of the instrument. Slightly rotate each screw starting with the horizontal adjustment and ending with vertical. Once again, maximize the CTS and EN readings. After reaching a maximal reading, record the CTS and EN values in the log book. Please record the wavelength and element under analysis as well.
5. Press (cont.). An absorbance reading will appear on the display. Locate the vertical adjustment knob for the burner. Hold a piece of white paper in the light path to determine the level of the light beam with respect to the burner, rotate the vertical adjustment knob as necessary to ensure that the burner is lowered completely out of the light path. Press (A/Z) to autozero the instruments
6. Slowly rotate the vertical adjustment knob to raise the burner into the light path. This will be apparent when a slightly positive absorbance reading appears on the display. Now rotate the knob to slightly lower the burner until the reading returns to zero. The light beam is now at the top of the burner, this would be at the very base of the flame if it were lit. The temperature is slightly lower at the base of the flame due to desolvation of the aerosol, the hottest, cleanest portion of the flame is slightly higher.
7. Atomic spectrometry requires completion of the desolvation process and vaporization of the individual atoms of analyte. The burner must be lowered so that the light beam will be higher in the flame. Rotate the knob an additional ¾ turn to achieve the optimum position.
8. Turn on the air and acetylene flow under supervision of the TA. Record the air and acetylene cylinder pressures in the log book.

   Note: Do not start the instrument if the acetylene cylinder pressure is below 100 Psi, or if air pressure is below 500 Psi.
9. Turn the "oxidant" switch on the instrument to air. Carefully under supervision of the TA, stand away from the burner and press the red "Ignite" button to light the burner. Record a start time in the instrument log book. Check the log book for the proper supply pressures and, as necessary, adjust the flow pressures for air and acetylene, record these in the log book. Consult the log book for the proper flow rates and, as necessary, adjust the flows for air and acetylene. Record these in the log book.
10. Aspirate deionized water. The instrument is now ready to run. Make sure that the instrument is aspirating deionized water whenever it is lit and a determination is not in progress. The water provides necessary cooling to the burner assembly. Failure to do this could result in damage to the instrument. Use a large beaker to hold the deionized water for aspiration.

Fill it completely and check it periodically to be sure that the sampling tube is in the liquid. The instrument needs about 15 to 20 minutes of warm-up to reach optimal stability.

II. Preparation of the standard solution and calibration of the instrument

1. Prepare the standard solution as determined in the pre-laboratory assignment or as directed by the TA.
2. Before beginning the calibration, the nebulizer should be checked for proper operation. Care must be excercised in adjusting the nebulizer.
3. Poor nebulization is probably the most likely source of poor result in this experiment. Please consult the TA while performing this operation.
   (a) Aspirate deionized water.
   (b) Slowly turn the nebulizer lock ring clockwise until it is well clear of the nebulizer adjustment knob.
   (c) Slowly turn the nebulizer adjustment knob counter clockwise until bubbles begin to appear at the end of the sampling tube.
   (d) Aspirate standard solution # 3 (The most concentration standard)
   (e) Slowly turn the nebulizer adjustment knob clockwise until the absorbance goes through a maximum and just begins to decrease. The insertion point at which absorbance changes marks the optimal setting. Slowly turns the adjustment knob counter-clockwise to obtain the maximum stable absorbance. When this is done, aspirate deionized water once again.
   (f) Lock the nebulizer adjustment knob in its final position by turning the nebulizer, locking the ring counter-clockwise while holding the nebulizer adjustment knob securely.
3. Please remember to keep aspirating deionized water. This is especially important between analysis of the standards and samples. Because of the high salt concentrations in these solutions, extended arpiration of them will lead to build-up within the nebuizer and on the burner. This, in turn, will lead to poor instrument operation and poor results.
4. In making absorbance measurements for AA and AE it is common to average the signal over a specified time interval. This is called integration. It is, likewise, routine to make measurements, that are actually averages of a collection of individual readings. Flame atomic spectroscopy, as well as plasma and furnace technique have inherently noisy components. The flame is not perfectly stable, nor is the nebulizer consistent over a short time frame. This noise can be very effectively diminished by the averaging technique. Press (Paramet. Entry), press

(Enter) to reach the integration time-screen. Enter the integration time of 3 seconds. The instrument will then request the number of replicates, enter 3. Each measurement made for the standards and the sample will now be an average of three second integrations.

5. Press (data) to enter the data acquisition mode where the multiple integration data points can be collected. Zero the spectrometer using deionized water, by pressing (A/Z).
6. Start the calibration with the extraction solution. This is the blank press (read) to make a measurement. The display will show each of the three replicates and then report a mean, absolute mean, standard deviation, SD and relative standard deviation, RSD. Record data in lab note book.
7. After measuring the extraction solution, measure each of the standard solutions in the same manner. Calibration measurement is now complete for magnesium.

III. Measurement of the Samples

1. Aspirate deionized water for atleast two minutes after calibration.
2. Autozero the instrument with deionized water.
3. Measure the absorbance of each and extract solution. To determine the precision of the instrument; choose one of the singular sample solutions, and measure its absorbance three times. Record data in lab note book.
4. Measure the absorbance of the unknown sample solution along with the prepared samples.
5. Aspirate deionized water.
6. Set the wavelength dial to 422.27 nm. This is the analytical wavelength for calcium. Press (energy) and rotate the wavelength control slightly so that the CTS and EN readings are at a maximum.
7. Repeat steps 4-6 of the calibration section II above for calcium.
8. Repeat steps 1-5 of this section for calcium.

   The section on AA is now complete. Proceed to AE.

IV. Instrumental set up for Atomic Emission

1. Aspirate deionized water.
2. Press (entry). Enter a lamp current of zero to shut off the lamp.
3. Press (EM) to put the instrument in emission mode.
4. Aspirate standard solution # 3. Press (gain) to adjust the detector for emission.
5. Aspirate deionized water.

V. Calibration and Measurement for Atomic Emission

1. Repeat steps 4-6 of the calibration section II above for calcium.
2. Measure only the emission of the unknown sample solution for comparison to AA data. Perform this measure in triplicate so that instrumental variance can also be compared.

The measurements are now complete. The instrument must run another 15 minutes while aspirating deionized water in order to clean the nebulizer and burner head.

The shut down the instrument, consult with the TA. First, remove the sampling tube from the water and allow it to run dry for about 30 seconds. Next, shut off the acetylene at cylinder valve. The instrument will shut down automatically when it loses acetylene pressure. Turn the gas control switch off. Turn off the instrument power switch and close the air cylinder valve. Record the stop time in the instrument log book.

Record any problems or observations about the instrument in the log book.

Data Reduction and Analysis

1. Construct separate calibration plots of absorbance verticle concentration for Ca and Mg. Construct a third plot of emission vs concentration for Ca, include the data for the extraction solution (the blank) on these plots. Perform linear regression for these plots. The plots should have data plotted as points only, with the linear regression line drawn through the points. Include the equation of the line on the plots. In the 'Results' section of the report, include a brief discussion concerning the linearity of these calibrations. Comparison of the linear regression y-intercept to the value (blank value) measured should be included in the discussion.
2. Use the calibration plots for AA of Ca and Mg to determine the concentrations in the drug samples. Include the unknown sand sample in this analysis, assume the sample weight for this sample to be exactly 0.5g. Do not report the concentration of the solutions. Report the concentrations of Mg and Ca in the drug samples.
3. Use the calibration plot for emission of Ca to calculate the concentration of Ca in the unknown sample solution. Once again, do not report a solution concentration. Report the concentration of Ca in the drug in μg/g. Assume a sample weight of exactly 0.5g.

Variance

When measurements are made, there are always indeterminate errors. It is, however, variance and not standard deviation that is propagated through any experiment or calculation. This is provided the variances are expressed as comparable quantities. Thus, when a series of events or operations is performed consecutively, the total variance introduced is the sum of the variance due to each operation. In an instrumental analysis, samples are collected, prepared for analysis, and then analysed with the instrument. The total variance (V total) in the sample analysis will be the sum of the variance for each operation.

$$V\ total = V\ sampling + V\ prep. + V\ instr.$$

Calculation of Variance

With the results from the AA analysis, Mg and Ca in the sand in µg/g, use the following definition to calculate the variance. Complete the calculation separately for Mg and Ca.

1. V total is the total variance of Mg or Ca in the four samples analysed. In order to calculate this, data for all the samples must be included and each data point must have the same measurement base. In order to achieve this, calculate the variance using only one point from each of triplicate measurements, plus the values measured for the sand sample measured singly and the unknown sample solution.

   The calculation will then include four data points.
2. V instr. is the variance due to the instrument. Calculate the variance using the concentration from the single solution that was measured three times. Calculate this value for both atomic absorption and emission. The value from AA will be used below. The value for AE will be used later to compare the two techniques.
3. (Vinstr. + Vprep.) is the variance due to the instrument plus that is due to the sample preparation. Calculate this, using the concentrations from the grid sample that was prepared and analysed three times.
4. Vprep. = (Vinstr. + Vprep.) – Vinstr.
5. Vsampling = Vtotal – (Vinstr. + Vprep.)

This type of data analysis is often called ANOVA, an acronym for analysis of variance. Since variance is additive in this fashion, its analysis is especially well-suited to this situation. It can aid in understanding how each of the steps in the analytical process affect the results obtained. It is hoped that this experiment will show the value as measuring the contribution of each analytical operation to the data produced. This experiment is a laboratory model of a coil sampling experiment. As such, some of the grids in the sand-box have been spiked to create a non-homogenous sampling situation. It is often the case that small regions of topsoil, like an individual farmer's field, are not homogenous with respect to soil nutrients like Ca and Mg. The same type of situation could arise in a manufacturing situation, such as pharmaceuticals, where a continuous production process feeds a batch packaging process. In either case, this in homogenous composition could have serious consequences. The farmer could improperly fertilize his field leading to poor yields.

A drug company could sell a lot of drug that is not uniform. In both of these cases with proper sampling and proper data analysis, the nature of the situation can be understood and appropriate steps can be taken.

Comparison of Absorption and Emission

Prepare a table comparing absorption and emission. The following values should be included : Sensitivity (The slope of the calibration curves), Vinstr. and concentration of Ca in the unknown sand sample.

Discussion

1. Explain the rationale behind the ANOVA calculations.
2. Comment on the relative magnitude of the different sources of variance. What calculations can be drawn from these values?
3. Compare, quantitatively, the variances obtained from the Mg and Ca data. In order to do so, you should convert the absolute values of variance to relative values based on the ratios of the variance for each step to the total variance. For example.
4. Discuss the two techniques of atomic absorption and emission, using the data obtained. Remember the instrument used as optimized for absorption measurements.
5. Discuss how the precision of their analysis could be improved. Relate the results of the ANOVA analysis to this discussion.
6. You are given the task of analysing 20 rail hopper cars of ore for Ca and Mg content. You have sufficient time and resources to collect and analyze 100 samples, although fewer samples would be preferable. You have no information concerning the uniformity of the ore within the cars or from car-to-car. Give a detailed description of how you would collect the samples.

Pre-Laboratory Assignment

1. Define variance (an equation is sufficient)
2. A series of standard solutions of magnesium are measured by atomic absorption. The following absorbances were collected:

   [Mg] in μg/ml Absorbance

   0.000.023

   0.200.075

   0.500.149

   1.000.273

A sand sample weighing 0.5081 g was treated as specified in the experiment. An absorbance of 0.089 was measured. What is the concentration, in μg/g, of magnesium in this sand sample?

3. Given a standard solution containing 50 μg/ml Ca and 10 μg/ml Mg specify, as a detailed procedure, how to prepare 100 ml each of the following standard solutions:

   Solution # [Mg] in μg/ml [Ca] μg/ml

   10.201.00

   20.502.50

   31.005.00

***Note*:** This dilution procedure will be used during the experiment.

4. A lot of an analytical reagent was analysed for iron. Five bottles out of the lot were sampled. For one of the bottles, five samples were analyzed. For the remaining bottles, one analysis was performed for each. The following results were obtained (Fe : in μg/g):

   Bottle # 1:5.08, 5.12, 5.03, 5.11, 5.17

   Bottle # 2:5.23

   Bottle # 3:5.10

   Bottle # 4:5.29

   Bottle # 5:5.01

   Calculate the mean iron content of this lot, in μg/g.

   Calculate the total variance observed for the lot.

   Calculate the variance due to sampling.

   Calculate on the uniformity of this lot of reagent with respect to iron.

Atomic Absorption and Emission Spectra

As we have noted in the section on the Bohr atom, isolated atoms can absorb and exit packets of electromagnetic radiation having discrete energies dictated by the detailed atomic structure of the atoms. When the corresponding light is passed through a prism of spectrograph it is separated spatially according to wavelength 1°.

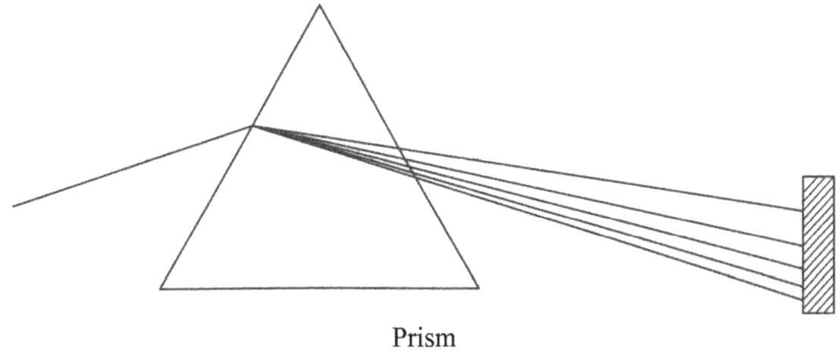

Prism

Continuum, Emission and Absorption Spectra

The corresponding spectrum may exhibit a continuum, or may have superposed on the continuum bright lines (an emission spectrum) or dark lines (an absorption spectrum).

Continuous Spectrum

Emission Spectrum

Absorption spectrum

Continuum, emission and absorption spectra

CHAPTER 14

FLAME PHOTOMETRY

Introduction

Flame photometry has been the proven standard method for the analysis of sodium and potassium for the last 70 years. The accurate and reproducible analyses of these elements are crucial in the clinical and many industrial fields.

Flame photometry (or) Flame emission spectroscopy in which a flame is used to excite atoms.

Emission spectroscopy, which deals with the examination of the energy emitted from a substance which when suitably excited, is an obvious instrumental approach for the determination of elements.

Emission of characteristic radiation by an element and the suitably correlation of emission intensity with the concentration of element forms the basis of flame photometry.

Theory

The underlying principle of FES may be explained when a liquid sample containing a metallic salt solution under investigation is introduced into a flame, the following steps normally take place in quick succession, namely.

(i) The solvent gets evaporated leaving behind the corresponding soil salt.

(ii) The solid salt undergoes vaporization and gets converted into its respective gaseous state and

(iii) The progressive dissociation of either a portion or all of the gaseous molecules give rise to free neutral atoms (or) radicals.

(iv) The resulting neutral atoms are excited by the thermal energy of the flame which are fairly unstable & hence instantly emit photons and eventually return to the ground state (i.e. the lower energy state).

The resulting emission spectrum caused by the emitted photons and its subsequent measurement forms the fundamental basis of FES.

Bohr's Equation

If we consider two quantized energy levels e.g. Higher as E_2 and lower as E_1, the radiation given out during the transition from E_2 to E_1 may be expressed by the following equation :

$$E_2 - E_1 = hv$$

where h = Plank's constant

v = Frequency of emitted light

where $$v = \frac{c}{\lambda}$$

C = velocity of light

λ = wavelength of the absorbed radiation

$$\therefore \quad E_2 - E_1 = \frac{hc}{\lambda} \quad \text{(or)}$$

$$\lambda = \frac{hc}{E_2 - E_1}$$

This equation is used for

1. Wavelength of the emitted radiation which is characteristic of the atoms of the particular element from which it was initially emitted.
2. Wavelength of radiation given out from a flame is indicative of the elements that might be present in that flame.
3. Intensity of radiation may quantify the exact amount of the element present.

Boitzmann Equation

The fraction of free atoms which are excited thermally, or in other words, the relationship between the ground state and the excited state quantum is exclusively represented by the Boitzmann equation.

$$\frac{N_1}{N_0} = \left(\frac{g_1}{g_0}\right) e^{-\Delta E / KT}$$

where N_1 = Number of atoms in the excited state (high energy level)

N_0 = Number of ground state atoms

$\frac{g_1}{g_0}$ = Ratio of statistical weights for ground and excited

E = Energy of excitation (= hv)

K = The Boltzmann's constant

T = Temperature (in Kelvin)

here 1. Fraction of atoms excited (N_1) solely depends upon the temperature of the flame (T).

2. Ratio $\frac{N_1}{N_0}$ is dependent upon the excitation energy (ΔE).

Therefore the fraction of atoms excited critically depends on the temperature of the flame thereby emphasizing the vital importance of controlling the temperature in flame emission spectroscopy (FES).

Principle

When a solution of metallic salt is sprayed on to a flame fine droplets are formed. Due to the thermal energy of the flame, the folvent in the droplets evaporate leaving behind fine residue which are converted to neutral atoms. These neutral atoms are converted to excited state atoms by the thermal energy of the flame. As the excited state is not stable, the excited atoms return to ground state, with the emission of radiation of specific wavelength. The wavelength of the radiation emitted is characteristic of the element and is used to identify the element (qualitative analysis). The intensity of the radiation emitted depends upon the concentration of the element analysed (quantitative analysis).

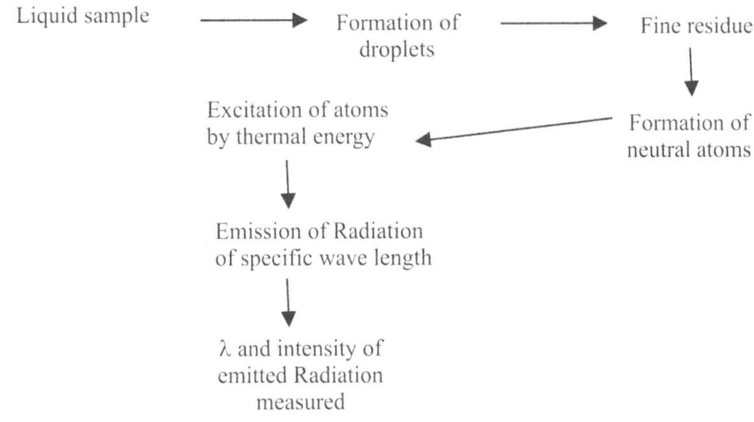

Sherwood Heritage

The model 100 developed by EEL in 1950, brought flame photometry to 50,000 laboratories world wide allowing for the first time the measurement of sodium and potassium to be made witn mixure rather than the lengthy and difficult gravimetric procedure used previously.

Starting with the model 100 Flame photometer for the past 50 years, a succession of instruments, developed in the UK, have advanced flame photometry incorporating for the first time; dual element read out model (150 1970); Internal standard reference (model 430 1970); Automatic ignition safety features (model 410 1985). There have been the products of a succession of companies; EEL, corning and from 1995 Sherwood Scientific Ltd.

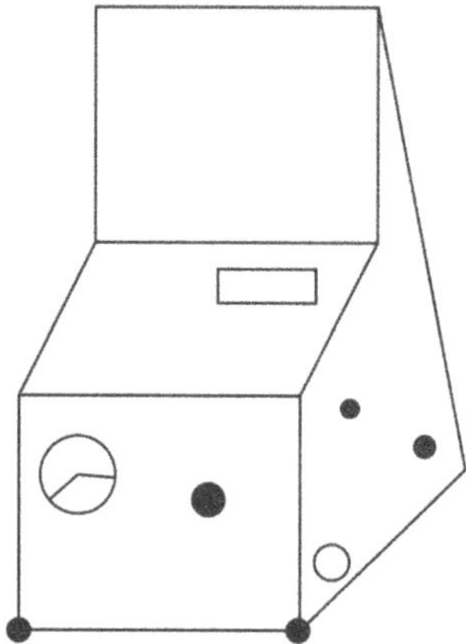

Components of a Modern Flame Photometer

The aqueous sample is aspirated into the nebuliser where it is vapourised and mixed with air and fuel in the mixing chamber. Here it encounters baffles designed to prevent all but the smallest aerosol mist reaching the flame. Larger droplets hit the baffles and are eliminated through the drain tube. This fine aerosol, intimately mixed with the gas, approaches the heat of the flame where the water content evaporates until only microscopic particles of hydroxides of oxides of the elements to be measured feed into the flame. Here they are thermally dissociated into molecules or atoms, electrons of which are energised by the heat from the flame. As the energised species pass into a cooler part of the flame, they lose energy in the form of light of characteristic wavelength as the atoms return to their “ground state”.

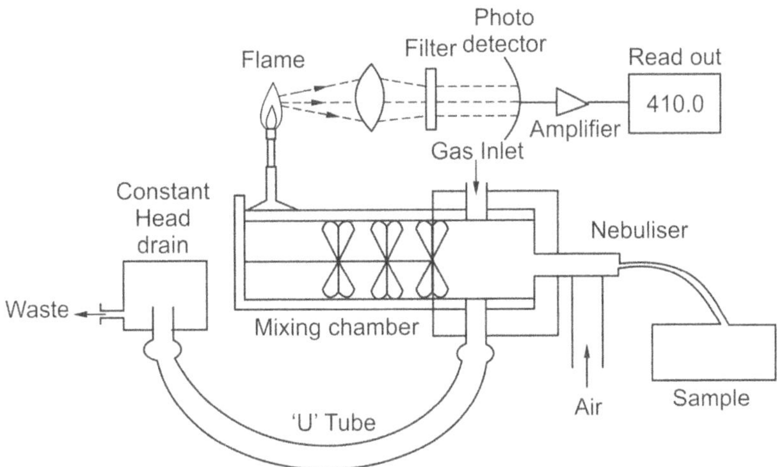

Experiment

Flame photometric Determination of Sodium

Note : A clean, labelled 100 ml volumetric flask for your unknown must be turned in at least one period prior to the day you are scheduled to do this experiment. Each student will have his own unknown, even if working in pairs.

Background

Flame photometry, more popularly called flame emission spectrometry, is a fast, simple and sensitive analytical method for the determination of trace metal ions in solution. Because of the very narrow and characteristic emission lines from the gas-phase atoms in the flame plasma, the method is relatively free of interference from other elements. Typical precision and accuracy for analysis of dilute aqueous solution are about $\pm$ 1-5%.

The method is suitable for many metallic elements, especially for those metals which are easily excited to higher energy levels at flame temperature, Na, K, Ca, Rb, Cs, Cu, Ba. Non metals generally do not produce isolated neutral atoms in a falme thus they are not suitable for determination by FES.

Flame photometry is an empirical method of analysis that is you must calibrate the method carefully. Many different experimental variables affect the intensity of the light emitted from the flame. Therefore careful and frequent calibration is necessary for good results.

Apparatus

Coleman Flame photometer, model 21, is used with a total consumption burner using natural gas and oxygen. Wavelenght isolation is by use of a simple interference filter.

Light from the flame is focussed on to the end of a fibre optic cable (a "light pipe") when the flame photometer. The electronic box therein converts the diode's output in a digital display.

Caution

Although the flame is quite small, it has so high a temperature that contact of the flesh with even the outer edge of the flame will instantly produce a third-degree burn. Except for lighting the flame, the hands should be kept completely out of the housing when even the flame is burning even if it has been turned very low between analysis.

Equipment

One 1000-ml volumetric flask, from your locker five 100-ml volumetric flasks checked out frm the TA, 10 ml and 25 ml volumetric pipes, or use a 50-ml burette.

Clean all equipment and rinse thoroughly with deionized water before and after use. Use deionized water for all solutions.

Reagents

Standard Sodium Stock Solution: 0.100 g Na^+ per L; dissolve 0.2542 g NaCl in 1.000 litre of deionized water (0.100 g/L = 100 mg / L = 100 ppm = 100 mg/ml). If you cannot weigh out exactly this amount, get it as you can, record the exact weight, and correct your concentrations accordingly.

Procedure

1. Pipette 10, 20, 30, 40 and 50 ml of the standard 100 ppm sodium solution into the first, second, third, fourth and fifth flasks, respectively. Dilute to the markwith water.
2. Use deionized water for the "blank".
3. Obtain the unknown from the instructor and dilute to the 100 ml mark with deionized water. Mix thoroughly.
4. Follow the instructions with the instrument and determine the emission intensity for each standard, the blank (deionized water), and the unknown.

Use of the Flame Photometer

1. When ready to take emission reading, call the TA to light the flame, stabilize the flame photometer, and to instruct you in its proper and safe usage.
2. Aspirate deionized water for at least 2 minutes to clean out and stabilize the unit. While aspirating deionized water, set the 'zero' knob in the read out unit to 0.0 units. There will be some bounce in the meter reading.

3. Aspirate the most concentrated standard solution, and use the GAIN knob to set the reading to 100.0 units. Recheck the 'zero' setting with deionized water and the 100 setting again with the most concentrated standard.
4. Now aspirate all the standards and unknown in turn, aspirating deionized water in between each one to clean the unit out. The burner shows a "memory effect".
5. Repeat steps 2-4 second time to get a good duplicate set of measurements. Repeat the whole sequence a third time if necessary to get a third set of values.
6. When done, aspirate deionized water for at least 2 minutes.
7. Call the TA to shut down the photometer.
8. Clean up your work areas.

Waste Disposal

All Na solutions can be safely disposed off by simply pouring down the drain and running some cold tap water to flash. Rinse out all glassware with deionized water.

Treatment of Data

Prepare a calibration curve by plotting the emission intensities as a function of Na concentration. Determine the concentration of sodium in the unknown sample by reading the concentration of the sample which corresponds to its emission intensity from the calibration curve. Report the concentration of sodium in ppm.

X-ray absorption

If an X-ray photon is absorbed in a solid, a core electron is excited to an empty state below the ionization threshold (X-ray excitation or above threshold. The X-ray absorption spectrum can be divided into near edge and extended fine structure. The X-ray absorption near-edge structure (XANES) is extended in the first 30-40 eV past the absorption edge, while the extended X-ray absorption fine structure (EXAPS) covers the photon energy range from about 40 eV to about 1000 eV past the edge. It is now well established that EXAFS is a consequence of the modification of the photoelectron final state due to scattering by the surrounding atoms (i) EXAFS spectroscopy has become a useful technique for investigating the local environment of specific atomic species in complex chemical system.

Core Excitation

The interpretation of XANES spectra is more complicated than 'EXAFS' spectra. So the observation of core excitation is a long standing theoretical problem. The formal theory of solid state excitation concentrates on the tightly bound limit of the Frekel – excitation and on the loosely bound limit of the wannier excitation. (ii) The Frenkel excitation is usually approximated by molecular cluster methods or even atomic excitation and the translational in variance of the lattice is neglected. (iii) On the other hand, the 'wannier excitation' limit is treated using the effective mass formulation. Note that from a solid state view point, the bound to bound transition to the collapsed final states are the atomic like Frenkel excitation. The appearance of the core excitation and its type is dependent on the core hole-excited electron interaction, on the type of chemical bond, and on the width of the band gap. Nevertheless, in the case XANES of insulators there have been arguments on whether the observed peaks are within the forbidden gap (core excition) or in the continuum because of the ambiguity in the position of absorption threshold. Note that in contrast to metals, which have a sharp density of states (DOS) cut off at fermi edge, the valence-band photo electron spectra of insulators do not have a sharp edge on side nearer the vacuum level. Consequently the photo emission curves for these compounds do not terminate abruptly at low photon energies and therefore it is difficult to obtain an exact value for the photoelectric threshold (iv).

Continuum Absorption

Non exitonic part of the XANES spectra is formed by the transitions to the unoccupied states above threshold. The procedures employed so far to calculate this part of the XANES spectra within an independent electron picture have been based on one of two approaches. Scattering formalism (v) (short range) or band structure calculations (vi) (long range), Because of excited core, atom of nuclear charge Z is virtually identical to an impurity of charge Z+1, the final sate wave function must correspond to an eigen state of the system in the presence if the core hole. Nevertheless, the X-ray absorption is a comple many particle process due to the change in potential when the core hole is created. So in correlated electronic systems like valence flucturating compounds where the ground or / and absorption final states are described by a mixing of atomic like configurations, the XANES spectra at threshold shows a splitting of localized atom like resonances due to multi electron configurations.

X-ray Spectroscopy

Several X-ray spectroscopies are of interest to geochemistry and environmental soil science. In the environmental and Soil Geochemistry group at Dart mouth, we principally use three of these techniques, X-ray absorption spectroscopy (XAS), X-ray photo electron spectroscopy (XPS), and synchrotron X-ray diffraction (S-XRD). The formation of each of these techniques is unique, but all of them use high energy X-ray sources to identify and characterize a wide variety of geological and environmental materials. Each of these techniques also takes advantage of the intense and continuously tunable X-ray produced at synchrotrons, large particle accelerators designed to produce a wide spectrum of light energies.

X-ray absorption spectroscopy (XAS)

X-ray photoelectron spectroscopy (XPS)

Synchrotron-Based X-ray diffraction (S-XRD)

A Brief overview of X-Ray Absorption Spectroscopy

X-ray absorption spectroscopy is an element –specific probe of the local structure (shortage) of elements in a sample. Interpretation of XAS spectra commonly uses standards with known structures, but can also be accomplished using theory to derive the structure of a material. In either case, the species of the materials is determined based on its unique local structure. An important advantage of this technique is its utility for heterogeneous sample, a wide variety of solid and liquids, including whole soils and liquids, can be examined directly and non-destructively. Additionally, since the local structure does not depend on long runge crystalline order, the structure of amorphous phases (and that of dissolved spaces) is easily achieved.

XAS is useful for concentrations from about 10ppm to major elements. As such, it is useful to special trace elements such as contaminants absorbed to pure minerals, soils and sediments, and is also a valuable tool for studying the mineralogical composition of the soil or sediment (especially when used in conjunction with other techniques such as X-ray diffraction).

X-ray absorption spectroscopy results from the absorption of a high energy X-ray by an atom in a sample. Their absorption occurs at a defined energy corresponding to the binding energy of the electron in the material. The ejected electron interacts with the surrounding atoms to produce the spectrum that is observed. Occasionally, the electron can be excited into vacant bound electronic states (unoccupied molecular orbital) near the valence band. As a result, distinct absorptions will result at these energies. Often these features are diagnostic of coordination and are of use for geochemistry. For example, the toxic chromate anion is tetrahedral and as a result has absorption feature just below the absorption edge (the so-called pre-edge) that is not present in the more benign Cr (III). As a result, the presence of this feature is diagnostic for the more toxic form of chromium.

Since the electron excited is usually the IS or 2p electrons, these energies are usually quite high (thousands of electron volts), this technique demands high energy (and tunable) X-ray excitation. As a result, it is done at synchrotron radiation facilites. There are 4 major synchrotron facilities in the US, and others in Europe, Asia and else where. These facilities provide a bright source that is required for these experiments to be useful at the concentrations needed for geo-chemical applications.

X-ray absorption spectroscopy is commonly divided into two spectral regions, the first is the X-ray absorption near edge structure (XANES) spectral region. XANES spectra are unique to the oxidation state and specification of the element of interest, and consequently is often used as a method to determine the oxidation state and coordination environment of materials. XANES spectra are commonly compared to standards to determine which species are present in an unknown sample. Once species are identified, their relative abundance is quantified using linear combination fitting (or other curve-fitting algorithms) using XANES standards to reconstruct the experimental data. It is important to note that XANES is sensitive to bonding environment as well as oxidation state. Consequently XANES is capable of discriminating species of similarly formed oxidation state but different coordination. For example, Arsenic (III) oxide is easily differentiated from Arsenic (III) sulphide, and octahedral Mo (VI) can be differentiated from tetrahedral Mo (VI).

The more distant region of the X-ray absorption spectrum is termed the extended X-ray absorption fine structure (EXAFS) region. EXAFS spectra are best described as a series of periodic sine waves that decay in intensity as the incident energy increases from the absorption edge. These sine waves result from the interaction of the elected photoelectron with the surrounding atomic environment. As such, their amplitude and phase depend on the local structure of excited atom. Since this interaction is well understood, theory is sufficiently advanced that the local structure of the excited atom can be determined by matching a theoretical spectrum to the environmental spectrum. This fitting yields many types of information, including the identity of neighboring atoms, their distance form the excited atom, the number of atoms in the shell, and the degree of disorder in the particular atomic shell (as expressed by the Debye, Waller factor). These distances and coordination numbers are diagnoste of a specific mineral or absorbate mineral interaction. Consequantly, the data are useful to identify and quantify major mineral phases, adsorption complexes, and crystallinity. Linear combination of EXAFS spectra using standards is also commonly used for quantitation for samples containing many species since it is quite difficult in practice to separate many species into their component shells.

A Brief Overview of X-ray Photoelectron Spectroscopy

XPS also used X-rays to excite electrons from molecular orbitals into the continuum. However conventional XPS does not measure absorption while scanning through the absorption edge as is done for XAS. Rather XPS is conducted by using a fixed energy source to excite electrons from the sample and then measuring their kinetic energy. Since their kinetic energy is dependent on their binding energy (and, strictly speaking, a correction factor called the work function), different chemical species can be identified based on their distinct binding energies. These experiments are commonly carried out with the Al (or) Mg anodes in the laboratory. These metals release X-rays when a high voltage is applied that is monochromatic and useful for XPS. However, synchrotron-based XPS (S-XPS) offers many benefits. Most importantly, since the excitation energy is variable, the kinetic energy of photons can be varied continuously. This is useful because the distance that an electron can travel through the solid (called the escape depth) varies with kinetic energy. Synchrotron based XPS remits the kinetic energy for oxygen orbital to be tuned to a value (typically about 50-100 eV) where the escape depth reaches minimum (about 1 monolayer or a few Å). Consequently, S-XPS is highly sensitive for surfaces. The incident energy can then be tuned to determine the thickness of any surface layers. S-XPS has other advantages over other methods. It affords superior resolution to conventional instruments, permitting the differentiation of similar chemical species. S-XPS also is useful for light elements (those with atomic number of Ca and lower) because they are difficult to analyze by XAS since their X-rays are too low in energy to pass through air as well. Therefore, elements such as A1, Si, N & C usually are analyzed by XPS. Fortunately, complementary XAS information can equally be obtained for these light elements concurrently to XPS in synchrotron-based XPS system.

It should be mentioned that there are limitations associated with this technique because it detects electrons. Since electrons do not pass through air, these experiments must be run in vacuum. This also means that samples must be dired (water evaporates in a vacuum). Their drying may impact the system or result in may chemical transformations. Also since this technique is highly surface sensitive it is less useful to analyze bulk properties; infact, it may make it impossible to identify anything but interferences on a dirty surface. Consequently, XPS is often done with clean, freshly cleaned single crystals.

A Brief Overview of Synchrotron-Based X-ray Diffraction

Synchrotron X-ray diffraction (S-XRD) is similar in design to conventional XRD. In it, X-rays are diffracted through a crystalline material, revealing the inter atomic spacing, atomic identities and positions of atoms within the crystal. Diffraction is the most fundamental means of determining structure of minerals and other even proteins, and it is especially useful to characterize environmental samples conventionally, XRD has several limitations. A key disadvantage of XRD is that it is limited to crystalline materials (since amorphous materials do not diffract). XRD also is time consuming and uses a large volume of sample. Fortunately, S-XRD is useful to circumvent these limitations. They offer exceptional resolution, even on very samples containing only a few grains of a particular mineral. This resolution and the excellent detection for S-XRD permit the identification and quantification of trace phases not possible using other means. Amorphous materials and thin films can also be analyzed thanks in part to the instrumental configuration of these instruments. Finally S-XRD can be collected over a large range of angles. Impossible with conventional instruments and invaluable when performing rietveld refinements. Rietveld refinements are used to determine the unit cell parameters and site occupancy for a powder XRD pattern given a crystal lattice. Such methods have proven invaluable for the study of things ranging from locating waters of hydration in zeolite, to arsenate substitution in sulphate minerals.

Absorption Spectroscopy and Time-Resolved Structural Dynamics

Since the construction of the 1st laser in the early 1960's time- resolved pump probe laser spectroscopy has become a key, if not essential, tool for understanding and unravelling the dynamics of molecular systems. In light induced reactions, monitoring the transition from ground state, to excited state (s), to products and the appearance and disappearance of transient chemical species; is a progression that is kinetically well-followed using lasers. However, getting time resolved structural information from transient absorption spectroscopy is a far less exact science, and in most cases will rely strongly on quantum calculations.

X-rays have long been used as a probe of structural information Power of X-ray diffraction has shown in resolving the structure of large biomolecules as well as the X-ray diffraction of a compound giving structural information, the absorption of X-ray will also allow us to determine the structure of a compound, but diffraction is best suited to well organized solids, XAS will give the same results in solid, liquid or gas. This gives great advantage as one can look at the structures of bio-systems in their natural environment, rather than in a restrictive lattice.

If one compares a movement the absorption of UV /VIS / IR radiation by a molecule, with the absorption of X-ray photons by a molecule, the difference in energy between these two regions of the electromagnetic spectrum gives the result the UV / VIS / IR photons and X-ray photons will probe two different types of transitions. The UV / VIS / IR photons, by exciting valence electrons, will probe electronic states of the molecule as a whole, the X-ray photons, being much higher in energy, will excite core electrons, probing the environment surrounding the atoms that make up the molecule.

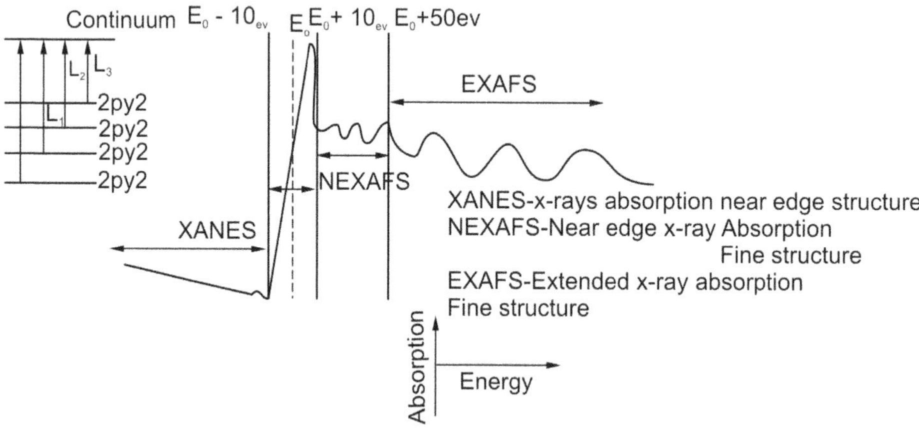

Figure shows an energy level diagram to illustrate core electron excitation by absorption of an X-ray photon, and a cartoon plot of an X-ray absorption spectrum. Examining the spectrum, as one increases energy, one sees that there is a sudden, sharp rise in absorption, which is followed by a series of oscillations. This sudden rise is known as the 'band edge'. It corresponds to the excitation of a core electron to and ionisation continuum. The energy E_0, marked on the spectrum, corresponds to the electron affinity of the electron excited, basically its binding energy, so for each of the different elements that make up any molecule, these band edges will beat different energies due to the signature nuclear changes of each element. The table below gives an idea of these energies for the most tightly bound electrons (The 1st electron) for a number of different elements. This band-edge, as can be seen from the energy level diagram, is called the K-edge.

Element	Atomic number	K-edge Binding energy/eV
Hydrogen	1	13.6
Helium	2	24.6
Potassium	19	3608.4
Calcium	20	4038.5
Titanium	22	4996
Iron	26	7122
Copper	29	8978
Rubidium	37	15200
Rothenium	44	22117

The oscillations that are seen after the band edge are interference patterns. Once the energy of X-ray photons are greater than E_0, the electron is no longer bound to the atom it was associated with. These interference patterns arise due to the interference between the outgoing electron wave, and the back scattered wave of the neighbouring atoms in the molecule. If one were looking at the X-ray absorption spectrum of an isolated atom, eg. Ar gas, one would not see such interference patterns. As can be seen from figure two, the nature of these oscillations are determined by a number of factors. This region of the absorption spectrum is known as the 'fine structure', by fourier analysis of the fine structure, one can get information about the nature of the environment surrounding a particular element in a molecule.

The fine structure is not the only region of the spectrum that can yield useful information on the element that one chooses to focus on. For example, as the energy of the band edge is determined by the binding energy of the electron excited, generally speaking as one increases the oxidation state of the element in question, one will see the band edge shift to higher energies as the electron becomes more and more tightly bound.

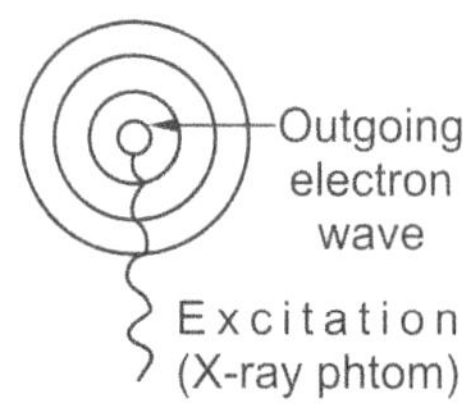

If there are no atoms bonded to, or coordinated to to the atom excited by the x-ray photon. The outgoing electron wave cannot back scatter. There will be no fine structure.

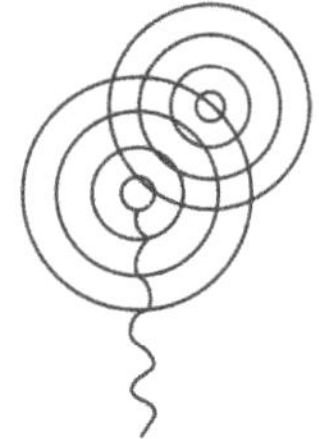

Back scattered electron wave inphase with outgoing wave gives rise to a peack in the EXAFS functions.

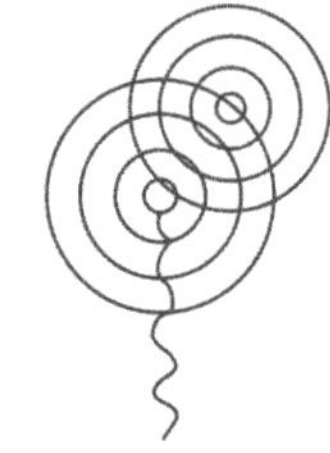

Back scattered electron wave out of phase with outgoing wave gives rise to a trough in the exacts function

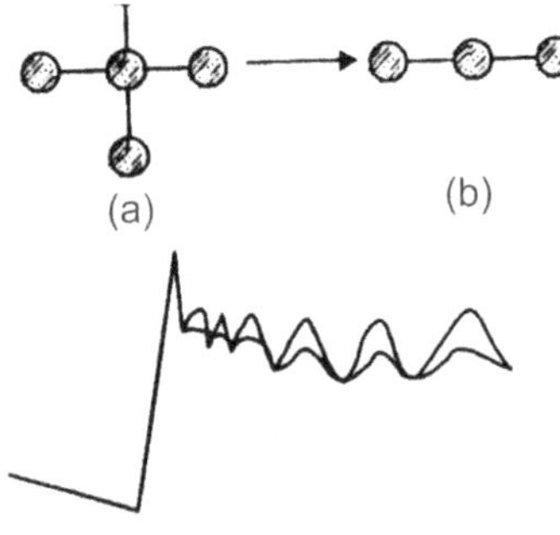

If the bond distance remains roughly the same but co-ordination number decreases (same co-ordinating atom), the amplitude of the XAFS Oscillations will decrease.

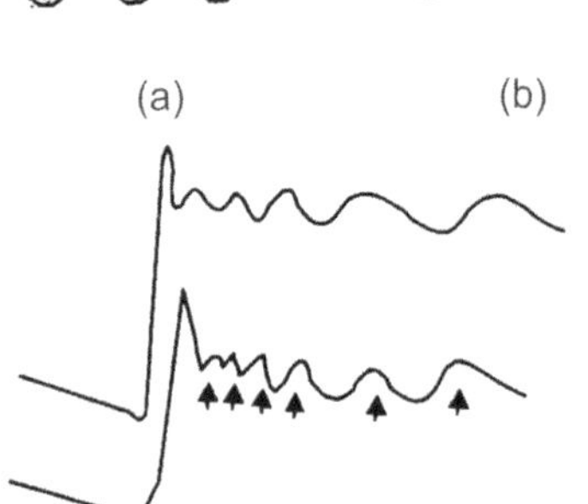

If the co-ordination number remains the same, but the bond length increases, the period of oscillation will decrease.

Fine-Structure – Electron Scattering

With the advent of short X-ray pulses from synchrotron sources, it has become possible, not only to use these techniques to obtain steady state structural measurements, but to use short X-ray pulses to probe the change in structure of a molecule, with respect to time, during a chemical reaction. In collaboration with Prof. Jorgen Larson, at beam line D611 at MA X AB, in Lund, currently in the process of setting up experiments to follow similar chemical and biological processes as currently followed already in this department using Laser pump and probe techniques, but using a short pulsed laser to excite the reaction/process and short pulsed X-rays, from the MAX II storage ring to monitor changes in the chemical structure of the reagents.

The initial work is focussing on monitoring the change of formal oxidation state that occurs upon laser excitation of a metal to ligand charge transfer (MLCT) state, within a number of different organometallic complexes, and thus following directly the laser induced oxidation of the metal centre. Depending on the system investigated, one can follow a number of different reduction processes.

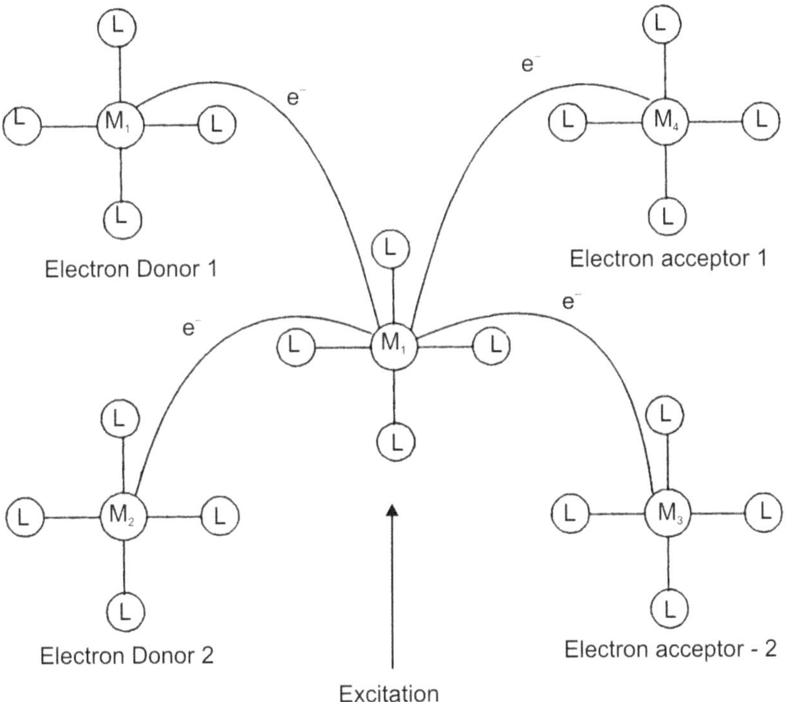

These processes can be examined using X-ray probes, by following the shift in the position of the band edge of the metal in the complex. The time resolution for such experiments, using standard. Detectors, due to the temporal width of the X-ray pulse, is of the order of 100 ps, but, taking advantage of X-ray streak camera technology , should be as low as 500 fs. We can then follow the structural rearrangement of the molecule after such excitation.

The systems where work is currently underway are complexes applicable to the research currently undertaken for the purpose of investigating methods of artificial photosynthesis and materials used in the dye sensitised solar cell research. In particular both RUN_3 and black dyes on TiO_2, probing the RuL edges and the O, M and L_3 edges; and reaction centers with Rhenium as the metal center, probing the ReM_4L_3 edges, where the Re is oxidised upon laser excitation and reduced by intramolecular electron transfer from a histidine moiety.

Hydrogen Emission and Absorption Series

The spectrum of hydrogen is particularly important in astronomy because most of the universe is made of hydrogen. Emission or absorption processes in hydrogen give rise to series, which are sequences of lines corresponding to atomic transitions, each ending or beginning with the same atomic state in Hydrogen. Thus, for example, the Balmer series involves transitions starting (for absorption) or ending (for emission) with the first excited state of hydrogen, while the lymen series involves transition that start or end with the ground state of hydrogen. The adjacent image illustrates the atomic transitions that produce these two series in emission.

Because of the deteails o hydrogen atomic structure, the Balmer Series is in the visible spectrum and the Lyman series is in the UV. The following image illustrates some of the transitions in the Balmer series.

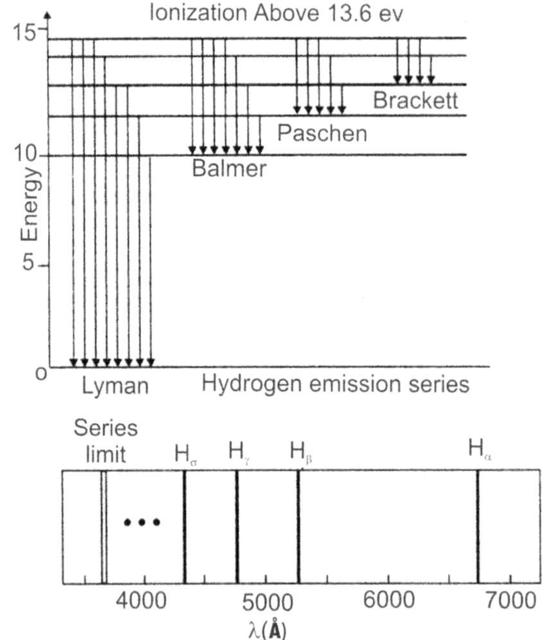

The Balmer spectrum of hydrogen

The balmer lines are designated by H with a great subscript in order of decreasing wavelength. Thus the longest wavelength Balmer transition is designated H with a subscript alpha, the second longest H with a subscript data, and so on.

Origin of Continuous, Emission and Absorption Spectra

The origin of these three types of spectra are illustrated in the following figure.

Sources of Continuous, Emission and Absorption Spectrum

Thus, emission spectra are produced by thin gases in which the atoms do not experience many collisions (because of the low density). The emission lines correspond to photons of discrete energies that are emitted when excited atomic states in the gas make transitions back to lower-lying levels.

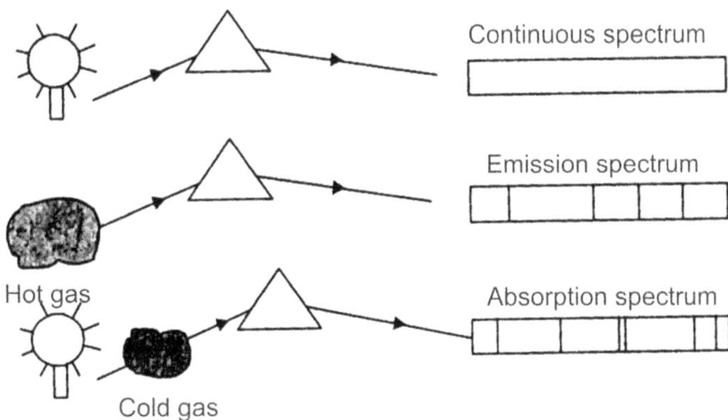

A continuum spectrum results when the gas pressures are higher. Generally solids, liquids or dense gases emit light at all wavelengths when heated.

An absorption spectrum occurs when light passes through a cold, dilute gas and atoms in the gas absorb at characteristic frequencies, since the re-emitted light is unlikely to be emitted in the same direction as the absorbed photons. This gives rise to dark lines (absence of light) in the spectrum.

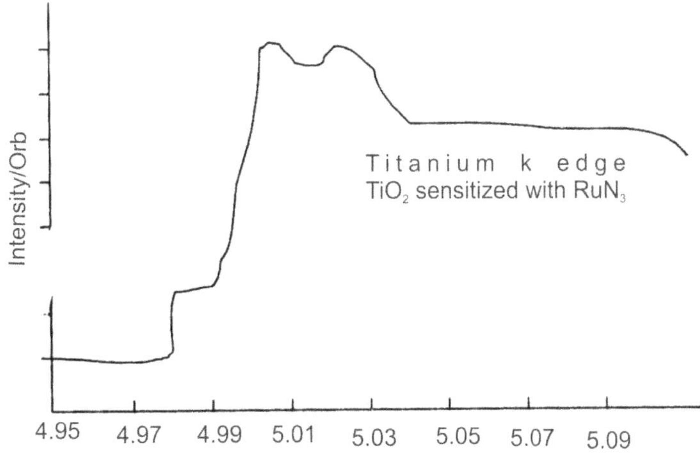

Instrumentation

1. Burner (with fuel and oxidant)
2. Filter / monochromator
3. Detector
4. Readout device

1. Burners

There are different burners available, which are used to spray the sample solution into fine droplets, mix with fuel and oxidant, so that a homogenous flame of stable intensity is obtained. The most common ones are Mecker Burner. Total consumption burner and laminar flow (premix) burner.

***Total Consumption Burner*:** The construction of a total consumption burner is simple and is shown in fig. In this the sample solution is aspirated through a capillary by the high pressure of fuel and capillary by the high pressure of fuel and capillary by the high pressure of fuel and oxidant and burnt at the tip of the burner.

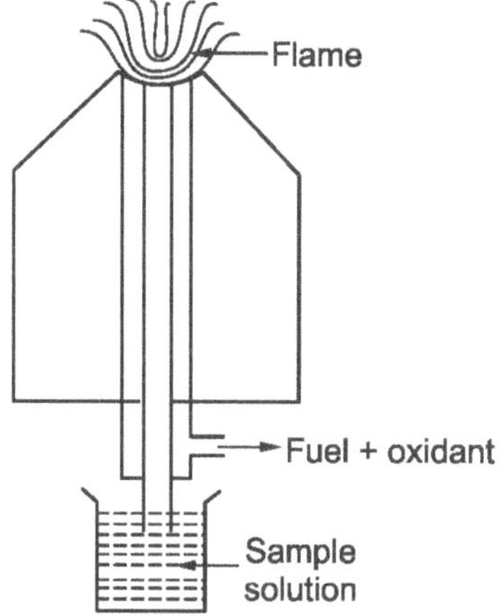

The advantage is that, the design is simple and the entire sample is consumed.

Demerits

As uniform and homogenous flame is not obtained, since droplet sizes vary, this leads to fluctuations in the flame intensity.

***Laminar Flow (Premix) Burner*:** This burner is the most widely used, because of its merits like uniformity in the flame intensity. In this type, the sample solution, fuel and oxidant are mixed before they reach the burner tip. Only few droplets of uniform size reaches the flame and the remaining are drained through an outlet at the bottom.

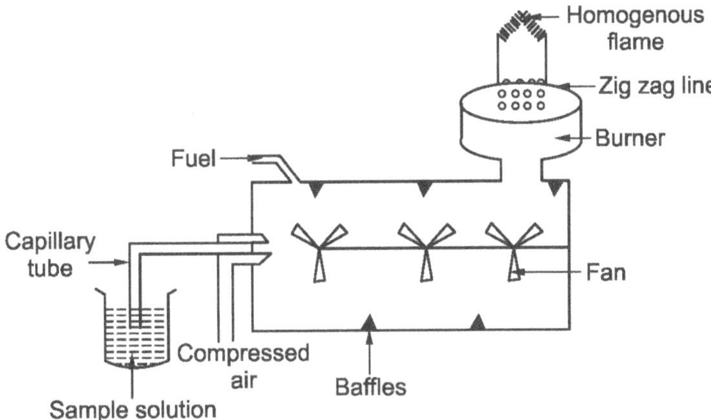

***Fuel and Oxidant*:** If the temperature of the flame is too low, it may not cause excitation of neutral atoms. If the temperature is too high, it may cause ionisation of atoms and thus sufficient population of atoms in excited state may not occur. Hence the temperature of the flame is critical. This makes it necessary to select deal combination of oxidant and fuel wihich gives the desired temperature in flame photometry

The different combinations of fuel and oxidant are used to get desired flame temperature. In most cases, a conventional flame photometer uses compressed air as oxidant and liquefied petroleum gas (LPG) as fuel.

Fuel	Flame temperature	
	Oxidant	
	Air	Oxygen
Propane	2100° C	2800° C
Hydrogen	1900° C	2800° C
Acetylene	2200° C	3000° C

***Filter Monochromator*:** In Flame photometry, the wavelength as well as intensity of the radiation emitted by the element has to be monitored. Hence a filter or monochromator is to be used. A detailed description of filters and monochromators is given below. Typically a simple flame photometer contains a filter wheel (containing several filters for either Ca, Li, Na or K) and when a particular element has to be analysed, the specific filter is selected.

The source of light gives radiation from 400 nm to 800 nm. This is polychromatic (heterochromatic) in nature (light of several wavelengths). In a colorimeter/ spectrometer we require only monochromator is used which converts polychromatic light into monochromatic light.

Filters are of two kinds. They are:

1. Absorption filters and
2. Interference filters

Monochromators are of two kinds:

1. Prism type (Dispersive type & Littrow type)
2. Grating type (Diffraction grating & transmission grating)

Filters

1. Absorption Filters

These filters are made up of glass, coated with pigments or they are made up of dyed gelatine. They absorb the unwanted radiation and transmit the rest of radiation which is required for colorimetry.

These filters can be selected according to the procedure given below :

1. Draw a filter wheel (Circle with 6 parts).
2. Write the colours (VIBGYOR) in clockwise (or) anticlockwise manner omitting indigo.
3. If the colour of the solution is red, we have to use green filter and if the colour of the solution is green, we have to use red filter. (The colour of the filter is opposite to the colour of the solution i.e. complimentary in nature).
4. Similarly, we can select the required filter in a colorimeter based upon the colour of the solution.

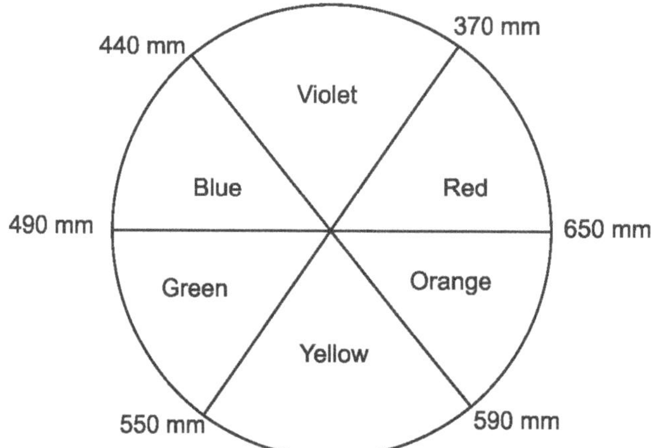

Merits

1. Simple in construction
2. Cheaper
3. Selection of filter is easy

Demerits

1. Less accurate since band pass is more (30 nm) (i.e. if we have to measure at 500 nm, radiation ranging from 470 nm to 530 nm falls on the sample). (Band pass is the difference in wavelengths between the point where the transmittance is one-half the maximum.
2. Intensity of radiation becomes less due to absorption by filters.

II. Interference Filters

This filter is otherwise known as Fabry-Perot filter. The features are:

1. It has dielectric spacer film made up of CaF_2, MgF_2 or SIO, between two parallel reflecting silver films.
2. The thickness of dielectric spacer film can be $\frac{1}{2}\lambda$. (Ist order), $2\frac{\lambda}{2}$ (2nd order) $3\frac{\lambda}{2}$ (3rd order), etc.
3. The mechanism is that, the radiation reflected by the 2nd film and the incoming radiation undergo constructive interference to give a monochromatic radiation, which is governed by the following equation:

$$\lambda = \frac{2nb}{m}$$

where λ = wavelength of light obtained

n = dielectric constant of layer material

b = layer thickness

m = order no (0, 1, 2, 3 etc)

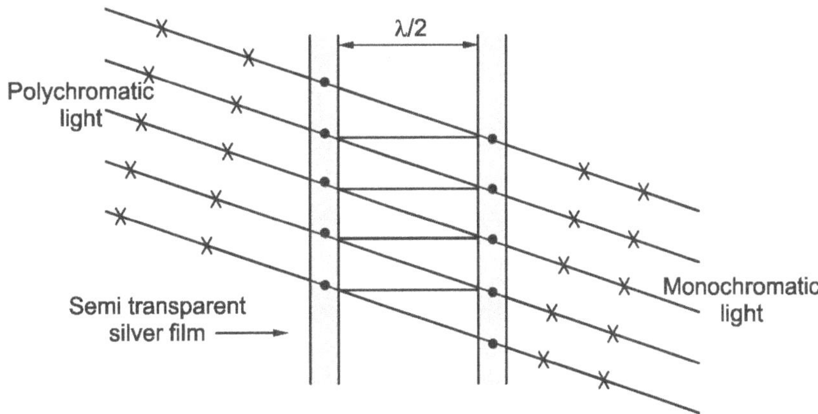

Interference Filter (Fabry-Perot)

4. Band pass is 10-15 nm. (i.e if we select 500 nm, the obtained radiation ranges from 490 nm to 510 nm).
5. Maximum transmission is 40%.

Merits

1. Inexpensive
2. Lower band pass when compared to absorption filters and hence more accurate.
3. Use of additional filter cuts off undesired wavelengths.

Demerits

1. Peak transmission is low, and becomes so when additional filters are used to cut off undesired wavelength.
2. The band pass is only 10-15 nm and hence higher resolution obtained with monochromators or gratings cannot be achieved.

***Monochromators*:** Monochromators are better and more efficient than filters in converting a polychromate light or heterochromatic light into monochromatic light. A monochromator has the following units.

1. Entrance slit (to get narrow source)
2. Collimator (to render light parallel)
3. Grating or prism (to disperse radiation)
4. Collimator (to reform the images of entrance slit)
5. Exit slit (to fall on sample cell)

1. Prims

The prisms disperse the light radiation into individual colours (or) wavelengths. These are found in inexpensive instruments. The band pass is lower than that of filters and hence it has better resolution. The resolution depends upon the size and refractive index of the prism. The material of the prism is normally glass.

The two types of prisms available:

(i) ***Refractive type*:** The (fig.) shows a prism, where the source of light, through entrance slit falls on a collimator. The parallel radiations from collimator are dispersed into different colours or wavelengths, and by using another collimator, the images of entrance slit are reformed. The reformed ones will be either Violet, Indigo, Blue, Green, Yellow, Orange or Red. The required radiation on exit slit can be selected by rotating the prism or by keeping the prism stationary and moving the exit slit.

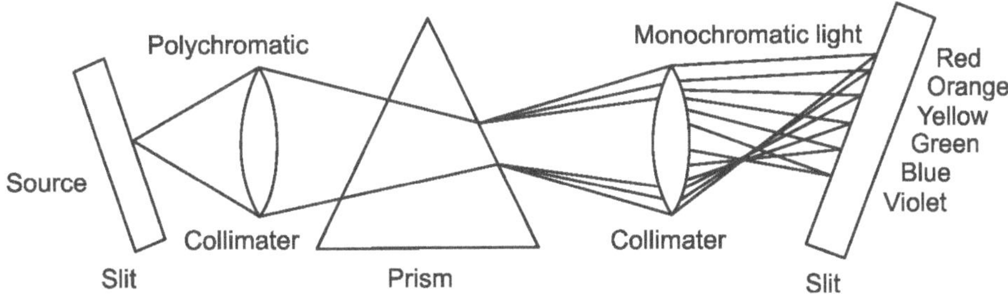

(ii) ***Reflective Type (Littrow Type Mounting)*:** The principle of working is similar to the refractive type except that, a reflective surface is present on one side of the prism. Hence the dispersed radiation gets reflected and can be collected on the same side as the source of light.

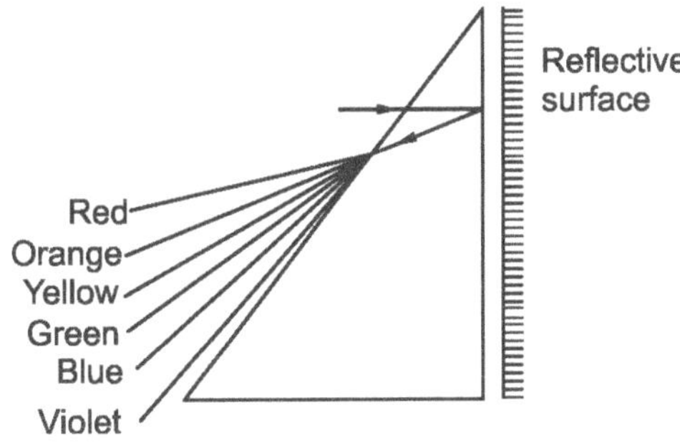

Littrow Type Mounting

2. Grating

Gratings are the most efficient ones in converting a polychromatic to monochromatic light in the real sense. As a resolution of 0.1 nm clould be achieved by using gratings. They are commonly used in spectrophotometers.

Gratings are of two types

(i) Diffraction grating

(ii) Transmission grating

(i) ***Diffraction grating*:** Gratings are nothing but rulings made on some materials like glass, quartz or alkyl halides, depending upon the instrument, whether it is visible for (or) IR spectrophotometer. The number of rulings per mm also ranges from 20 grooves or lines per mm for IR spectrophotometer to 3600 grooves or made per mm from visible spectrometer.

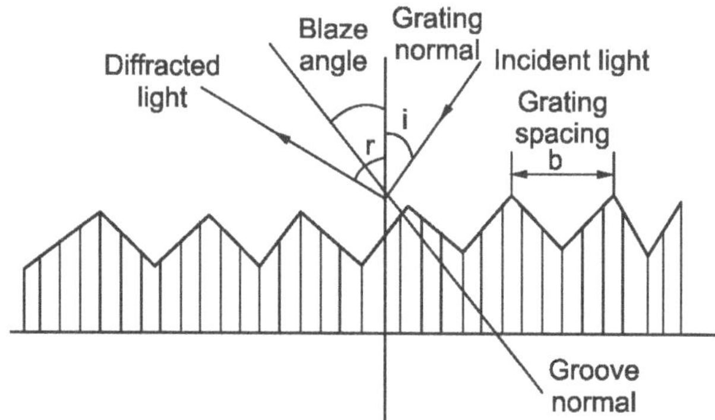

These gratings are replica made from master gratings, by coating the original master grating with epoxy resin and are removed after stetting. To make the surface reflective, a deposit of aluminium is made on the surface.

The mechanism is that diffraction produces reinforcement. The rays which are incident upon the grating gets reinforced with the reflected rays and hence the resulting radiation has wavelength which is governed by th equation.

$$m\lambda = b\,(\sin i \pm \sin r)$$

where λ = wavelength of light produced

b = grating spacing

i = angle of incidence

r = angle of reflection

m = order (0, 1, 2, 3 etc)

The band pass of these gratings are 0.1 nm, which means they are most efficient and hence gratings are preferred.

(ii) ***Transmission Grating*:** Transmission grating is similar to diffraction grating, but refraction takes place instead or reflection, refraction produces reinforcement. This occurs when radiation transmitted through grating reinforces with the partially refracted radiation.

The wavelength of radiation produced by transmission gratings can be expressed by the following equation.

$$\lambda = \frac{d\sin\theta}{m}$$

where λ = wavelength of radiation produced

d = 1/lines per cm

m = order no. (0, 1, 2, 3 etc)

θ = angle of deflection (or) diffraction

A light radiation at any angle θ or any order can be collected and used in the instrument by either moving the grating and fixing the slit or moving the slit and keeping the grating constant.

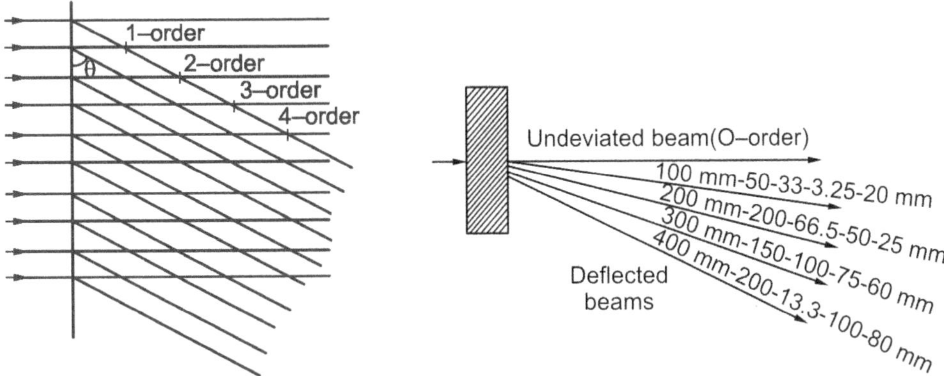

3. Detector

The radiation emitted by the element is mostly in the visible region. Hence conventional detectors like photovoltaic cell (or) phototubes can be used. In a flame spectrophotometer, photomultiplier tube is used as detector.

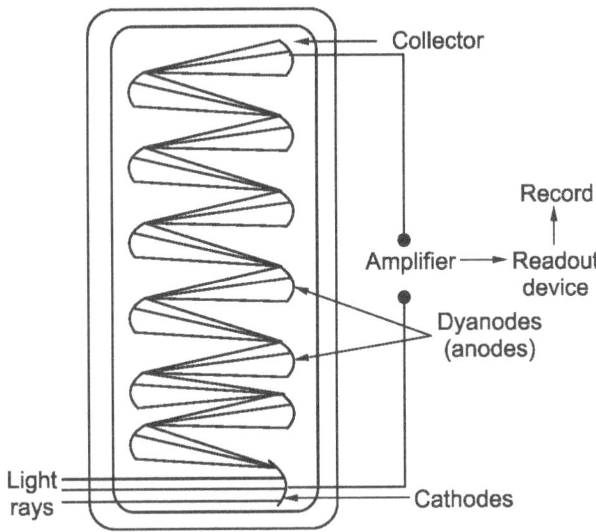

Photomultiplier Tubes (PMT)

This type of detector is the most sensitive of all the detectors expensive and used in sophisticated instruments. The principle employed in this detector is that, multiplication of photoelectrons by secondary emission of electrons. This is achieved by using a photo cathode and a series of anodes (dyanodes). Upto 10 dyanodes are used each dyanode is maintained at 75-100 V higher than the preceding one. At each stage the electron emission is multiplied by a factor of 9 or 5 due to secondary emission of electrons and hence an overall factor of 10^6 is achieved.

PMT can detect very weak signals, even 200 times weaker than that could be done using photo-voltaic cell. Hence it is useful in fluorescence measurements. PMT should be shielded from stray light in order to have accurate results.

4. Readout Device

The signal from the detector is shown as response in the digital readout device. The readings are displayed in an arbitrary scale (% Flame intensity)

There are two types of flame photometers that are used in flame emission spectroscopy (FES), namely:

(a) Simple Flame Photometer, and

(b) Internal Standard Flame Photometer

***Simple Flame Photometer*:** The line-sketch of a simple flame photometer is as follows.

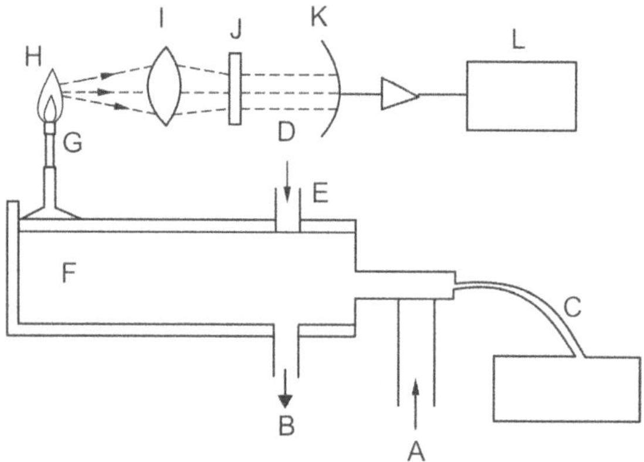

A = Inlet for compressed air

B = Drain outlet (to maintain constant pressure head in the mixing chamber)

C = Liquid sample (sucked into the Nebulizer)

D = Inlet for Fuel-Gas to the Laminar-Flow-burner

E = Nebulizer to atomize the liquid sample

F = Mixing chamber for Fuel gas, compressed air, and atomized liquid-sample

G = Burner

H = Flame

I = Convex lens

J = Optical filter to transmit only a strong line of the element, and

K = Photo cell

L = Amplifier to amplify the feeble electrical impulse and a building direct readout device.

In general, Flame photometers are designed and intended mainly for carrying out the array of elements like : Sodium, Potassium, Calcium and Lithium that possess the ability to give out an easily excited flame spectrum having sufficient intensity for rapid detection by a photocell.

Procedure

The compressed and filtered air (A) is first introduced into a Nebulizer (E) which creates a negative pressure (Suction) enabling the liquid sample (C) to gain entry into the atomizer (E). Thus, it mixes with the stream of air as a fine droplet (mist) which goes into the burner (G). The fuel gas (D) introduced into the mixing chambers (F) at a given pressure gets in touch with the air and the mixture is ignited. Consequently, the radiation from the resulting flame (H) is made to pass through a convex lens (I) and ultimately an optical filter (J) that allows specifically the radiation characteristic of the element under examination to pass through the photocell (K). Finally the output, from the photocell is adequately amplified (L) and subsequently measured on an appropriate sensitive digital-read out device.

***Internal Standard Flame Photometer*:** The Layout of an internal standard flame photometer is illustrated as follows.

A = Inlet for compressed air

B = Inlet for Acetylene (Fuel-gas)

C = Liquid sample sucked in by an atomizer

D = Flame

E = Mirror

F = An optical filter to allow the transmission of only one strong line of the element.

G = Amplifier to amplify the weak electrical current

H = A null detector to record the intensity of the element under study and the internal standard (Lithium)

I = A calibrated potentiometer

J_1	=	Lines due to the 'sample'
J_2	=	Lines due to the internal standard 'Lithium' and
K_1 & K_2	=	Photocells to convert light energy to electrical impulse.

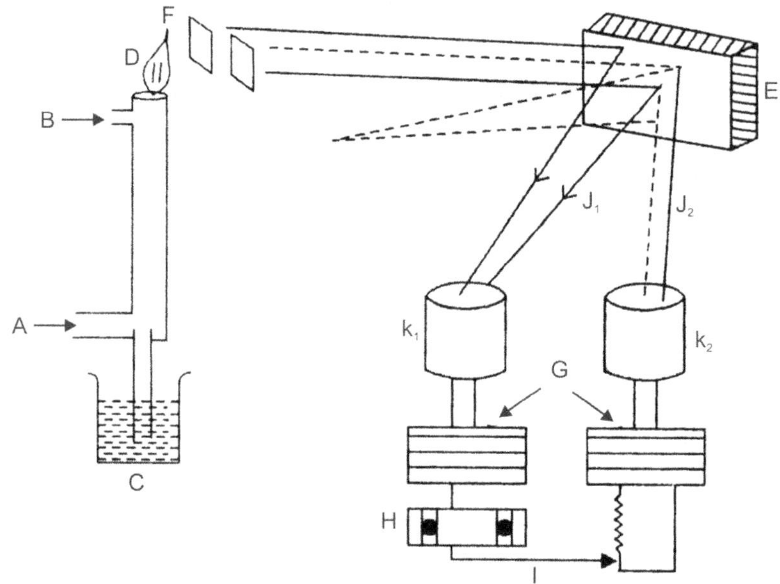

The use of an internal standard flame photometer not only eliminates the visible effects of momentary fluctuations in the flame characteristics produced by variation in either the oxidant or under full pressure, but also the errors caused due to differences in surface tension and in viscosity are minimized to a great extent.

Procedure

In this particular instance 'Lithium' is employed as an internal standard and an equal concentration is added simultaneously to the sample and the standard solutions. The sample (C) solution having the internal standard (Lithium) is sucked in by an atomizer and a fine spray is thereby introduced into the flame (D). The radiation thus emitted is subsequently passed through a filter (F) and then collected by a mirror (E). The emitted radiation reflected from the mirror is split up into two parts : The first part is caused due to the internal standard (Lithium), where as the second part arises due to the element under examination. Bothe these lines J_1 and J_2 are passed through the respective photocells K_1 and K_2 whereby the light energy is transformed into the electrical impulses. These electricl impulses are usually very weak and feeble and hence, they are duly amplified by a suitable amplifier (G) individually and are subsequently introduced into the common detecting device (H) i.e. a 'null detector' – so as to enable it to record the intensity of the element under investigation and also the internal standard (Lithium) accurately using a calibrated potentiometer (I).

In short, an internal standard flame photometer provides a direct and simultaneous result with respect to the ratio of intensities.

Pharmaceutical Applications of Flame Photometry

1. **Qualitative Analysis**

   Flame photometry is used to identify the elements in a given sample solution. This is done by a technique called as peak matching, where at least 3 peaks of emission spectrum should match when sample and standard spectra are recorded. For example, 'Ca' emits radiation at 422nm, 554nm and 626nm. If the spectrum of the sample shows emission maximum at these wavelengths, then the sample can be identified by using the standard.

2. **Quantitative analysis**

   Flame photometry is mostly used to determine the concentration of the elements belonging to group IA and group IIA elements. Most often, the concentration or the amount of elements like Li, Ca, Na or K in sample can be determined.

   The following are some of the quantitative applications:

   (a) Concentration of calcium in serum.

   (b) Concentration of Calcium, Sodium, Potassium in Urine.

   (c) Amount of Sodium, Potassium, Calcium and Magnesium in IV fluids, oral rehydration salts.

   (d) Assay of potassium chloride in syrup.

   (e) Concentration of Lithium in serum for therapeutic drug monitoring.

The concentration or the amount of elements can be determined by any one of the following methods:

(a) Direct curve method

(b) Calibration curve method

(c) Standard addition method

(d) Internal standard method

(a) ***Direct Comparison Method*****:** In this method, the % flame intensity (% F, I) of a standard solution and sample solution is compared. The merits of this method are less time is required for the estimation and more standards need not be prepared. The demerit is that, it is subject to more errors, especially when the concentration of the sample and the standard are in the non-linear region of calibration range.

Concentration of ion in sample solution

$$= \frac{\%\text{ F.I of sample}}{\%\text{ F.I standard}} \times \text{Conc.of ion in standard}$$

(b) ***Calibration Curve Method*****:** In this method, a series of standard solutions of the element to be estimated, is prepared and a calibration curve of concentration i.e. % F.I is mde. From this calibration curve, the concentration of sample solution is determined from its % F.I. The detailed procedure is as follows : (for determination of Sodium)

(i) Prepare a stock solution of Sodium Chloride solution (1000 μg/ml).

(ii) From the stock solution, prepare a series of standard solutions of Sodium (10, 20, 30, 40 and 50 μg/ml).

(iii) Select the Sodium filter in the instrument.

(iv) Set the air pressure of 0.4-0.5 kg/sq. cm and set the flame in the burner.

(v) Use distilled water (or demineralised water) and set to % F.I.

(vi) Set 100% F.I (or full scale in the instrument) by using the maximum concentration of standard solution in the calibration region (50 μg/ml).

(C) ***Standard Addition Method*****:** In this method, the region sample solution is divided into aliquots and to each, increasing concentrations of standard solution of the same element is added. The % E.I of sample solution as well as those of sample solution to which standard solutions where added were determined.

A calibration curve as shown in figure is constructed, with negative X-axis. The line when intrapolated, meets at the negative X-axis, which is the concentration of the ion present in the given sample solution.

Procedure

This method is used, when the interfering elements cannot be removed or difficult to be removed from the sample matrix. Standard addition method overcomes physical or anionic interferences, but cannot avoid cationic interference e.g. standard addition method is used in the estimation of Calcium in μg chloride for dialysis.

Let us assume that the concentration of calcium in the given sample is X μg/ml. Pipette out 5ml aliquots of sample solution into each of four 10 ml standard flames. To the flasks, add respectively 5 ml of 10 μg/ml, and 40 μg/ml of standard solution of calcium ions.

Determine the % F.I of sample solution (X μg/ml)as well as those of (X + 10 μg/ml), (X + 20 μg/ml), (X + 30 μg/ml) and (X + 40 μg/ml).

Plot a calibration curve as shown in figure. Intrapolate the line to meet negative X-axis (miorror image of X-axis) which is the concentration of the sample ion in the given sample solution.

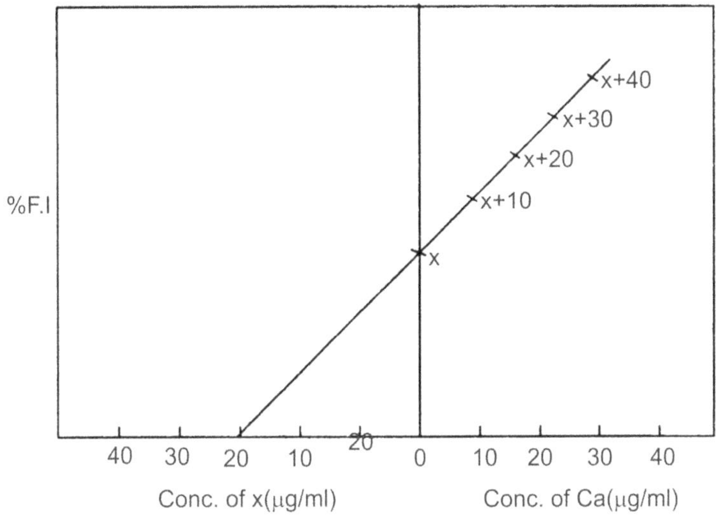

(d) *Internal Standard Method*: Internal standard method is used to avoid or minimise the errors due to fluctuations in the flame intensity, errors in atomising the sample solution due to high viscosity, etc.

In this method, a known concentration of a different element is added to standard solution as weel as to sample solution. The following example will illustrate the procedure adopted in internal standard method.

e.g. Estimation of Ca in unknown sample.

1. Add known concentrations of strontium to various standard solutions of Ca and to sample solution.
2. Measure the F.I of standard and sample at 227 nm for Ca 260 nm for strontium, simultaneously (since double flame photometer is used).

3. Plot a graph of conc. of Ca (Vs) $1_{227}/1_{260}$ for standard solution.
4. Concentration corresponding to 1227/1260 of sample is read from the graph.

A few typical examples of 'Flame-emission spectroscopy' are given.

Assay of Sodium, Potassium and Calcium in Blood Serum and Water

(i) ***Standard Potassium and sodium solutions, approximately 500 PPM*:** Weigh accurately 0.95 g of dried KCl and 1.25 g of dried NaCl into separate 1-litre volumetric flasks. Dissolve in water and dilute to the mark.

(ii) ***Standard Calcium solution, approximately 500 PPM*:** Weigh accurately 1.25 g of $CaCO_3$, which has been dried at 110^0 C into a 500 ml beaker. Add about 200 ml of distilled water and 10 ml of conc. HCL. Cover the beaker with a watch – glass during addition of acid to prevent loss of solution as CO_2 is evolved. After the solution is complete, transfer it quantitatively into a 1-litre volumetric flask and dilute to the mark with distilled water.

(iii) ***Radiation Buffer for Sodium determination*:** Prepare a saturated solution with reagent grade $CaCl_2$, KCl, $MgCl_2$ in that order.

(iv) ***Radiation buffer for Potassium determination*:** Prepare a saturated solution with reagent-grade NaCl, $Cacl_2$ and $MgCl_2$ in that order.

(v) ***Radiation buffer for Calcium determination*:** Prepare a saturated solution with reagent grade NaCl, KCl, $MgCl_2$ in that order.

Procedure

(a) ***Preparation of Working Curves*:** Transfer 5 mt of the appropriate radiation buffer to each series of 100 ml volumetric flasks. Add a volume of the standard solution which will cover a concentration ranging between 0-100 PPM. Dilute to 100 ml with distilled water and mix well, measure the emission intensity of these samples by taking at least three readings for each. Between each set of measurements, aspirate distilled water through the burner. Correct the average values for background luminosity and prepare a working curve from this data.

(b) ***Analysis of Blood Serum/Water Sample*:** Prepare aliquot portions of the sample as described in the above step. If necessary, use a standard to calibrate the response of the spectrometer to the working curve. Then measure the emission intensity for the unknown. After correcting the data for background, determine the concentration by comparison with the working curve.

Assay of Barium, Potassium and Sodium in Calcium Acetate

The technique of flame emission spectroscopy is used to determine the concentration of Ba, K and Na ions by measuring the intensity of emission at a specific wavelength by the atomic vaour of the element generated from calcium acetate. i.e. by introducing its solution into a flame.

***For Emission Measurements*:** Introduce water into the atomic vapour generator, adjust the instrument reading to zero, introduce the most concentrated solution into the generator and adjust the sensitivity to give a suitable reading. Again introduce water or the prescribed solution into the generator and when the reading is constant readout, if necessary, to zero.

Method of Standard Addition

The various steps are as follows:

1. Place in each of not fewer than three similar graduated flasks equal volumes of the solution of the substance being examined, prepared as followed:
   (a) Prepare a 5% w/v solution and use $BaSO_4$ solution ASP* (Dissolve 1.778 g of $BaCl_2$ in sufficient water to produce 1000 ml. Dilute it with water so that 1 ml contains 1 mg of Ba), suitably diluted with water to prepare the standard solution.
   (b) Prepare a 1.25% w/v solution and use potassium solution ASP** (Dissolve 1.144 g of KCl, previously dried at 100^0 C to 105^0 C for 3 hrs. in sufficient water to produce 1000 ml (It contains 600 mg of K in 1 ml). Suitably dilute with water to produce the standard solution.
   (c) Prepare a 10% w/v solution and use sodium ASP** (Dissolve 0.5084 g of NaCl, previously dried at 100^0 to 105^0 for 3 hrs, in sufficient water to produce 1000 ml; It contains 200 mcg of Na in 1 ml). Suitably dilute with water, to prepare the standard solution.
2. Add to all but one of these flasks a measured quantity of the specified standard solution to produce a series of solutions containing increasing amounts of the element being determined.
3. Dilute the contents of each flask to the required volume with water.
4. After havin calibrated the instrument as directed above, introduce each solution into the generator three times and record the steady reading. If the generator is a flame, wash the apparatus thoroughly with water. If a furnace is used, fire it after each introduction.
5. Plot the mean of the readings against concentration on a graph. The axes of which intersect at zero added element and zero reading.

6. Extrapolate the straight line joining until it meets the extrapolated concentration axis. The difference between this point and intersection of the axes represents the concentration of the element (e.g. Mg, K, Na) being determined in the solution of the substance being examined.

Limits of Elements Present in Calcium Acetate Sample

Mg : Not more than 500 PPM of mg

K : Not more than 0.1% of K and

Na : Not more than 0.5 5% of Na

Special Applications

1. **Waters**

   Water usually contains Ca, Fe, Mg, Si, sodium and sometimes Al and K in the form of bicarbonates, chlorides, hydroxides, nitrates and sulphates. Small amounts of nickel, strontium are also present in sea water. Industrial wastes have been found to contain elements peculiar to the plant operation. Because of very low concentration of most of the components, the analysis of fresh water by flame spectrometry is very difficult and that is why, a prior concentration step is needed.

   The cations are usually isolated by making use of cation exchange results and then eluted with o.2 N HCl.

2. **Glasses**

   The sodium and potassium contents in glass melt have successfully been determined by 'Williums' and 'Adams' in 1956.

   Aluminium can be extracted as tetra alkyl boron tetrafluoride complex.

3. **Cements**

   The presence or absence of certain elements greatly affects the quality of cement.

   For the determination of sodium (Na_2O) and potassium (K_2O), the cement samples are compared against a series of standards containing 630 μg/ml of CaO in 5 : 95 HCl. This method can be also be used for Mn and Li. A mixed series of standards, also containing the same quantities of CaO and HCl is used to prepare the working curve. 'Li' cannot be determined by internal standard method, because it is a constituent of the cement. Flame photometry may, however, be used for the separate determination of Li, along with other alkali metals.

   In order to eliminate the effects of sulphate, Silica, Al and Ca compensatory standards are necessary for the determination of Mg and Sr.

4. Biological Fluids and Tissues

The speed and sensitivity of flame spectrometry is ideally suitable for problems in biology and medicine e.g. Na and K^+ in minute quantities in biological fluids can be determined.

Flame spectrometry provides the first insight into the incidence of pathological disturbances.

In determination of potassium, cool air gas flames are preferred, because of minimum ionisation. The amount of potassium present in most body fluids is less than sodium and hence a series of standards of potassium are prepared with a fixed amount of sodium in each series. Readings on both elements are then taken and estimation of potassium is then carried out by working curve for potassium corresponding to the content of sodium found.

5. Petroleum Products

Flame spectrometry has also been used in the determination of tetramethyl lead (TEL) and manganese in gasoline stocks accurately by Gilbert (1951) and Smith (1955) respectively. In order to avoid evaporation losses, speed is necessary in handling the gasoline samples. The Mn samples can be compared against a standard calibration curve, if the sample is very dilute.

Metal additives in lubricating oils can be determined by making use of flame photometry by diluting known amount of the unknown sample with an organic solvent and than atomizing the mixture into a suitable flame.

For example: For the determination of 'B', a suitable solvent is 1 : 1 clears naphtha (or benzene) – isopropyl alcohol. The standards used for Li, K, Ca, Sr, Ba are metal (Lead or Mn) naphthenates.

6. Metallurgical Products

Flame emission spectroscopy has also been applied with some success to the analysis of metallurgical products.

For example: Alkali and alkaline earth metals are determined in a number of metallurgical products, catalysts, alloys and high purity metals.

7. Agronomic Materials

FES can be used rapidly and accurately for the determination of Sodium and Potassium in agronomy. Calcium and Mg can also be determined but only after removing or separating interferants.

Interference and Remedies

Although flame photometry is simple in operation, it has some demerits due to various types of interferences.

The radiation intensity may not accurately represent the sample concentration because of the presence of other materials in the sample. These materials result in an interference in the analytical procedure. It is only through adequate control of this interference that flame photometry would provide good analytical results. Following are the more commonly encountered interference processes in flame photometry.

1. **Background absorption**

   This occurs due to the sample matrix, flame itself, scattering, absorption by similar alkali halides etc.

   Remedy : Use of gratings will avoid or minimise these interferences.

2. **Spectral line Interferences**

   The first type of special interference arise when two elements or compounds may exhibit different spectra but their spectra may partly overlap and both are emitting at some particular wavelength in this case, the detector cannot make distinction between the sources of radiation and will record the total signal. Thus an incorrect answer will be obtained. This type of interference is more common at high flame temperatures because numerous spectral lines are produced at high temperatures.

   Atomic line interference, occurs due to the presence of other cations, which can emit radiation in the same region of emission by that of the element under analysis. This is also called as cation-cation interference (or) molecular spectral interference.

   ***For example*:**

   (a) Orange band of Ca – 593-622 nm interference with Na doublet 589 and 589.6 nm and Ba line at 553.6 nm

   Iron 329.7 nm interferes with copper 324.8 nm.

   (b) Aluminium interferes with emission of Ca and Mg.

   (c) Na and K mixtures interfere with each other.

   Remedy

   1. Extraction of interfering material.
   2. Calibration curve of interfering material
   3. Use of gratings instead of prisms/filters

3. **Vapourisation Interference**

   Chemical type, which occurs due to presence of some acids, by affecting the dissociation with other metals.

   Physical type, due to high viscosity e.g. Dextrose, Sucrose (interference with atomisation)

   ***Overcome by*:**

1. Choice of flames, burners, atomisers and additives.
2. **Additives**

Releasing agents: Add few PPM of Lanthalium / Strontium as ionisation suppressant to overcome interference due to PO_4.

***Chelation/Masking*:** Add EDTA to mask Ca in the presence of PO4 (cation-anion interference).

4. **Ionisation Interference**

More ionisation depopulates neutral atoms both in ground state and excited state. Hence it decreases the sensitivity of the method.

***Remedy*:** Add excess of easily ionisable ions like K, Cs, Strontium excited state, hence it decreases the sensitivity of the method.

***Remedy*:** Add excess of easily ionisable ions like K, Ca, Sr, as suppressants to the sample and standard solution (100-1000 μg/ml). These have lower ionisation potential (< 7.5 eV), and hence they are preferentially ionised over the elements to be analysed.

Factors that influence the Intensity of emitted Radiation in a Flame Photometer

A number of factors will influence the intensity of light emission from a given solution. Some of these are as follows :

(a) ***Viscosity*:** The addition of a substance which increases the viscosity of the solution (e.g. Sucrose) decreases the intensity of light emission. This decrease results in due to a reduction in the efficiency of atomization.

(b) ***Presence of Acids*:** When an acid is present in the sample solution, this decreases the light intensity. This decrease arises due to the disturbance of the initial dissociation equilibrium.

(c) ***Presence of Other Metals*:** If other metals are present, these also alter the intensity of emitted radiation. In order to remove this defect, special filters are used which will absorb radiation due to the element which is to be emitted in the sample solution.

Limitations of Flame Photometry

(i) Although flame photometry is a means of determining the total metal content present in a sample, it does not provide information about the molecular form of the metal present in the original sample.

(ii) Flame photometry cannot be used for the direct detection as well as for the determination of the inert gases.

(iii) Only liquid samples may be used. In some cases, lengthy steps are necessary to prepare liquid samples.

(iv) Flame photometry cannot be used for the direct determination of all metal atoms. There is a limitation on the number of elements that can be analysed by this method.

CHAPTER 15

MASS SPECTROSCOPY

Introduction

Mass spectrometry has been described as the smallest scale in the world, not because of its size but because of the size of the things it weighs.

Mass spectrometry, also called Mass Spectroscopy, is an instrumental approach that allows for the Mass measurement of molecules. In this technique, the sample is converted into rapidly moving positive ions and ion fragments by bombardment of compound to be investigated, the ions are then separated and characterised. Hence the mass spectroscopy deals with the study of the charged molecules and fragment ions produced from a sample exposed to ionising conditions and also of the relative intensity spectrum which results from the correlation of the ions with their mass to charge ratio (mass number) m/e.

The five basic parts of any mass spectrometer are a vacuum system, a sample introduction device, an ionisation source, a mass analyser, and an ion detector. Combining these parts, a mass spectrometer determines the molecular weight of chemical compounds by ionising, separating and measuring molecular ions according to their mass to charge ratio.

The ions are generated in the ionisation source by inducing either the loss or the gain of the charge (e.g. electron election, protonation or deprotonation). Once the ions are formed in the gas phase they can be electrostatically directed into a mass analyser, separated according to mass and finally detected. The result of ionisation, ion separation, detection is a mass spectrum that can provide molecular weight or even structural information.

Mass spectrometers have become pivotal for a wide range of applications in the analysis of inorganic, organic and bio-organic chemicals, Examples include:

- dating or geological samples
- drug testing and drug discovery
- Process monitoring in the petroleum, chemical and pharmaceutical industries.
- Surface analysis and structural identification of unknown.

Further, mass spectrometry identification of unknown and has recently had significant advances in its application to molecular biology, where it is now possible to analyse proteins, DNA and even viruses.

History of Mass Spectrometry

Today's mass spectrometer is based on the chemical work performed by Sir J.J. Thomson of the Cavendish Laboratory of the university of Cambridge. Thomson's research which led to the discovery of the electron in 1897, also led to the first mass spectrometer while he was measuring the effects of electric and magnetic fields on ions generated by residual gases in cathode ray tubes. Thomson noticed that the ions move through parabolic trajectories proportional to their "Mass to Charge" ratios.

The time period from the late 1930's to the early 1970's was a time of great achievement in the field of mass spectrometry. By the end of the world war I, the work of Francis W. Aston and Arthur J. Dempster brought improved higher accuracy mass spectrometers into reality. Later, Alfred Neir incorporated these developments along with the advances in vacuum technology and electronics to greatly decrease the size of mass spectrometers.

In 1946, William E. Stephens proposed the concept of time-of-flight analysers, which also separated ions by measuring velocities as the ions move in a straight path towards a collector. The other analyser in use today. The quadrupole analyser, was developed in the mid-1950's by Woltgang Paul. This analyser is capable of separating ions with an oscillating electrical field further increasing the utility of mass spectrometers. Another Paul innovation was the quadrupole ion trap, which is a device specially designed to trap and measure ions.

Two techniques developed in the mid 1980's electrospray ionisation (ESI) and matrix assisted laser desorption/ionisation (MALDI), have had a significant impact on the capabilities of mass spectrometry. ESI is the production of highly charged droplets that are treated with dry gas or heat to facilitate evaporation, which eventually eject the ions in the gas phase. ESI was first conceived by Malcolm Dole in the 1960's yet, by incorporating technology that has become available over the years, John Fenn put ESI into use for biomolecule analysis in the 1980's. MALDI was developed by Tanaka etal. (Japan) as well as by Franj Hillenkamp and Michael molecules from a solid or liquid matrix containing a highly UV-absorbing substance.

Both ESI and MALDI have allowed for sophisticated applications of mass spectrometry to the fields of biology and medicine.

The limitations of mass spectrometry have yet to be defined as larger and more complex molecules are being successfully characterised.

Applications, that were once inconceivable are in wide use today include ; sequencing of peptides and proteins, studies of noncovalent complexes and immunological molecules, DNA sequencing and the analysis of intact viruses.

In the 1990's mass spectrometry hit the mainstream chemistry and bio-chemistry Laboratories with commercially available, high performance instruments.

Principle

The evolution of mass spectrometry has been marked by an over increasing demand for its application to problems of increasing difficulty such as biomolecule analysis and the coincidental development of computer technology. New developments in the technology have created a complex array of instruments, but the basic components of all mass spectrometersare essentially the same. These components may be best understood by tracing the ion's path through them. First, an ion source ionises the molecule of interest, then a mass analyser differentiate the ions according to their mass-to-charge ratio and finally, a detector measures the ions beam current. Each of these elements exist in many forms and is combined to produce a wide variety of mass spectrometers with specialized characteristics.

Mass spectra is also called a positive ion spectra or line spectra. Unlike other kinds of spectroscopy, we do not use any electromagnetic radiation for excitation, and there is no ground or excited state. In this electron bombardment is used to convert a neutral molecule to a positive charged one.

The basic principles on which mass spectrometry is based comprises the following:

(i) A substance in the gaseous or vapour state when subjected to high voltage electric current is made to lose electrons and form positively charged ions (cations) i.e. a beam of cations from the specimen is generated.

(ii) These ions can be deflected by means of magnetic (or) electrical fields.

(iii) The deflection of the ions will depend on their mass, charge and velocity i.e. a spectrum according to mass to charge ratios of ions is produced.

(iv) Consequently their abundances and relative masses can be recorded.

Machanism of Cation Production

An electron impact technique is utilised to produce ions. The sample in the vaporised condition is introduced under low pressure into a tube called ion source where the entering molecules are bombarded with a beam of electrons emitted from a hot tungsten or rhenium wire. If the energy of the bombarding electrons is less than the ionisation potential of the sample molecules (about 10 eV in organic molecules) no change takes place in the molecules.

When the energy of the bombarding electrons is increased just above the ionisation potential, possibility increases that there will be a collision between sample and electron.

The molecular ion is called parent ion and is usually designated as M^+, it is positively charged with an unpaired electron.

$$M + e^+ \rightarrow M^+ + 2e^-$$

e.g. $$CH_3 - OH + e^- \rightarrow CH_3 - OH^+ + 2e^-$$

The ion produced is a radical cation. However, If the energy of the bombarding electron is further increased, some of their excess energy will be transferred to the molecular ions which will bring further fragmentation of the sample molecules.

The electrical potential of the bombarding electrons which is just high enough to initiate fragmentation is called appearance potential. The magnitude of the appearance potential is equal to or greater than the sum of the dissociation energy of the fragmented bond and the ionisation. When the bombarding electrons have a very high energy, more than one bond in the molecule can be broken.

In actual practice, a voltage of 70 eV is used to accelerate the electrons so that there is enough energy to break and bond in the sample molecules.

The set of ions (fragment ions or daughter ions) are analysed in such a way that a signal is obtained for each value of m/e that is represented.

The intensity of each signal represents the relative abundance of the ion producing the signal.

The largest peak in the structure is called the base peak and its intensity is taken as 100. The intensities of other peaks are represented relative to the base peak.

Theory

The m/e value of the parent ion is equal to the molecular mass of the compound. In few cases, the parent ion peak may be the base peak and can be easily recognised. In most of the cases, parent ion peak is not the base peak and is often of very small abundance.

The molecular ion peak may not be confused with the base peak. The base peak has 100% abundance. Mass spectrum of a compound is a plot which represents the intensities of the signals at various m/e values. It is highly characteristic of a compound. No two compounds can have exactly similar mass spectra. A single mass spectrum is equivalent to dozens of physical properties of that compound for revealing the structure.

Consider a molecule M, which is bombarded with a beam of electrons. This is ionised as follows :

$$M^+ e^- \rightarrow M+ + 2e^-$$

M^+ is an ionised molecule

e^- is an electron

The ions are then accelerated in an electric field at voltage V. If this is the condition, the energy given to each particle is eV and this is equal to the kinetic energy which is equal to ½ m^2.

$$\frac{1}{2}m^2 = eV \quad \text{..... (i)}$$

$$v^2 = \frac{2eV}{m}$$

$$V = \sqrt{\frac{2eV}{m}}$$

v = Velocity of the particle

m = Mass

e = The charge on an electron

V = The accelerating voltage

All the particles possess the same energy eV.

Also, the particles have the same energy eV.

As the value of 'm' varies from particle to particle the velocity 'v' also changes such that 1/2 mV^2 remains a constant.

For a particle of mass m_1 velocity V_1

$$\frac{1}{2}m_1V_1^2 = eV$$

Similarly for a particle of mass m_2, velocity V_2

$$\frac{1}{2}m_2V_2^2 = eV$$

For particles m_3, m_4 .... of velocities V_3, V_4....

$$\frac{1}{2}m_2V_3^2 = eV$$

From the above equations – we have

$$\frac{1}{2}m_1V_1^2 = \frac{1}{2}m_2v_2^2 = \frac{1}{2}m_2v_3^2 = \text{so on}$$

It follows that the velocity of different particles will vary, depending on the mass of the particles.

After the charged particles have been accelerated by an applied voltage, they enter a magnetic field H.

The field attracts the particles and they move in a circle around it. This attractive force, due to magnet is HeV, whereas the balancing centrifugal force of the particle is mv^2/r.

When the particle starts moving uniformly around the circular path, the two forces become equal i.e.

$$\frac{mv^2}{r} = HeV$$

$$\frac{1}{r} = \frac{HeV}{mv^2}$$

$$r = \frac{mV}{He}$$

r = radius of the circular path of the particle

$$r = \frac{m}{eH}\left(\frac{2eV}{m}\right)^{\frac{1}{2}} \qquad \left[\because V = \sqrt{\frac{2eV}{m}}\right]$$

On squaring both sides

$$r^2 = \frac{m^2}{e^2H^2} \cdot \frac{2eV}{m}$$

$$r^2 = \frac{m}{e} \cdot \frac{2V}{H^2}$$

$$r = \left[\left(\frac{2V}{H^2}\right) \cdot \left(\frac{m}{e}\right)\right]^{\frac{1}{2}}$$

$$\therefore \qquad \frac{m}{e} = \frac{H^2r^2}{2v}$$

From these equations it follows that the radius of the circular path of particules depends on the accelerating voltage V, the magnetic field H, and the ratio m/e.

As e, v, and H are constant,

It means that the radius of the ionised molecule depends on m, its mass.

$$r = \left[\left(\frac{2V}{H^2}\right) \cdot \left(\frac{m}{e}\right)\right]^{\frac{1}{2}}$$

It is basis of separation of particles according to their masses.

Based on the theory, the mass spectrometer is designed to perform three basic functions.

(i) To vaporise compounds of varying volatility.

(ii) To produce ions from the neutral compounds in the vapour phase.

(iii) The separate ions according to their mass over charge ratio and to record them.

The plot of m/e values taken along abscissa and their relative intensities along the ordinate is called the mass spectrum.

Fundamental Aspects of Mass Spectroscopy

(a) ***The Sample*:** If organic, the sample must have an obtainable vapour pressure of atleast 10^{-7} mm Hg. In general the higher the vapour pressure, the more easily the mass spectrum is obtained.

(b) ***Ions*:** Ions must be prepared from the sample molecules. Ionisation is usually affected by electron bombardment of the sample vapour. The electrons possess sufficient energy (50-100 eV) to induce rupture of any bond which might be present in the molecule.

(c) ***Positive ions*:** The positive ions are more analysed. The positive ions are used because of the fact that they are usually more abundant than the negative ions by factor 102-104.

Ion mass analysis is accomplished by injecting the positive ions into a magnetic field where they will assume a circular path whose radius is determined by m/e ratio.

It is common to use the word ‘mass’ when referring an ion rather than the more current mass / charge ratio, because of the fact that singly charged ions predominate.

(d) ***The mass spectrum*:** The mass spectrum is magnetically scanned by varying the magnetic field in a precise manner, causing the mass separated ion beams to impinge upon a collector electrode in order of mass sequence. The ions are usually bent through an angle of 60^0, 90^0 or 180^0.

(e) ***Electrostatic scanning*:** In which the magnetic field strength is held constant and the energy of the injected ions is varied in a controlled manner, has also been used.

(f) ***Mass analysis*:** Mass analysis can also be accomplished by injecting the ions into a linear drift region, which is free of all electric and magnetic fields. The velocity of the ions is proportional to their mass and a usable mass separation is after the ions have flown for a distance of 30 cm or more.

(g) ***The mass spectrum*:** The mass spectrum usually consists of a role of chart paper of varying length depending upon the length of mass range scanned. Galvanometers and photosensitive paper or common pen and ink recorders have been used to produce the record. The choice depends upon the rapidity by which one wishes to scan the spectrum. In sone instruments the mass spectral recording is produced by allowing the mass separated ions beam to stike an emulsion of a glass photographic plate placed within the vacuum system of mass spectrometer. Subsequent photographic development of the plate provides a permanent recording of mass spectrum.

A strip chart recording may also be prepared from photographic plate by passing it through a recording densitometer. It is, however, more convenient to record the mass spectrum on magnetic tapes.

Components of Mass Spectrometer

A mass spectrometer is an instrument that is used for the determination of constitution of materials. The main spectrometers used for the investigation of any compound may vary in their types but all contain components to perform the following functions :-

1. Ionisation of the sample.
2. Acceleration of the ions by an electric field.
3. Dispersion of the ions according to their mass to charge ratio.
4. Detection of the ions and production of a corresponding electric signal.

To perform the above functions all mass spectrometers generally contain the following components:

1. The inlet system (or) sample handling system for sample introduction

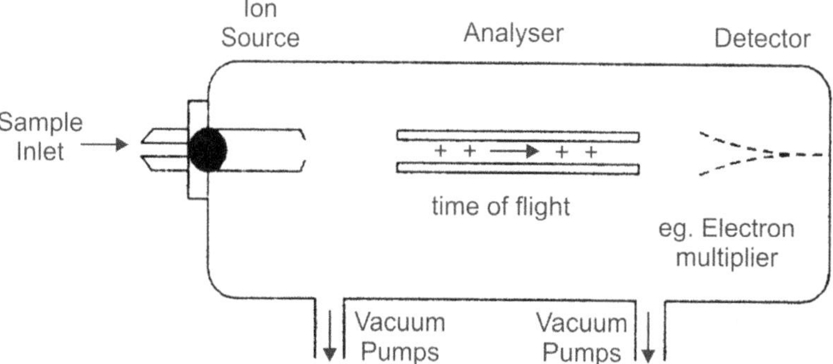

Components of a Mass Spectrometer

2. The ion source (or) ionisation chamber
3. The electrostatic accelerating system.
4. The ion separator (or) mass analyser
5. The ion collector (the detector and read out system).

Components of a Mass Spectrometer

1. Sample introduction (or) Sample handling System

Mass spectrometers are extremely sensitive instruments and only very small amounts of the sample are needed. A sample size of about 1μ mole is required.

As a mass spectrometer should have a vapour sample and to ensure that the sample enters the ionisation chamber at a constant rate, the sample is converted into gaseous state in the inlet system. To achieve this the inlet system is usually heated.

The sample inlet is the interface between the sample and the mass spectrometer.

The rate at which the sample is introduced into an ionisation chamber must remain constant so that the relative abundances of different species in mass spectrum can be determined.

There are a number of methods for introducing sample into the ionisation source, the choice depending upon the physical properties such as melting and boiling points. So to handle different types of materials, different inlet sample systems are employed.

***Gases*:** If the sample is a gas or a volatile liquid, it is best handled by allowing it to diffuse into a previously evacuated glass or metal bulb which communicates with the ion source via a tiny orifice, called pinhole or molecular leak. Most gases are introduced from a 1-5 lit reservoir into an evacuated volume contained between valves in the inlet system. The pressure of the sample in the reservoir should be about 1-2 orders of magnitude greater than that within ionisation chamber to maintain a steady flow through the pin hole into the chamber. A volume of 1-2 cm^3 is frequently used, although much smaller volumes can be employed. A 'leak' of sintered glass or metal maintains a constant flow of sample into the ion source which is at much lower pressure than the sample. i.e. ranges from 30 to 50 torr. Gas inlet systems may be either cold or heated. Gaseous samples are thus readily handled by expansion of a small volume into an expansion reservoir of large volume, upto 5 litres. The pressure ranges from 10^{-3} to 10^{-1} torr. The pinhole has a diameter of about 0.013 to 0.050 mm in a gold foil.

***Liquids*:** Liquids are handled by hypodermic needle injection through a silicone rubber dam. Boiling below 150°C is required for liquids, a suitable quantity of the sample is evaporated into an evacuated reservoir at room temperature and the vapour is expanded into the reservoir. If the sample is less volatile and thermally stable, the sample and reservoir may be heated. As the reservoir has low pressure, it draws liquid immediately and vaporises instantly.

***Solids*:** For metals and semiconductors, a spark source is used by making use of some special equipment. Organic solids that cannot be handled as vapours are introduced directly into the source by means of a probe which is a stainless steel rod, 6 mm in diameter and 25 cm long, bearing a cup at its top to hold the sample.

There are two approaches for introducing sample.

(a) ***Direct insertion technique*:** One approach to introducing sample is by placing a sample on a probe which is then inserted, usually through a vacuum lock, into the ionisation region of the mass spectrometer. The sample can then be heated to facilitate thermal desorption or undrgo any number of high energy desorption processes used to achieve vaporization and ionisation.

(b) ***Capillary infusion*:** Capillary infusion is often used because it can efficiently introduce small quantities of a sample into a mass spectrometer without destroying the vacuum. Capillary columns are routinely used to interface the ionisation source of a mass spectrometer with other separation techniques, including Gas Chromatography (GC), Liquid chromatography (LC).

Gas chromatography and liquid chromatography can serve to separate a solution into its different components prior to mass analysis. When mass spectrometry is used as a detector for these chromatography techniques the extra information that mass analysis provides can be very valuable for compound identification.

2. Ion Source (or) Ionisation Chamber

***Ionisation*:** Ionisation is the act of placing a charge on a neutral molecule.

From the inlet system, the sample is introduced into the ionisation chamber. In this chamber, a beam of electrons is put across the molecules of the samples. If the electron beam is moving slowly, the molecules remain intact, although ionised. If the electron beam is accelerated by a high voltage (upto 100 V) on the collector, the energy of the electrons will be increased. Then the collisions between electrons and molecules result in the production of well defined fragments. Each fragment carries a definite positive charge and moves through the instrument as a charged molecule.

***Note*:** There are chances that fragments may recombine to form such molecules which might not be present in the original sample. The recombination of the fragments can be avoided by maintaining the system at low pressure and thus decreasing the number of collisions between fragments of molecules inside the cell.

***Necessity for ionisation*:** Since gaseous ions can only be utilized by the mass analyser, hence analysis is effectively limited to samples that are either gases or have appreciable vapour pressure. Non volatile solids are first converted into gases by pyrolysis induced by intense thermal or electrical energy and then studied.

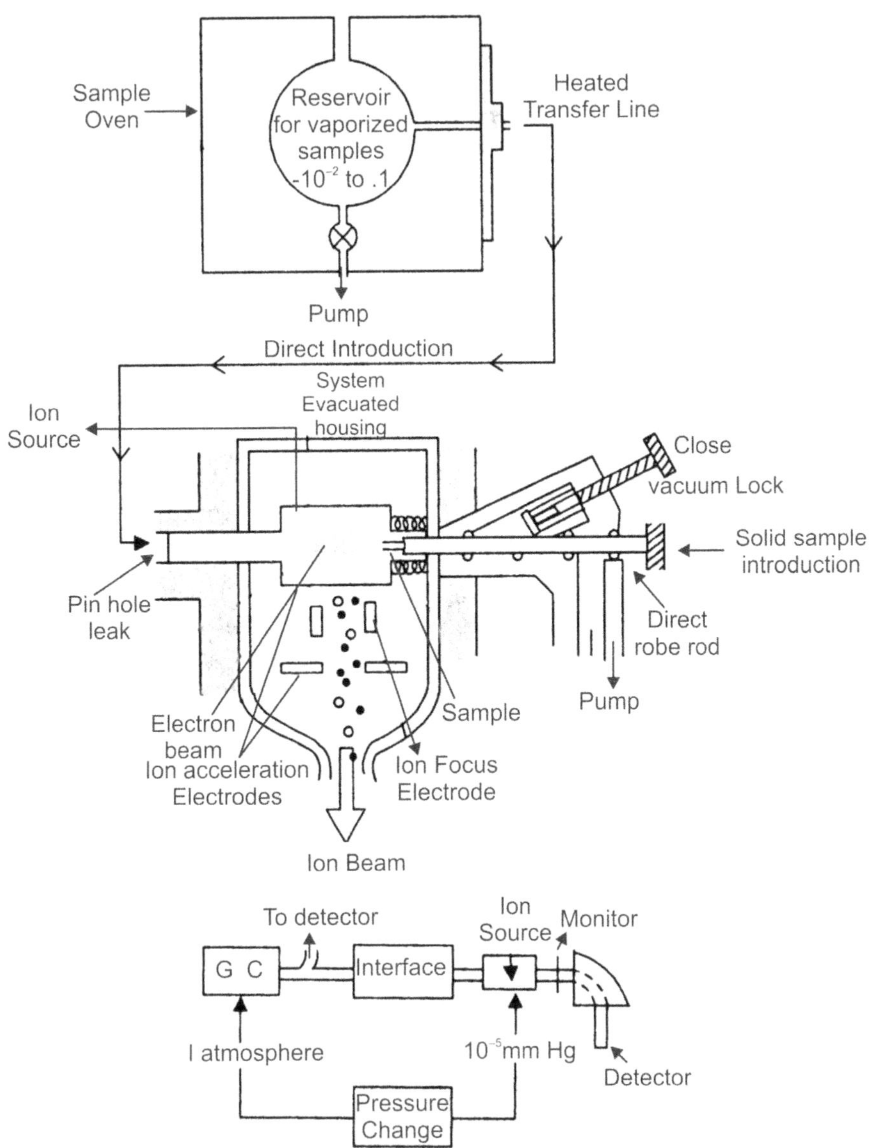

GC – MS Combination

Various ion sources are employed in mass spectrometers.

They are as follows :

(a) Electron ionisation (or) Electron Bombardment and Electron impact

Electron ionisation plays an important role in the routine analysis of small molecules. In fast, databases containing over 100,000 electron ionisation mass spectra are used daily by thousands of chemists. These data bases, combined with current computer storage capacity and searching algorithms, allow for rapid comparison with known mass spectra, thus facilitating the structural determination of small molecules.

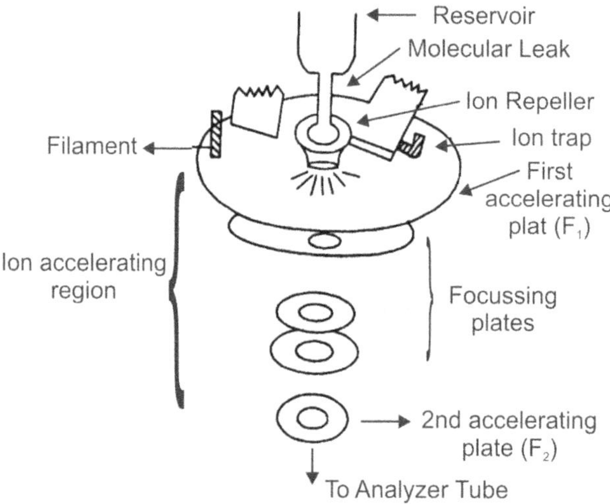

Components of Ion Source Mass Spectrometer

The vapourised sample is introduced under low pressure into the ion source tube and the sample molecules are bombarded with a beam of electrons emitted from a hot tungsten or rhenium wire.

An ion source contains:

(a) ion repellers

(b) acceleration plates

(c) ion focussing plates

A small electrostatic field is applied between the repeller electrode and the first accelerating plate so that ions generated are forced into the ion generating region. A potential of 1000-2000 volts is used to accelerate the ions through a slit system so that a narrow beam of fast moving ions is formed.

The electron ionisation technique is straight forward. The sample must be delivered as a gas which is usually accomplished by heating the sample to vaporize it off of the probe. Once in the gas phase, the compound passes into an electron of nearly homogenous energy (70 eV), typically causing electron ejection and some degree of fragmentation. Then these ions are withdrawn by the electric field which exists between the repeller plate and 1st accelerating plate then the focussing plate focus the ion beam and the 2nd accelerating plate gives a final acceleration to the ions.

The energy of the electron beam is controlled by the potential on anode (or) electron trap. If the energy of the electron beam is low, there occurs only the production of singly charged molecular ions, resulting in a mass spectrum having almost a single peak corresponding to the mass of the origin molecule.

$$M + e^- \rightarrow M^+ + 2e^-$$

If the energy of the electron beam is increased, this yields highly excited ion which may produce fragments if it is complex or may knock out the second electron.

$$M^+ + e^- \rightarrow M^{2+} + 2e^-$$

$$M^{2+} + e^- \rightarrow M^{3+} + 2e^-$$

Generally, the electron beam is given an energy in the range of 50.8 eV which gives the most reproducible results.

The potential between repeller plate and first accelerator plate is small and should be sufficient only to remove the positive ions from the electron beam. In this way, the positive ions will pass through slit with variable but small kinetic energy. Generally, most of acceleration is achieved between the 1st and 2nd acceleration electrodes which differ in potential from a hundred to thousand volts. In most spectrometers, the potential between the accelerator slits provides the means, whereby particle of a particular mass is focused on the collector.

At a given accelerating voltage, all singly charged ions possess the same kinetic energy defined by the following equations : -

$$\text{Kinetic energy} = \frac{1}{2}mv^2 = eV$$

$$V = \sqrt{2v.\frac{e}{m}}$$

m = mass of the ion

v = velocity

This indicates electrons move with velocities determined to a good degree of approximation by their charge to mass ratio e/m.

For accurate mass measurements, a monoenergentic beam of ions is required for the proper separation of the ions.

Electron ionization is most useful for compounds below a molecular weight of 400 Daltons since larger molecular tend to thermally degrade during ionization.

While Electron ionization is one of the most widely used methods of ionization in mass spectrometry, the principal problems associated with it include excessive fragmentation in the ionization source, the inviolability of large molecules and thermal decomposition during vaporization.

Electron ionization is principally used as a detector for gas chromatography (GC / Ms) in a wide variety of areas including synthetic organic chemistry, hydrocarbons analysis, pharmaceutical compounds and drugs of abuse (for example it is widely used in the Olympic drug testing program), and environmental studies such as water testing.

Disadvantages

1. The electron impact process is not efficient.
2. The sample should be in the vapour state.
3. All back ground gases also undergo ionisation with the same efficiency as the sample.
4. When the energy of the impinging electrons is decreased to a value near the ionization energy. It increases the molecular ion intensity but greatly reduces the absolute ion intensity.
5. Molecules which are unstable with respect to electrons impact, do not show molecular ion peaks in their mass spectra.

In order to overcome these defects, the following types of ion sources are also employed.

(b) ***Knudsen Cell*:** This cell is used for thermodynamic studies and for special analysis of solids and also for low vapour pressure liquids.

This cell employs the thermal and electron bombardment excitation. The sample is put into a crucible. On heating, the sample is vaporised through a small effusion orifice into mass spectrometer ion source, which is traversed by the electron beam.

The temperature is adjusted continuously ambient to 2500° C.

(c) ***Electro spray ionization*:** Electro spray ionization is the one of the most exciting ionization techniques to arrive. Electro spray ionization generates ions directly from solution (usually an aqueous or aqueous / organic solvent system) by creating a fine spray of highly charged droplets in the presence of a strong electron field (typically 3.5 kV).

As the droplet decreases in size, the electric charge density on its surface increases. The mutual repulsion between like charges on this surface becomes so great that it exceeds the forces of surface tension, and ions begin to leave the droplet through what is known as a "Taylor Cone". The ions are then electrostatically directed into the mass analyser. Vaporization of these charged droplets results in the production of single or multiple charged gaseous ions.

The number of charges retained by an analyte can depend on such factors as the composition and pH of the electrosprayed solvent as well as the chemical nature of the sample. For small molecules ($<$ 200 Daltons) ESI typically generates singly (or) doubly charged ions, while for large molecules ($>$ 2000 Daltons) the ESI process typically gives rise to a series of multiple – charged species. Because mass spectrometers measure the mass-to-charged ratio, the resultant ESI mass spectrum contains multiple peaks corresponding to the different charged states.

ESI allows for very sensitive analysis of small, large and labile molecules such as peptides, proteins, organometallics, oligosaccharides, and polymers.

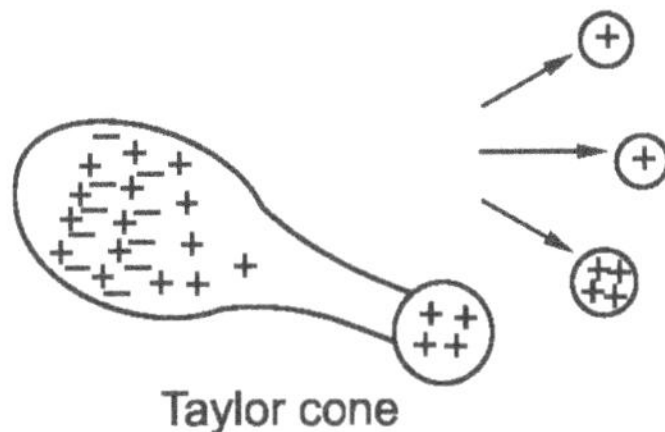

Another advantage of ESI-MS is that ions are formed directly from solution (usually in aqueous or aqueous/organic solvent system), a feature that has established the technique as a convenient mass detector for liquid chromatography also known as HPLC. While past attempts to couple LC with MS resulted in limited success. ESI has made liquid chromatography mass spectrometry routine, adding a new dimension to the capabilities of liquid chromatography characterization.

In fact, using electrospray ionisation mass spectroscopy as a detector or liquid chromatography was one of its obvious applications.

(d) ***Matrix-Assisted Laser Desorption/Ionization (MALDI)*****:** Matrix-assisted laser desorption / ionization mass spectrometry (MALDI-MS), first introduced in1988 by Tanaka and independently by Hillenkamp and karas, has become a wide spread analytical tool for peptides, proteins and most other bio-molecules (oligonucleotides, carbohydrates, natural products and lipids.)

The efficient and directed energy transfer during a Matrix-Assisted laser-induced desorption event provides high ion yields of the intact analyte, and allows for the measurement of compounds with high accuracy and sub-picomole sensitivity.

Examples of Matrices used in MALDI

MALDI provides for the non destructive vapourisation and ionization of both large and small bio-molecules.

In MALDI analysis, the analyte is first co-crystallized with a large molar excess of a matrix compound, usually a UV-absorbing weak organic acid, after which pulse vapourization of the matrix which carries the analyte with it. The matrix therefore plays a key role by strongly absorbing the laser light energy and causing, indirectly, the analyte to vaporize. The matrix also serves as a proton donor and receptor, acting to ionize the analyte in both positive and negative ionization modes, respectively.

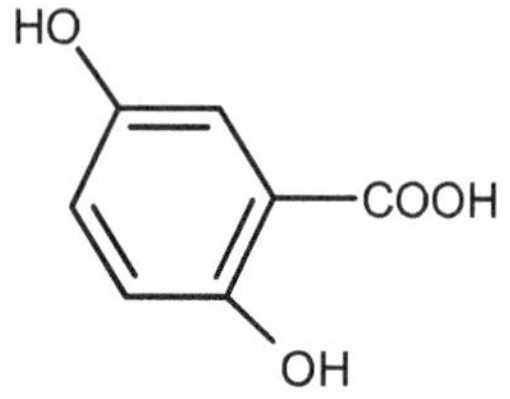

→ HO, COOH, OH

2, 5 dihydroxy
Benzoic acid

For peptides,
Small proteins
and oligonucleotides

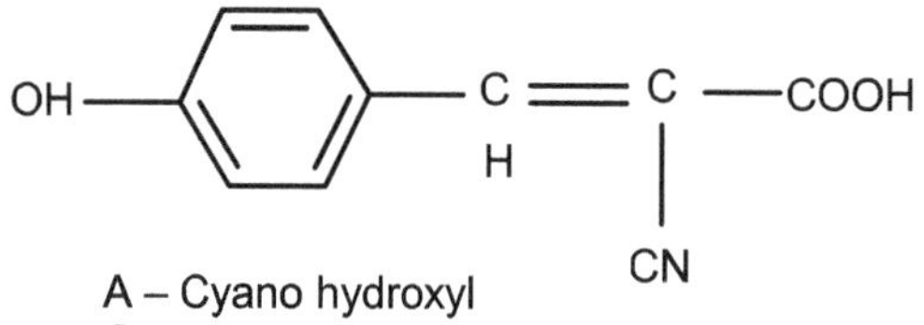

→ OH — C = C — COOH, H, CN

A – Cyano hydroxyl
Cinnamic acid

For peptides
and
glycopeptides

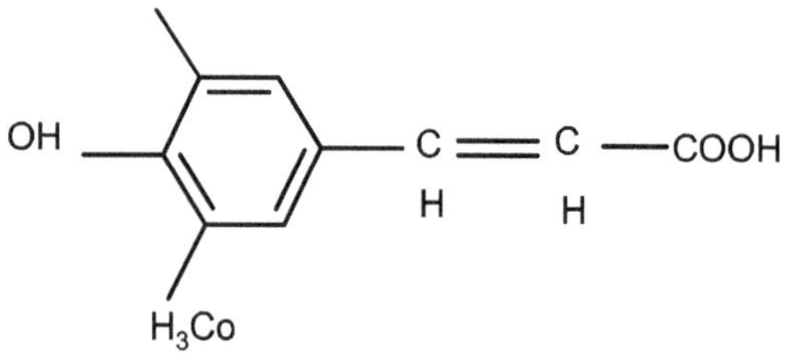

→ OH — C = C — COOH, H, H, H_3Co

3, 5 dimethoxy – 4 hydroxy
Cinnamic acid
(sinapinic acid)

For peptides
and Proteins

MALDI has had its biggest impact on the field of protein research. The ability to generate MALDI-MS data on whole proteins and proteolytic fragments is extremely useful for protein identification and characterization. For example, a protein can often be unambiguously identified by the accurate MALDI mass analysis of its constituent peptides (produced by either chemical or enzymatic treatment of the sample). As the human genome nears completion, it can be argued that the characterization of genomic proteins (a field of research also known as "proteomics") is the most important application of modern mass spectrometry.

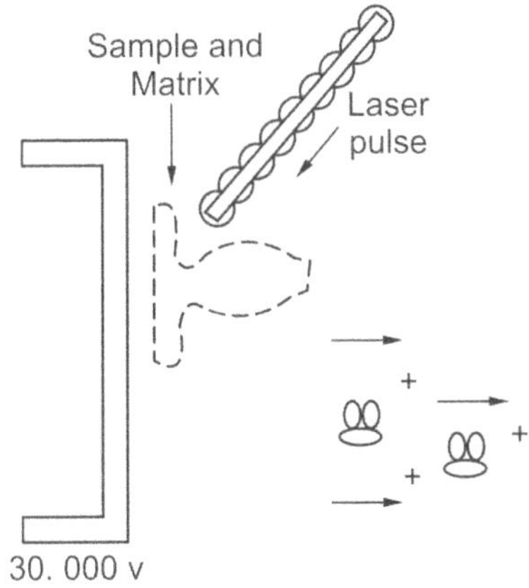

Formation of Ions by Mtrix Assisted Laser Desorption (MALDI)

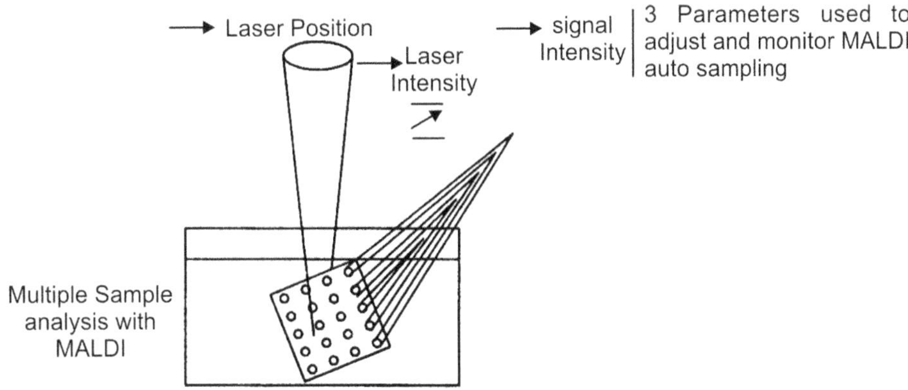

The MALDI Sample plate can be used for multi-sample preparation and automated sample analysis

(e) ***Atmospheric Pressure Chemical Ionisation (APCI)*:**

Similar to electrospray ionisation, liquid effluent is introduced directly into the Atmospheric Pressure Chemical ionization source, however the similarity with electrospray stops there.

The APCI source contains a heated vaporizer which facilitates rapid desolvation / vaporization of the droplets. Vaporised sample molecules are carried through an ion molecule reaction region at atmospheric pressure. The ionization occurs through a corona discharge, creating reagent ions from the solvent vapour. Chemical ionisation of sample molecules is very efficient at atmospheric pressure due to the high collision frequency. Proton transfer (protonation MH^+ reactions) occurs in the positive mode, and either electron transfer or proton transfer (proton loss, [M – H] -) in the negative mode. The moderating influence of the solvent clusters on the reagent ions, and of the high gas pressure, reduces fragmentation during ionization and results in primarily molecular ions.

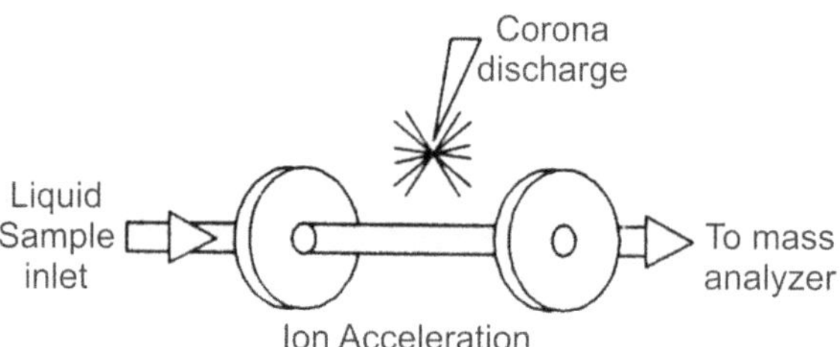

Atmospheric Pressure Chemical Ionization

APCI is widely used in the pharmaceutical industry to analysis relatively non-polar, semi-volatile samples of less than 1200 Daltons and it is an especially good ionization source for liquid chromatography.

(f) ***Surface Ionization*:** In this method, the solid sample to be studied by mass spectrometer is coated on a ribbon filament. When the filament is heated to 2000°C, there are chances that a positive ion may evaporate instead of a neutral molecule. This situation is expressed mathematically as follows :-

$$\frac{M}{M^2} \alpha \exp\left(\frac{1-W}{kT}\right)$$

I = Ionization potential of the sample material (non-volatile)

W = Work function of the ribbon (tungsten) filament

For conversion of neutral molecules into positively charged ions, the ionization potential of the sample material must be below the work function of the filament material.

This technique is very useful for such inorganic materials that possess low ionization potentials (3-6- eV). This method is superior because there is no ionization of the background gases in the mass spectrometer. This technique cannot be employed for organic compounds having ionization potentials of 7 – 16 eV.

In this, ions are produced directly.

(g) ***Spark source ionization***: In it a high voltage radio frequency is passed between electrodes one of which is made of the sample material or contains the sample.

In this method the inorganic substances to be analysed are formed into two electrodes held on small movable vises. When a potential (100 KV) is applied, and a discharge initiated, the positive ions are produced and evaporated. The energy spread of the positive ion beam is very broad and, therefore, it is controlled by the ion optics. In order to maintain adequate resolution, double focussing analysers are used.

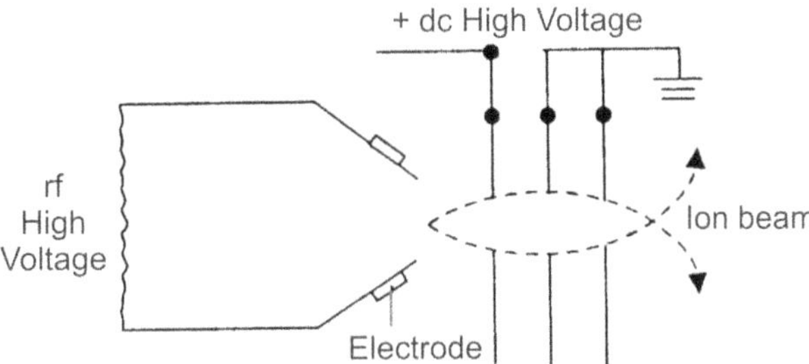

Advantages of Spark source ionization

1. Its detection sensitivity is very high.
2. It has non selectivity.

Its mass spectrum will exhibit all elements in the sample with the same detection sensitivity.

(h) ***Fast Atom Bombardment (FAB)***: This ionization technique is a soft ionization method that typically requires the use of a direct insertion probe for sample introduction and a high energy beam of xenon atoms or cesium ions to sputter the sample and matrix from the probe's surface. The matrix, such as m-nitrobenzyl alcohol, is used to dissolve the sample and facilitate dissorption as well as ionization.

The FAB matrix is a non volatile liquid materal that serves to constantly replenish the surface with new sample as the incident ion beam bombards this source. The matrix also serves to minimize sample damage from the high energy particle beam by absorbing most of the incident energy and the matrix is believed to facilitate the ionization process.

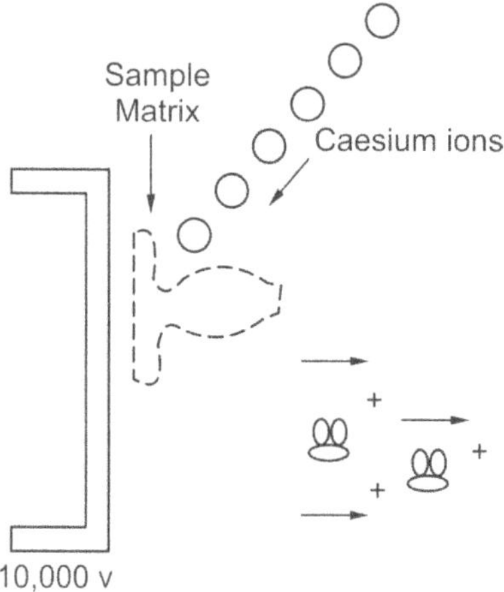

Fast Atom Bombardment

(i) ***Chemical Ionization*** **(CI):** In chemical ionization technique a reaction gas like methane is introduced along the sample to be analysed by mass spectrometer in the ionization chamber. The chemical ionization process is also initiated with a reagent gas such as isobutene or ammonia, which is initially ionized by electron ionization. When a beam of electrons is passed through the ionization, a high gas pressure in the ionization source results in the propagation of ion – molecule reactions between the reagent gas ions and reagent gas neutrals, i.e. the reaction gas undergoes ionization to produce ions which further react with neutral molecules to form products. The products so formed are chemical reactive species and some of these ions can interact with the sample molecules to form positive ions.

Chemical ionization is applied to samples similar to those analysed by electron ionization and is primarily used to enhance the abundance of the molecular ion. The Chemical ionization uses ion-molecule reactions in the gas phase to produce ions from the sample molecule.

(j) ***Inductivity Coupled Plasma Ionization (ICP)*****:** Inductively coupled plasma (ICP) is used in mass spectrometry as an ionization source where gaseous ions, the plasma, are produced by inductive coupling of high-frequency energy to a gas flow of argon. An aerosol of a nebulized analyte solution is injected into the center of the plasma where the aerosol droplets are vaporised and ionized. The plasma is operated in atmospheric pressure and then the elemental ions generated from the high energy ICP source are directed into the vacuum of the mass analyser for mass analysis.

ICP-MS has rapidly gained a significant role in elemental analysis. It is an important high-performance tool for many applications including materials science, environmental analysis, the electronic industry, nuclear technology, biology and medicine.

3. **Electrostatic Accelerating system**

The positive ions formed in the ionization chamber are withdrawn by the electric field which exists between the first accelerator plate and the second repeller plate. A strong electrostatic field between these plates is of 400-4000V accelerates the ions masses m_1, m_2, m_3 ... to their final velocities. The ions which escape through the slit consist of a collimated ribbon of ions having velocities and kinetic energies:

$$eV = \frac{1}{2}m_1v_1^2 = \frac{1}{2}m_2v_2^2 = \frac{1}{2}m_3v_3^2$$

Whenever the mass spectrometer is started to record the spectrum, the second accelerator is charged to an initial potential of 4000 volts. Then this charge is permitted to leak off to ground at a controlled rate over a period of 25 minutes.

4. **Mass Analyzers**

Immediately following ionization, gas phase ions enter a region of the mass spectrometer as the mass analyser. The analyser separates ions according to their masses. The mass analyser is used to separate ions within a selected range of m/e ratios.

The mass analyser must have the following characteristics : -

(i) It should have a high resolution.

(ii) It must have a high rate of transmission of ions.

The analyser is an important part of the instrument because of the role it plays in the instrument's accuracy and mass range. Ions are typically separated by magnetic fields, electric fields or by measuring the time it takes an ion to travel a fixed distance.

There are several possible ways of separating ions according to mass number. Based on the way they sort out the ions, mass spectrometers are differentiated.

(a) ***Signal focussing magnetic deflection*****:** In single focussing type of instruments, there is only one analyser sector and the dispersed ions arrive at the ion collector through a fine slit system at the end of the analyser tube. This is the most common type of separator.

It has a horse shoe shaped glass tube which is evacuated.

Sample in the form of vapour is allowed through sample inlet. This sample is bombarded with electron beam at 70eV. This knocks off one electron from every molecule. These molecules become positively charged, they are accelerated by accelerating plates which have also positive charge. These accelerated molecules travel in a straight path. Because of the application of either electric or magnetic field, they travel in curved path, when they travel in curved path, the positively charged molecular ions are separated according to their masses.

$$\left(\frac{m}{e} \alpha \, r^2\right)$$

The radius of the path depends upon their velocity and mass and also on field strength. Particles of different mass can be focussed on the exit slit by varying their velocity via the accelerating potential or the field.

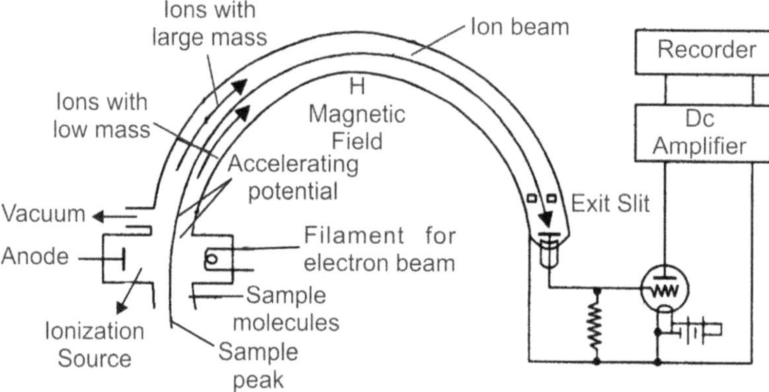

Single Focussing Mass Spectrometer (or) Magnetic Deflection Mass Spectrometer

Resolution is the important specification of mass spectrometer. The ability of a mass spectrometer to separate ions of different mass to charge ratio is called the resolving power.

There are two types of magnetic deflection mass spectrometers :

(a) ***Low Resolution*****:** Low resolution instruments are those that separate unit masses up to m/e 2000.

Unit mass or low resolution spectra are obtained from these instruments.

(b) ***High Resolution*****:** It can separate two ions differing in masses by atleast one part in 10,000 to 15,000. An instrument with 10,000 resolution is capable of separating on ion of mass 50,000 from one of mass 499.95.

This important class of mass spectrometer can measure the mass of an ion with sufficient accuracy to determine the atomic composition.

At a given accelerating voltage V, all the singly charged ions are given the same kinetic energy defined by the relation:

$$\text{Kinetic energy} = \frac{1}{2}mv^2 = eV$$

The charged particle possess a magnetic force in magnetic field H, is

$$F = HeV$$

It results in a circular trajectory radius from counter balancing centrifugal force.

$$He\,V = \frac{mv^2}{r}$$

$$r = \frac{mv^2}{HeV} \qquad \therefore r = \frac{mv}{He} \qquad .....(2)$$

H is magnetic field strength

A homogenous beam of ions diverging from a slit can be brought to focus by a magnetic field in a shape of sector and this forms the basis of the magnetic sector mass spectrometer.

In order, to focus the equation (2) indicates that they must have some or equal momentum mv.

$$\frac{m}{e} = \frac{H^2r^2}{2V} \qquad .....(3)$$

$$R = \frac{1}{H} = \frac{1}{H}\frac{\sqrt{2Vm}}{e} \qquad .....(4)$$

This equation indicates that every species of ion, characterised by a particular value of m/e will follow its own curve.

Although equation (3) pertains to ions, only those with a particular radii will be collected.

For most of the spectrometers, H and r are maintained fixed so that the mass particle which is colleced is inversely proportional to V.

(b) ***Double Focussing Magnetic Sector Mass Analyser*:** In order to improve resolution, single sector magenetic instruments have been replaced with double-sector instruments by combining the magnetic mass analyser with an electrostatic analyzer. i.e., the beam can also be rendered isoenergetic by means of an electrostatic sector.

According to equation $m/e = H^2r^2/2V$ all ions enter the magnetic field with the same kinetic energy i.e. all the ions with same m/e ratio should passess the same velocity. This is not quite correct because the ions vary in initial energy and therefore leave the electron beam with variable energies. So that the energy is reduced before the ions are allowed to enter the magnetic field, one can achieve much better focussing.

While passing through the annular space between two concentric electrodes, the beam of electrons assumes a circular trajectory.

The energy is determined from the relation,

$$\frac{1}{2}mv^2 = \frac{eEr}{2}$$

r = radius

E = applied field

Electric sector also called energy filter is used in conjunction with a magnetic sector, i.e. one that focuses the ions both in energy and in mass.

Electric sector acts as a kinetic energy filter allowing only ions of a particular kinetic energy to pass through its field, irrespective of their mass-to charge ratio. Given a radius of curvature R, and a field E, applied between two curved plates, the equation $R = 2V/E$ allows one to determine that only ions of energy V will be allowed to pass.

Thus the addition of an electric sector allows only ions of uniform kinetic energy to reach the detector, thereby increasing the resolution of the two-sector instrument to 100,000.

Magnetic double focussing instrumentation is commonly used with FAB and EI ionisation, however they are not widely used for electrospray and MALDI ionization sources primarily because of higher cost of these instruments.

There are two double focus designs:

1. **Nier Johnson Design**

   It makes use of 90° sectors with an intermediate slit.

2. **Mattauch Herzog Geometry**

   It makes use of an electric sector with an angle of 31°50. At this angle, the effect of the sector is to colliminate the ion beam, analogous to forming an optical virtual image at infinity. This means all ions enter the magnetic field at normal incidence.

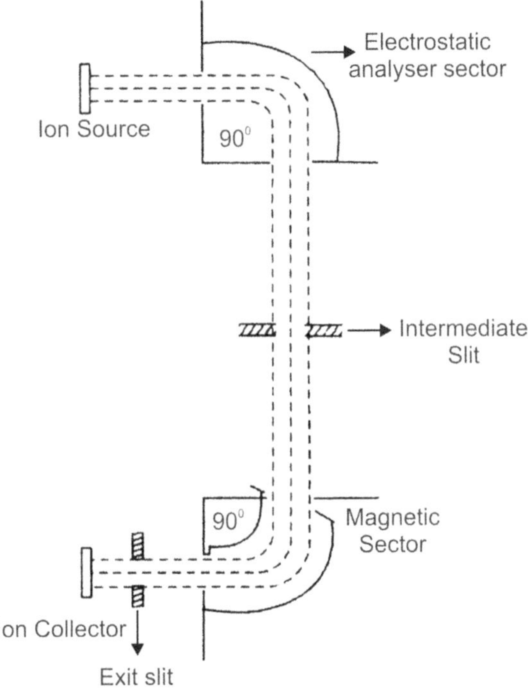

Nier Johnson Design

The resolution of this spectrometer is very high, there is a slow transmission of ions, i.e., the ion currents are slow. So that Double focussing instruments are used wherever high resolution is required i.e. upto 90000.

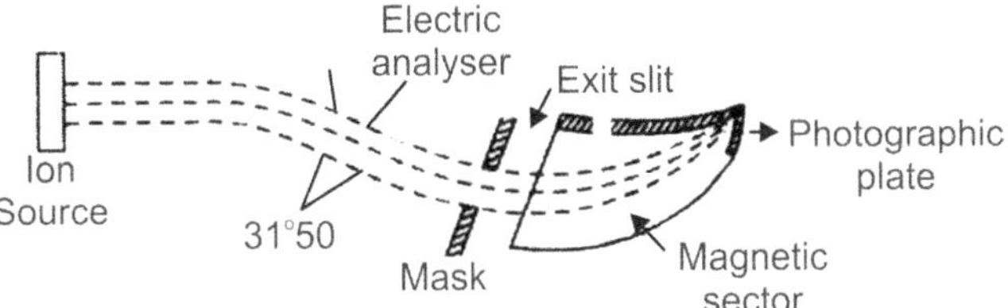

Mattauch Herzog Geometry

The passing of ion beam through two sectors results in velocity focussing as well as direction focussing. Hence focussing of an ion beam containing ions of same mass travelling with different speeds in the same direction and direction focussing are both achieved.

This is generally used to determine precise molecular weights.

(c) ***Cycloidal focussing*:** In cycloidal focussing ions while passing through crossed magnetic and electric fields will produce a cycloidal path. The small radius of curvature allows the use of smaller magnet without reducing the resolution or range.

(d) ***Time-of-flight (TOF) analyser*:** A time-of-flight analyser is one of the simplest mass analysing devices and is commonly used with MALDI. Time-of-flight analysis is based on accelerating a set of ions to a detector with the same amount of energy. Because the ions have the same energy, yet a different mass, the ions reach the detector at different times.

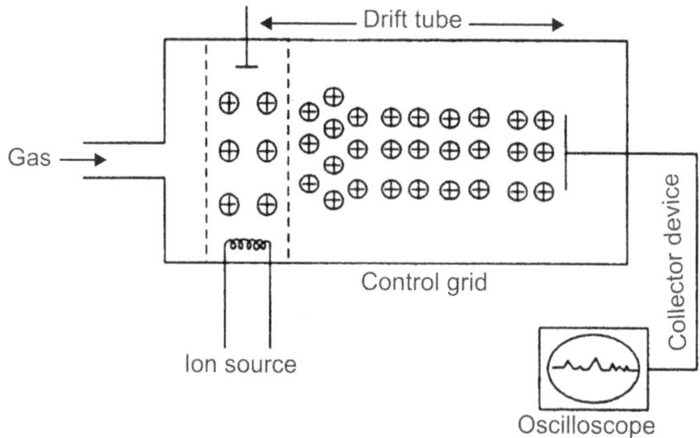

Time of Flight Mass Spectrometer

It has been observed that all ions leave the acceleration field with different velocities, depending on their masses. The smaller ions reach the detector first because of their greater velocity and the given distance. The measurement of this time of flight forms the basis for the non-magnetic separtator and the mass is determined at the ions' time of arrival.

If the ions are permitted to enter the drift tube continuously, the time required for the ions to travel in a non magnetic separator can't be measured. The problem is solved by inserting a control grid in the electron beam.

The arrival time of an ion at the detector is dependent upon the mass charge and kinetic energy of the ion.

Since kinetic energy is equal to ½ mv^2

$$v = \left(\frac{2KE}{m}\right)^{\frac{1}{2}}$$

Ions will travel a given distance d within a time t where K it is dependant upon their m/e.

$$t = K\sqrt{\frac{m}{e}}$$

K = proportionality constant, it depends on the length of the flight path.

The values of are generally in micro seconds. Elaborate electronics devices are used for measure these short times. Oscilloscopes are employed to display the spectrum.

(e) ***Radio Frequency Analyser*:** In this type, an assembly of grids are employed to select ions according to their velocities. The alternate grids are connected to a radio frequency source whereas the remaining grids are connected together to a steady potential.

The ions which are in phase with the rf field acquire a velocity, say V1

$$V = s\,f$$

f = frequency of the field

s = spacing between adjacent grids in centimetres.

In front of the Radio frequency analyser, an energy selector is adjusted.

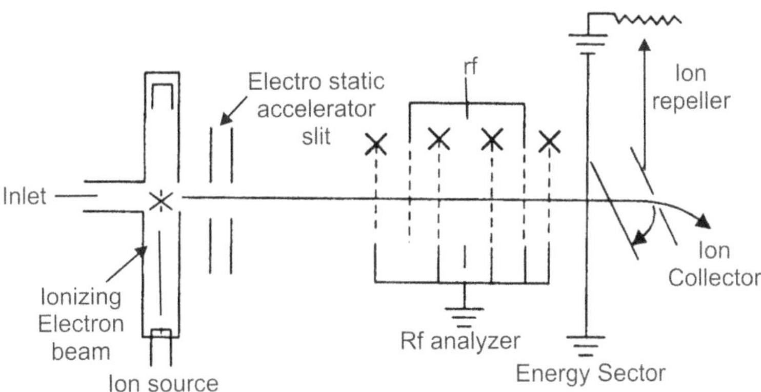

RF : Mass Spectrometer

A positive voltage is applied to the ion repeller which will repel all those ions which have received less than a specified fraction of the total available energy.

The mass spectrum will be obtained by varying the frequency of the rf section of the analyser.

$$\frac{m}{e} = 0.266 \frac{V}{S^2 f^2}$$

Its mass range is from 2 to 100.

(f) ***Tandem Mass Spectrometry*:** Tandem mass spectrometry (abbreviated MS^n – where n refers to the number of generations of fragment ions being analysed) allows one to induce fragmentation and mass analyse the fragment ions. This is accomplished by collisionally generating fragments from a selected ion and then mass analysing the fragment ions.

Fragmentation can be achieved by inducing ion/molecule collisions by a process known as collision-induced dissociation (CID) also known as collision – activated dissociation (CAD). Co, induced dissociation is accomplished by selecting an ion of interest with a mass analyser and introducing that ion into a collision cell gas. The selected ion then collides with a collision gas (argon (or) helium) resulting in fragmentation.

The fragments are then analysed to obtain a fragment ion spectrum. The abbreviation Ms^n is applied to processes which analyse beyond the initial ions (MS) to the fragment ions (MS^2) and subsequent generations of fragment ions(MS^3, MS^4 and ....)

This type of analysis if primarily used for obtaining structural information.

(g) ***Quadrupole Mass Analysers*:** The quadrupole analyser is a device in which ions can be resolved according to their m/e ratio without the need of heavy magnet.

Quadrupoles are four precisely parallel metallic rods with a direct current (DC) voltage and a superimposed radio-frequency potential. And by scanning a pre-selected radio-frequency field, one can effectively scan a mass range. The beam shoots down the centre of the array. A circular orifice rather than a slit is used as an centre of the array. A circular orifice rather that a slit is used as an inlet. Diagonally opposite poles of de source and also to a radio – frequency oscillator.

Quadrupole mass analysers have been used in conjunction with electron ionization sources since the 1950's and the most common mass spectrometer in existence today.

Quadrupoles have three primary advantages. First, they are tolerant of relatively poor vacuums (-5×10^{-5} torr), which make them well suited for electrospray ionization since the ions are produced under atmospheric pressure conditions.

Secondly, Quadrupoles are now capable of routinely analysing up to a m/e of 3000, which is useful because electrospray ionization of proteins and other biomolecules commonly produces a charge distribution below m/e 3000.

Finally the relatively low cost of Quadrupole mass spectrometers makes them attractive as electro-spray analysers.

Considering these mutual beneficial features, most of the successful commercial electrospary instruments have been coupled with Quadrupole mass analysers.

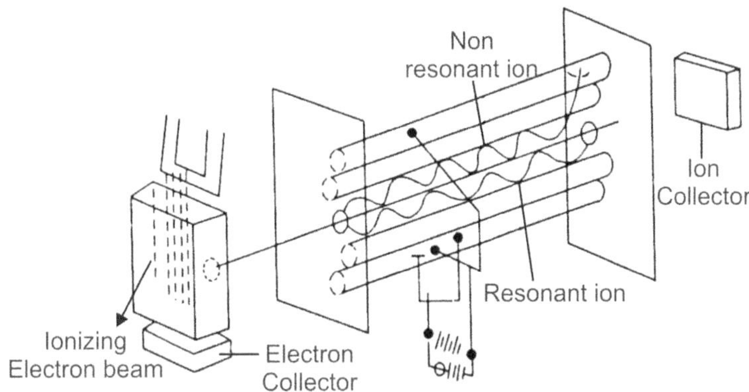

Quadrupole Mass Spectrometer

Quadrupoles are used up to several hundred mass numbers

Unit resolution of the order of 400-500 can be achieved. In Quadrupoles the resolution is proportional to the mass number.

(h) ***Quadrupole ion trap Analyser*****:** The Quadrupole ion trap mass analyser was conceived of at the same time as the quadrupole mass analyser and by the same person. Nobel Prize winner Wolfgang Paul.

The physics behind these ion separators is very similar.

In an ion trap the ions are trapped in a radio frequency quadrupole field. One method of using anion trap for mass spectrometry is to generate ions externally with Electrospray which are then injected into the trapping volume. The ions are then ejected and detected or the radio frequency field is scanned.

Further, it is also possible to isolate one ion species by ejecting all others from the trap. The isolated ions can subsequently be fragmented by collisional activation and the fragments detected to generate a fragmentation spectrum.

The primary advantage of Quadrupole ion trap is that multiple collison induced dissociation experiments can be performed without having multiple analysers.

Other important advantages include in compact size and the ability to trap and accumulate ions to increase the signal-to-noise ratio of a measurement.

Quadrupole ion traps have been utilized in many applications yet predominantly in electrospray ionisation for the analysis of peptides and small molecules.

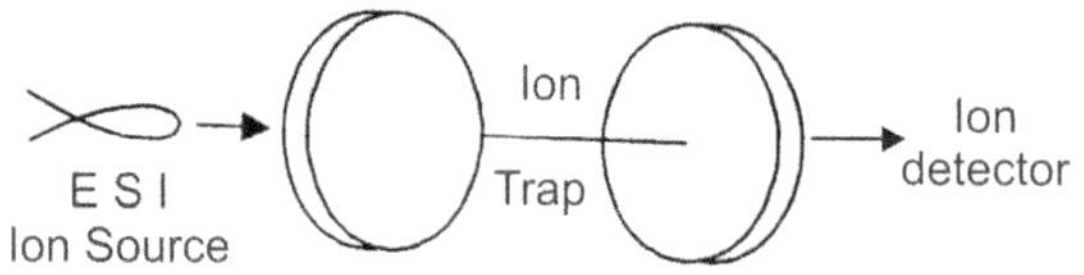

Ion
Trap
E S I
Ion Source
Ion
detector

Ions inside an ion trap mass analyser can be mass analysed to produce a mass spectrum. (or) Particular ion can be trapped inside and made to undergo collisions to produce fragmentation information.

(i) ***Fourier-Transform Mass Spectrometry (FTMS)*:** Fourier transform ion cyclotron resonance mass spectrometry (FTMS) offers two distinct advantages; high resolution and the ability to tandem MS experiments.

This analyser is particularly suitable for study of ion molecule reactions.

This was first introduced in 1974 by Comisorow and Marshall. FTMS is based on the principle of a charged particle to orbiting in the presence of a magnetic field. While the ions are orbiting, a radio frequency signal is used to excite them and as a result of this radio frequency excitation, the ions produce a detectable electron current on the cell in which they are trapped.

The time-dependent image current can be Fourier – transformed to obtain the component frequencies of the different ions which correspond to their m/e – Coupled to ESI and MALDI, FTMS has potential in becoming an important research tool offering high accuracy with errors as low as $\pm$ 0.0014.

Ions are formed by electron impact in a region of crossed magnetic and electric fields, causing them to follow cycloidal trajectories, drifting away from the point of formation in a direction perpendicular to both fields with a velocity of

$$v_d = \frac{E}{H}$$

Ions are detected by subjecting them to weak high frequency ac field and resonance frequency v_c at which energy is absorbed.

The resonance frequency

$$v_c = \frac{He}{2\pi m}$$

(ii) ***Omegatron analyser*:** This is less elaborate form of Ion Cyclotar resonance spectrometer, lacking the drift potential is omegatron.

Resonance ions are collected at a detector electrode

It is used mostly as a residual gas analyser.

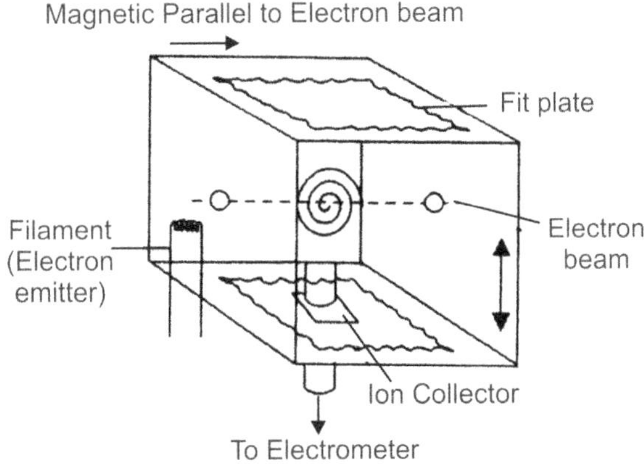

Omegatron Mass Analyser

5. Ion Collector (Detector and Readout System)

***Ion detection*:** Once the ion passes through the mass analyser it is then detected by the ion detector, the final element of the mass spectrometer.

The detector allows a spectrometer to generate a signal current from incident ions by generating secondary electrons, which are further amplified.

Alternatively, some detectors operate by inducing a current generated by a moving charge.

Among the detectors described, the electron multiplier and scintillation counter are the most commonly used and convert the kinetic energy of incident ions into a cascade of secondary electrons.

(a) ***Faraday Cup*:** A Faraday Cup operates on the basic principle that a change in charge on a metal plate results in a flow of electrons and therefore creates a current. One ion striking the dynode surface of the Faraday Cup (a dynode is a secondary emitting material, usually BeO, Gap or CSSb) induces several secondary electrons to be ejected and temporarily displaced. This temporary emission of electrons induces a current in the cup and provides for a small amplification of signal when an ion strikes the cup.

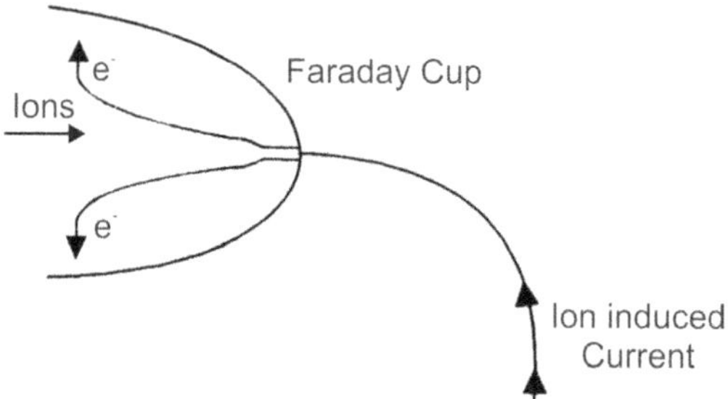

The detector is the least sensitive and used in spectrometers in which great sensitivity is not required. It is cup shaped (in order to reduce the chances of escape of secondary electrons liberated by ion impact) and consists of an insulated conductor directly connected to an electrometer amplifier.

(b) ***Electron multiplier*:** An electron multiplier is one of the most common means of detecting ions, achieving high sensitivity by extending the principle used with a Faraday Cup. For ion currents below 10^{-15} ampere, an Electron multiplier is necessarr. In this, the ion beam after travelling through an analyser, strikes Be-Cu electron multiplier. This results in the production of secondary electrons which are made to move under the influence of a magnetic field to follow circular paths causing them to hit the same electrode of Be-Cu electron multiplier but at a different point. Then the emitted electrons from Be-Cu electron multiplier are allowed to follow a series of semi-circular jumps between a pair of glass plates coated with a high resistance metallic film. Then, an electron gradient is maintained along the lengths of these plates to produce the required acceleration.

The Faraday Cup uses one dynode, but in an electron multiplier a series of dynodes are maintained at ever increasing potentials. Ions strike the dynode surface resulting in the emission of electrons. These secondary electrons are then attracted to the next dynode where more secondary electrons are generated, ultimately resulting in a cascade of electrons.

The magnetic field is maintained with the help of small permanent magnets.

With the help of Electron multiplier detectors, the rapid scanning of peaks, occurring across the collector slit can be made.

Typical amplification (or) current gain of an electron multiplier is one million.

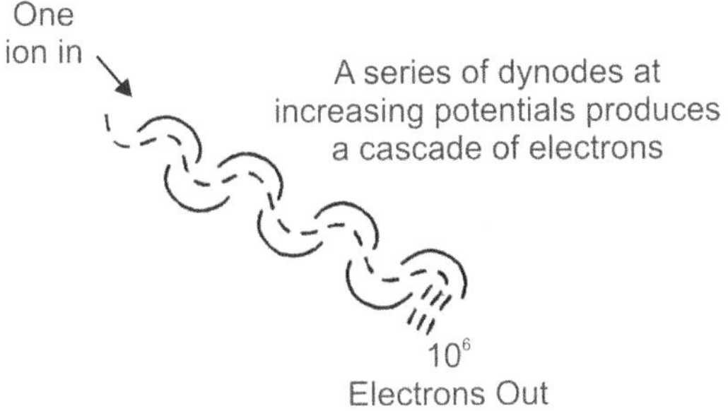

(c) Photomultiplier Conversion Dynode

(Scintillation Counting (or) Daly Detector)

The Photomultiplier conversion dynode detector is similar to an electron multiplier where the ions initially strike or dynode, resulting in the emission of electrons. However, with the photomultiplier conversion, dynode detector electrons the strike a phosphorus screen. The phosphorus screen, much like the screen on a television set, releases photons once an electron strikes. These photons are then detected by a photomultiplier, while operating with a colliding action much like an electron multiplier.

The primary advantage of the conversion dynode set up is that the photomultiplier tube is sealed in vacuum (photons pass through sealed glass), unexposed to the internal environment of the mass spectrometer. Thus the possibility of contamination is removed.

A five year or greater life time is typical and with sensitivity similar to electron multipliers, photo multiplier conversion dynode detectors are becoming more widely used in mass spectrometers.

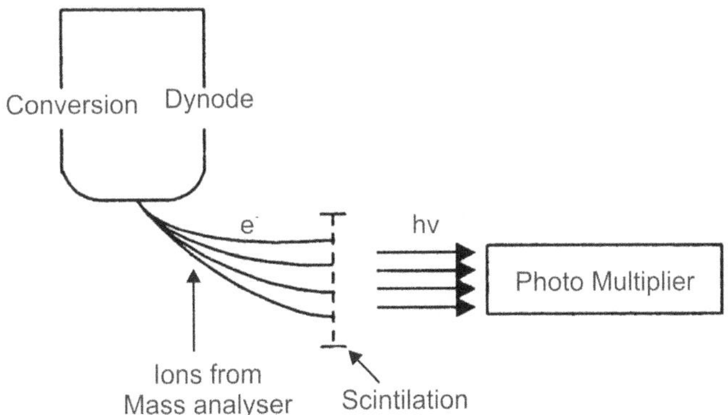

***Read out system*:** The read out display usually possesses a direct writing recording oscillograph which has 3.5 galvanometers with relative sensitivities of 1, 3, 10, 30 and 100.

This method is cheap, easy to operate and reliable. But it requires manual manipulation which has to be done in counting each mass number.

Important Technical Adjuncts in Mass Spectrometry

1. Vacuum system

All mass spectrometers require a vacuum. A vacuum is necessary to permit ions to reach the detector without colliding with other gaseous molecules. Such collosions would reduce the resolution and sensitivity of the instrument by increasing the kinetic energy distribution of the ions inducing fragmentation, or by preventing the ions from reaching the detector.

Coupling any sample source to a mass spectrometer requires that the sample (at atmospheric pressure 760 torr) be transferred into a region of high vacuum (10^{-6} torr) without compromising the later. The billion fold difference in pressure between the atmosphere and the high vacuum was one of the first problems faced by the originators of mass spectrometry.

Various mechanical configurations are now used to maintain the vacuum in a mass spectrometer while introducing the sample into the vacuum chamber. One method is to introduce the sample in small quantities through a capillary column (or) through a small orifice directly into the instrument. A second method is to initially evacuate the sample chamber through a vacuum lock.

Once a moderate vacuum in achieved (10^{-13} torr) by the vacuum lock in a prechamber, the sample can be introduced into the main vacuum chamber on the mass spectrometer. This method is directly employed with the direct insertion probes used with MALDI and FAB.

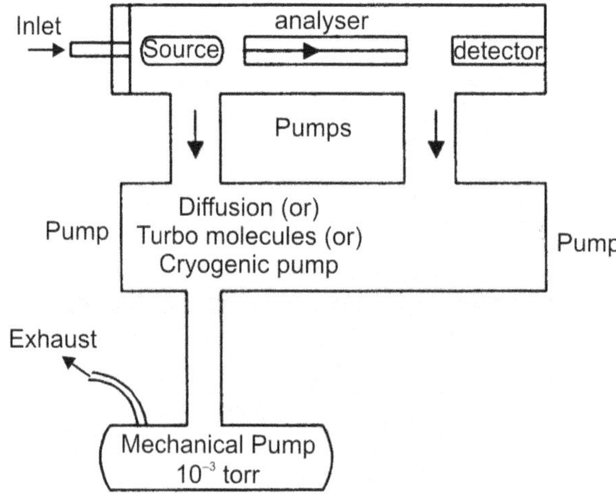

Mass Spectrometer with Vacuum System

In the figure a mass spectrometer is with three alternative pumping systems. All three systems are capable of producing a very high vacuum, and are all backed by a mechanical pump. The mechanical pump serves as a general workshorse for most mass spectrometers and allows for an initial vacuum is achieved, the other pumping systems can be activated to obtain pressures as low as 10^{-9} torr.

A well maintained vacuum is essential to the function of a mass spectrometer. Once the vacuum is compromised, sensitivity and resolution will be reduced. Also, at higher pressures the high voltage used in the instrument may discharge to ground, which can damage the instrument and or the computer system running the instrument. Such a breakdown, which may arise from a extreme leak, is basically an implosion, and can seriously damage a mass spectrometer by destroying electrostatic lenser, coating the optics with pump oil, and damaging the detector.

In general, maintaining a high vacuum is crucial to obtaining high quality spectra.

2. Computers and Software

The introduction of small computers for Laboratory work during the 1960s, entirely altered the manner in which mass spectrometry was performed. Once computers were interfaced with mass spectrometers, it was possible to rapidly perform the analyses.

It is the introduction of faster processors and larger storage capacities, that has helped launch a new era in mass spectrometry.

Automation is now possible allowing for thousands of samples to be analysed in a single day.

Researchers have also been developed mass spectra data bases which can be accessed to quickly identify organic compounds.

Software package have helped make the mass spectrometer more user friendly as well as expanding the instrument's capabilities.

Recording of a Mass Spectrogram

In a mass spectrometer, the sample is introduced into the ionization chamber very slowly to produce positive mass particles i.e. fragmented into different masses.

Then the accelerating voltage is adjusted to a high voltage to accelerate the mass particles to a high velocity. Under these conditions, only particles with lowest mass numbers will be deflected by the magnet. Therefore, only particles with the lowest mass numbers reach the collector and are counted. The numbers reaching the collector simultaneously increase. When accelerating voltage becomes zero, the record of the distribution of the masses in the sample is complete and is presented as a mass spectrogram, according to m/e ratio of ions.

The sequence in which the particles hit the detector, follows the equation:

$$\frac{m}{e} = H^2r^2/2V$$

From the above equation, if accelerating voltage (V) decreases, m increases, provided all other variables are constant under experimental conditions.

Therefore, the mass spectrum of a particular compound is a graphical record of its fragmentation pattern.

The mass spectrum is presented in two ways:

(a) Bar graph (b) % table

The mass spectrogram is generally represented by a bar graph in which intensity on the ordinate is plotted against m/e ratio on the abscissa but this method is cumbersome. Therefore, the data are often represented by a graph which plots relative abundance on the ordinate and m/e ratio on the abscissa. The relative abundance of the fragment is given as the percent intensity of a given peak relative to the most intense peak in the spectrum. The most intense peak in the spectrum is given a value of 100% and is called the base peak. The other peaks are then reported as the % of the base peak. It gives a quick idea of mass number and % abundances.

The time required to obtain a complete mass spectrum depends on the particular instrument. The time varies from 20 min to 1 second.

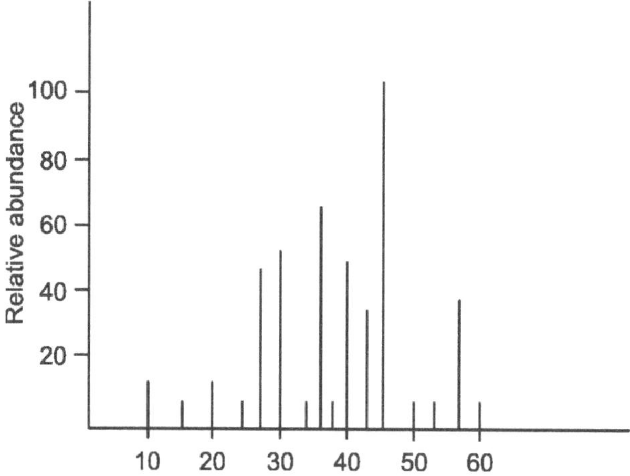

Resolution of a Mass Spectrometer

The abilityof a mass spectrometer to distinguish between ions of nearly equal masses is termed as the resolution of the instrument.

For many inorganic and organic applications, the resolution is expressed as,

$$\text{Resolution} = \frac{m}{\Delta m}$$

m & Δm are the mass number of two neighbouring peaks of equal intensity in the mass spectrum.

e.g. a resolution of 533 is necessary to distinguish oxygen of mass 31.9988 from sulphur of mass 32.06.

For most of the routine mixture analysis, the resolving powers below 1000 are used.

The resolution of the instrument is generally decreased due to the following factors :

1. Distribution of kinetic energies produced in the electron beam.
2. Variation in the accelerating voltage.
3. Variation in the magnetic field.
4. Poorly Collimated ion beam.
5. Space charge on the ion beam.
6. Width of the ion beam as determined by the slits.
7. Pressure in the spectrometer.

Types of Ions produced in a Mass Spectrometer

1. Molecular Ion or Parent peak

When a sample substance is bombarded with electrons of energies of 10 – 15 eV usually removes one electron from the molecule of the organic compound in the vapour phase. It results in the formation of molecular ion.

This will give rise to a very simple mass spectrum with essentially all of the ions appearing in one peak called parent peak.

The higher occupied orbital of aromatic system and non-bonding electron orbitals on oxygen and nitrogen atoms readily lose one electron.

In organic compounds, there is generally a small peak appearing one mass unit higher than the parent peak (M + 1) due to small but observable abundance of C and H in these compounds. Again, if the same molecule has two heavy isotopes, there is an even smaller peak at M + 2, Chlorine and Bromine yield abnormally high M + 2 peaks.

If a molecule contains a –electron system, the stability of the molecular ion is increased more than a molecule ion having a bond. i.e.

-bond.

Following order:

Unbranched hydrocarbons > ketones > amines > esters > ethers >

If a molecule yields the parent peak due to molecular ion, the exact molecular weight can be calculated i.e. the mass of the parent ion gives the molecular mass of the sample.

In a mass spectrum, it is important to locate the molecular ion at the high mass region of the spectrum. The stability of the molecular ion decides it relative abundance. The peak intensity of the molecular ion differs from one compound to another.

In some cases, parent ion peak is not formed which means that the rate of decomposition of parent ion is too high for its detection i.e. the rate of decomposition of the molecular ion increases with the molecular size in the homologous series. Larger molecular ion provides more possible reaction pathways for detection.

$$M \xrightarrow{-e} M^{+}(g) + 2e$$

2. **Base peak**

   If an electron beam of energy of 70 eV is used in a mass spectrometer, the molecular ion is produced by the loss of a single electron which undergoes splitting to form many fragments, and the parent peak in mass spectrum is called the base peak and the heights of all other peaks are measure with respect to it. Generally the ion abundance are expressed in terms of percent of the base peak.

3. **Dissociation Process**

   The molecular ion produced in the mass spectrometer is generally left with considerable excess energy. This energy is rapidly lost by the molecular ion resulting in one or more cleavages in it with or without rearrangement. One of the fragment retains the charge whereas the remaining fragments may be stable molecules or radicals. Cleavage is favoured at branched carbon atoms. In a homologous series, the extent of cleavage increases with molecular weight.

   The interpretation of mass spectra rests upon the fact that at sufficient energy each molecular species ionizes to form a unique, reproducible, and often a predictable pattern. This is called cracking (or) fragment pattern. The resulting fragments are a fraction o the relative strength of the bonds within the molecules, the component atoms, the molecular weight of the compound and the ionization potential.

A mass spectrum is a theoretical plot of m/e on horizontal axis vs intensity of the peaks on the vertical axis. The height of the peak indicates the relative abundance, whereas the position gives the mass number of particles. The most intense peak (base peak) in any given spectrum is arbitrarily assigned a value of 100 and other peaks are reported as percentages of this.

It is generally advisable when analysing mass spectra to assign a mass number to each peak, to deduce from the mass number the possible species involved and finally to examine the possible method by which this species could be formed.

It should be kept in mind that cracking pattern of a given molecular species, the highest mass detected, is usually that of the ionized molecule. This peak is called the parent peak and mass is parent mass.

$$M^+ \rightarrow M_1^+ + M_2 \text{ (or) } M + e^- -> M_1^+ + M_2 + 2e^-$$

Many of the peaks in mass spectrum are due to fragmentations. Fragment peaks give information regarding molecular structure because it is specific to the structure of the molecule.

4. ***Rearrangement ions***

In some cases, fragments are observed which are not a part of the original molecule. These are known as rearrangement ions which are formed from the molecular ion by redistribution of atoms or groups of atoms at the moment of decomposition of the molecular ions.

In many cases rearrangement takes place with respect to hydrogen. In hydrocarbons, the rearrangement is non-specific and unpredictable, whereas in hetero-atoms rearrangement is specific and this may result in a very intense peak.

5. ***Multiple charged Ions***

In mass spectrometer, the ions are generally carrying a single positive charge. However, sometimes double or even triple charged ions are found in the mass spectrum. These ions are recorded at a half or a third of the m/e value of the singly charged ions. The formation of these multiple charged ions are common in heteroaromatic molecules.

6. ***Negative ions***

In addition to positive ions, negative ions may be formed from electron bombardment of the sample. The formation of negative ions is very rare but these can be produced in three ways.

1. $AB + e \rightarrow A + B^-$ (Dissociation resonance capture)
2. $AB + e \rightarrow AB^-$ (Resonance capture)
3. $AB + e \rightarrow A^+ + B^- + e^-$ (Ion pair production)

The negative ions are focussed by reversing the fields in the mass spectrometer. These are not useful in structural determinations e.g. O^-, OH^-, C_2H^- are negative ions formed in spectrum.

7. Meta-stable ions

The life time of an ion may be so small that it undergoes decomposition during its passage between the source and collector units in the spectrometer.

The ions resulting from the decomposition between the source region and the magnetic analyzer are called metastable ions.

Metastable peaks can be easily determined in a mass spectrum. Some important characteristics of these peaks are:

1. They do not necessarily occur at the integral m/e values.
2. These are much broader than the normal peaks.
3. These are of relatively low abundance.

These are useful in studying the mechanism of fragmentation. However, these are not used for the study of structure.

The metastable ion formed in the ion source, that spontaneously decompose during their passage through the spectrometer. If the ion decomposes further into a neutral fragment and a stable ion, before being accelerated, it will not be possible to detect because a normal peak should be shown in the spectrum.

This is

$$M_1^+ \rightarrow M_2^+ + \text{Neutral fragment}$$

If, however the metastable ion is accelerated before decomposition takes place, a part of KE of M_1^+ will be lost on decomposition, and the resulting ion, labelled M^+, will have less momentum than is normally associated with ion M_2^+, and is recorded as a lower mass number. The process of decomposition during flight is known as a metastable transition, provided that it takes place between the exit of the ion source and the entrance to the magnetic field.

Thus if an ion M_1 fragments after acceleration, but before entering the magnetic field, it will have been accelerated as mass M_1 but dispersed in the magnetic field as M_2.

The resulting ion current will be recorded as a low intensity broad peak at apparent mass M^+.

$$M^* = \frac{M_2^2}{M_1}$$

The peak caused by ion current corresponding to mass M^* is called metastable peak.

M is mass of parent ion

M_2 is mass of daughter (metastable) ion

M_3 is mass of neutral fragment

M^* is apparent mass of the metastable ion.

Measurement of the mass of the metastable peak gives information that M is derived directly from M1 by loss of a neutral fragment.

Interpretation of Mass Spectra

By understanding the ionization process which occurs before the ions are reaching the collector, we interpret the mass spectrum.

One basic approach is to observe fragmentation patterns and then tries to explain how and why they have occurred. This approach is very useful in relating spectra to structure.

General approaches used to arrive at the molecular formula are :

1. **The exact molecular weight**

   Mass spectrometer can be used to determine the molecular weight of a pure compound from the identification of the parent peak. From the molecular weight, one can determine the molecular formula.

2. **The Isotope effects**

   Mass spectrometer can be used to determine the distribution of naturally occurring isotopes. Molecules having heavy isotopes will exhibit peaks in a mass spectrum at m/e one (or) more units higher than normal i.e., there will be small peaks at M + 1 and M + 2. From the heights, an exact molecular weight can be calculated. From the molecular weight value, one could quickly decide the molecular formula.

3. Nitrogen Rule

This rule was given by Beynon. It states that if the molecular weight of an organic susbstance is even, the number of nitrogen atoms in the molecule is even. If the molecular weight is odd, the number of nitrogen atoms in the molecule is even. This rule also states that all fragment ions formed by cleavage of one bond have odd mass if they have even number of nitrogen atoms but even mass if they have an odd number of nitrogen atoms. This is applied to compounds having covalent bonds and the molecular weight to be used in the sum of most abundant isotopes.

4. Ring Rule

If the molecular formula is known by mass spectrometer, one may calculate the number of "unsaturated sites" from the ring rule.

According to this rule the number of unsaturated sites R, is equal to a the number of rings in the molecule plus the number of double bonds twice the number of triple bonds.

The ring rule for molecule CwHxNyOz may be stated as

$$R = W + 1 + \frac{y - x}{2}$$

From the above rules mass spectra can be interpreted as follows :

1. Firstly, a single electron is removed and no other band is affected i.e., we get five ion radical with mass equal to the molecular weight. It is known as parent ion i.e. M peak. The strong peak in the spectrum is called base peak and other peaks are expressed in terms of % of the base peak.
2. Secondly, a single bond can split and produce principle fragments.
3. Thirdly, a cleavage with rearrangement of hydrogen atom or a larger group can occur.
4. Fourthly, two electrons may get lost and give rise to an ion apparent m/e ½ of true value.
5. After establishing the parent ion peak, i.e., M, the fragment peaks, we should measure M + 1 and M + 2 peaks i.e., isotopic peaks. This will give the number of C, N, O atoms.

M + 1 peak due to 1.1% of ^{13}C in normal Carbon + 0.4% ^{15}N in normal Nitrogen.

M + 2 peak is due to ^{18}O isotope of oxygen and due to SI and S. Fluorine and iodine are monoisotopic, but chlorine as ^{35}Cl, ^{37}Cl in 3 : 1 ratio, while bromine has ^{79}Br, ^{81}Br in 1 : 1 ratio. For chlorine, the pattern will comprise peaks spaced 2 masses apart.

Applications

Mass spectrometry is being applied to a wide variety of questions include protein structure, drug metabolism, flavour and smell chemistry, petroleum and petro-chemicals, organic fossils, inherited metabolic diseases, atmospheric chemistry, the analysis of respiratory gases, viral identification, forensics, and many other specialized subjects.

1. **Atomic Masses**

   The discovery of isotopes with the first mass spectrometer answered the question about the integer value of atoms. (e.g. carbon-12, Nitrogen-14).

   These measurements were originally undertaken by Francis W. Aston and repeated with increasing precision by succeeding generations of scientists.

   Since those original experiments, mass spectroscopy and nuclear physics have combined to determine isotopic masses to a high degree of accuracy.

   The mass unit now used is defined such that the mass of the C-12 isotope is exactly 12 atomic mass units (amu).

2. **Geochronology and Geochemistry**

   Mass spectrometers capable of measuring isotopic ratios allow the composition of elements to be determined in which one or more isotopes result from radioactive decay. The age of the rock from which the element has been obtained can be determined if the amount of the parent element can be measured and certain requirements on the environmental history of the rock are met.

   The use of isotopes has also proven to be especially valuable in understanding the origin and nature of the solar system. A great body of evidence now suggests that meteorites are objects that solidified very early in the history of the solar system. Extinct radioactivities of elements with various half lives have been identified that set limits on the time between the synthesis of the elements and their condensation.

3. **Accelerator MS and dating materials**

   The particle accelerators used in nuclear physics can be viewed as mass spectrometers to rather distorted forms, but the three principal elements – the ion source, analyzer, and detector are always present. Accelerator MS was applied in measuring cosmogonic isotopes, the radio isotopes produced by cosmic rays incident on the Earth or planetary objects. These isotopes are exceedingly rare, having corresponding terrestrial element, which is an isotopic ratio far beyond the capabilities of normal mass spectrometers. The advantage of the large, high energy accelerator mass spectrometer is the great detector selectivity that results from ions having 1,000 times more energy than any previously available machine could provide. Conventional mass spectrometers have difficulty measuring abundances less than one hundred – thousandth of the reference isotope, because interfering ions are scattered into the analyzer location where the low abundance isotope is to be sought. Extremes of high vacuum and antiscattering precautions can improve this by a factor of 10, but not the factor of 100 million that is required. An accelerator suffers from this defect to an even greater degree, and large quantities of "trash" ions are found at the expected analyzer location of the cosmogenic isotope. The ability of certain kinds of nuclear particle detectors to identify the relevant ion unambiguously, enables the accelerator mass spectrometer to overcome this shortcoming and functions as a powerful analytical tool.

The accelerator method has opened lines of investigation that had previously been inaccessible. There is improvement of radio carbon dating which is strong motivation for inventors. Scientists are now able to make age determinations from much smaller samples and to make age determinations from much smaller samples and to make them much more rapidly than by radioactive counting, but C-14 proved to be a considerably more difficult problem for instrumental development than the other cosmogenic isotopes. The method was applied almost immediately to analyses involving Beryllium-10, chlorine-36, with aluminium-26, calcium-41, iodine-129 following soon after, notable achievements resulted from all five. Cosmic rays striking the atmosphere are a strong source of beryllium-10, carbon-14, Cl-36 which are deposited in rain and snow, when their migration may be followed. These isotopes have proved useful in determining the ags and irradiation histories of meteorites and lunar samples. There have been extensive studies of beryllium-10 in cores of polar ice and ocean sediments that give unique information about the intensity of cosmic rays over the past few million years.

4. Organic Chemistry

Mass spectrometry has a critical role in organic chemistry. With a high-resolution mass spectrometer it is possible to carry out mass measurements on the molecular ion or any other ion in the spectrum to an accuracy of approximately one part in one million. This mass provides the best index for determining ionic formulas. Once the formula is known, it is possible to deduce the total rings and double bonds making up the molecular structure and to begin to speculate on possible structural formulas. In order to deduce structural formulas from molecular formulas, it is also essential to study the fragment ion in the mass spectrum.

Using a computer coupled to a high resolution mass spectrometer, about 1000 mass peaks per minute can be plotted at a resolving power of upto 20,000. Accurate measurements can be made on each peak, and peak heights and ion compositions can be printed out in the form of an 'element map' to aid in the interpretation of the spectrum. It is also possible for the computer to carry out many of the logical steps in reducing the data that leads to structural elucidation.

Continuous sampling of the materials contained in a reaction vessel, followed by analysis with mass spectrometer has been used to identify and measure the quantity of intermediate species formed during a reaction as a function of time. This kind of analysis is important, both in suggesting the mechanism by which the overall reaction takes place and in mechanism by which the overall reaction takes place and in enabling the detailed kinetics of reactions to be resolved.

5. Combinatorial Chemistry

Combinatorial chemistry is used to create large populations of molecules or libraries, whereby the generation of huge number of compounds increases the probability that they will find novel compounds of significant therapeutic (or) commercial value. While many fields of research have been influenced by this approach, the largest investment has come from the pharmaceutical, biotechnology, and agrochemical arena. In the field of drug development, combinatorial chemistry represents a convergence of chemistry and biology, made possible by fundamental advances in automation, such as that of mass spectrometry.

Mass spectrometry is playing an increasingly important role in the molecular characterization and activity of combinatorial libraries. Crucial to distinguishing the most active component for obtaining structure activity relationships of compounds in a library, is an efficient qualitative and quantitative assay. Toward this end, electrospray ionization and MALDI-MS have been useful for qualitative, and more recently, the quantitative screening of combinatorial libraries. Moreover, the development of these two techniques has significantly extended MS application towards a wide variety of challenging problems in drug discovery and toward the identification of effective ligand-receptor binding, new catalysts and enzyme inhibitors. In addition because mass spectrometry does not involve chromophores or radiolabelling, ir provides a variable alternative to existing analytical techniques which typically require extensive sample preparation and optimization time out disposal of biohazardous waste or require a significant amount of sample.

6. **Biochemistry**

Mass spectrometry has emerged as an important tool in bio-chemical research. Now, the commercial availability of MS instruments which offer picomole to altomole sensitivity and enable the analysis of biological fluids with a minimum amount of sample preparation has made the routine analysis of a large variety of compounds including : proteins, peptides, carbohydrates, oligonucleotides, natural products, drugs and drug metabolites.

Extending beyond simple molecular weight characterization, the mild ionization methods can be applied to many new applications, including protein-protein interactions, dynamic rival analysis, high sensitivity protein sequencing, routine DNA sequencing, protein folding, high through put analysis in combinatorial chemistry and drug discovery.

Both electrospray and MALDI-MS are sensitive tools for mass measurement and can provide surprisingly large amounts of other information as well. Initially, both methods are used to obtain accurate M.W. information on molecules that were traditionally difficult or impossible to analyse (i.e. proteins, oligonucleotides and carbohydrates).

The ability to analyse complex mixtures has made electrospray and MALDI very useful for the examination of proteolytic digests, an application otherwise known as protein mass mapping. Through the application of sequence specific proteases, protein mass mapping allows for the identification of protein primary structure. Performing mass analysis on the resulting proteolytic fragments thus yields information on fragment mass with accuracy approaching $\pm$ 5 ppm, or $\pm$ 0.05 Da for a 1,000 Da peptide.

The characterization of genomic proteins for proteomics is arguably the most important application of modern mass spectrometry where the primary tools are proteases and computer facilitated data analysis. As a result of generating intact ions, the molecular weight information on the peptides / proteins are quite unambiguous. Sequence specific enzymes can then provide protein fragments that can be associated with proteins within a database by correlating observed and predicted fragment masses. With the availability of the human genome sequence identification of the proteins can be quickly determined simply by measuring the mass of proteolytic fragments.

Protein mass mapping has also been used for studying higher order protein structure by combining limited proteolytic digestion, mass analysis and computer facilitated data analysis. In the analysis or protein structure, enzymes are used to initially cleave surface accessible regions of the protein or protein complex. These initial cleavage sites are then identified using accurate mass measurements combined with the protein's known structure and the known specificity of the enzyme. This approach has also been used to examine viral protein capsid structure by utilizing computer based sequence searching.

Mass spectrometry can be used as a tool to observe complexes in the gas phase taken from an aqueous environment, thereby providing insights into specific non-covalent associations in solution. The selectivity of mass spectrometry may eventually help avoid impurity problems associated with immunoaffinity procedures and also facilitate drug screening e.g. the observation of the haemoglobin in complex, DNA Duplex, cell surface carbohydrate association, catalytic antibody – inhibitor interactions and the analysis of whole viruses.

7. Peptide and DNA sequencing

An important goal of mass spectrometry is the routine acquisition of complete sequence information from bio-polymers. ESI and MALDI have realized this goal. More specifically ESI tandem MS has been routinely used to generate fragment ions from a selected precursor ion by initiating ion/molecule which can then be mass analysed and used to obtain sequence information. ESI tandem MS has been successfully applied to the sequencing of small oligonucleotides.

MALDI-MS is playing an equally exciting role in biopolymer sequencing, used in conjunction with enzymatic or chemical digestion to generate sequence – specific ladders for proteins and oligonucleotides. This process is also known as ladder sequencing. Protein that has undergone a stepwise degradation in which ladder generating chemistry produces a family of sequence – defining peptide fragments that differ from the next by one amino acid. Once the mixture of peptides is obtained, MALDI-MS analysis is performed to generate a mass spectral sequence ladder.

8. Small Bio-molecule characterization with sleep-inducing potential

The sensitivity of modern mass spectrometry was applied to the study of sleep, a fresh purely chemical approach was taken in attempting to identify molecules of the CNS.

Cerebro spinal fluid analysis began with preparative liquid chromatography fraction collection. These experiments produced U.V. data on each fraction to determine any differences between subjects at various points in their sleep cycle. Even though the compound associated with this absorbance was only present in small amounts, partial characterization was initially obtained by performing exact mass measurements and tadem mass analysis. Using a tadem mass spectrometry and ESI mass analysis on the fractions associated with the differences in the chromatogram produced a significant ion at m/z 282. Mass spectroscopy will play an increasing large role in studying other attributes of human behavious such as hunger and pain and other.

9. Viruses

Mass spectrometry is offering a new perspective on the solution and gas-phase properties of viruses. Viruses are particles designed to transport genes between hosts and the cells of a host. The broad application of mass spectrometry to viral structure provides unique insights into many biological processes, including viral antibody binding, protein-protein interactions, and protein dynamics. Mass measuring viral proteins is now routine and since viruses are typically well characterized, in that the capsiol protein and DNA of RNA sequences are known, identifying a virus based on the mass of the protein and enzymatic digestion fragments is relatively straight forward.

Using mass spectrometry, it is also possible to identify viral protein post – translation modifications and have even been recently used to study viral protein dynamics. Mass spectrometry has also been applied on a global scale via the mass measurement of entire intact viruses.

Identification of viral mutants typically requires sequencing part or all of the genome to determine the nature of the mutation. Automated DNA sequencing is a well established method for identifying mutant proteins and is used to pinpoint specific regions that undergo mutation. The mass spectrometry used to identify mutant proteins consists of enzymatic digestion of proteins followed by mass analysis of there resulting peptide mixture. By comparing differences in the mass of peptides that are released by such treatment, one is able to identify peptides in which amino acid differences occur. This information defines the regions containing a mutation and, in cases when nucleotide sequencing is required, significantly narrows the region of the genome that must be sequenced. Accurate mass measurements and tandem mass spectrometry can then be used to definitely identity the aminoacid substitution.

10. Preparative Mass Spectrometry

In the early 1940's E.O. Lawrence developed a mass spectrometry – based separation approach to enrich radioactive uranium U-235 from the natural isotopic distribution of Uranium. This method used calutron mass spectrometers to separate ions according to their m/e ratio and once separated the ions were collected.

This preparative mass spectrometry approach applied to the purification of radioactive U-235, which was then used to construct the first nuclear weapon. Since those early experiments, more efficient means of generating and separating uranium isotopes have been established, yet separating compounds based on mass is certainly an intriguing idea which has not lost its appeal. In these experiments a monodisperse polymer was generated and collected from a synthetically derived polydisperse version of the polymer. This simple example serves to illustrate the potential of using Es This simple example serves to illustrate the potential of using ESMS as a preparative tool for molecular separation and purification.

11. Forensics

Electrospray ionization and MALDI mass spectrometry have been used to examine evidence in a wide variety of criminal cases.

12. Space probes

Future space exploration, addressing the question of whether life exists elsewhere in the solar system, will rely on the mass spectrometer to produce spectra of those molecules characteristic of life, such as aminoacids. An unmanned spacecraft equipped with a mass spectrometer has already been used and more missions are being planned to Mars to help learn about its surface and atmosphere, and to determine whether life once existed there.

13. Small Mass Spectrometers

Just as mass spectrometers measure incredibly small molecules allowing them to be called "the smallest scale in the world" the instruments themselves are also getting smaller. Many research groups are actively pursuing the miniaturization of mass spectrometers for a new field known as microfluidics. Smaller instrumentation will help to facilitate a wide variety of tasks such as in space exploration, forensics, environmental studies, explosives detection, combinatorial chemistry, as well as biochemistry.

General Applications

Qualitative Applications

***Molecular weight determination*:** The molecular weight of compound that can be easily volatilized can be calculated easily and the method requires the identification of the molecular ion peak the mass of which gives the molecular weight to atleast the nearest whole number and accuracy that cannot be realized by other molecular weight measurements.

***Determination of molecular formula*:** If it is possible to identify the molecular ion peak, the molecular formulae can be determined from the mass spectrum either partially (or) exactly. By making use of high resolution instrument capable of detecting mass differences of a few thousand of unit, it is possible to derive a unique formula for compound from the exact mass of the ion peak.

Quantitative applications

***Quantitative analysis of Mixtures*:** In this, the spectra are recorded for each component. From a careful inspection of the individual mass spectra, known or suspected to be present in the mixture, it is possible to select analysis peaks on the basis of intensity and freedom from interference by the presence of both components. The sensitivity is usually given in terms of the heights of the analysis peak per unit pressure-obtained by dividing the peak height of the analysis peak by the pressure of the pure compound in the sample reservoir.

If the components of the mixture give spectra, with atleast one peak, whose height is due entirely to the presence of one component, the calculation of sample of compositions can be simplified.

***Isotopic abundance*:** The isotopic abundance of easily vaporisable elements can be determined using mass spectrometer. When this information is coupled with the precise isotopic mass determination, values of the atomic weights of the elements may be obtained.

***Isotopic dilution method*:** Mass spectrometry is used to determine the amount of a component of a complicated mixture from which it cannot be separated quantitatively. By this method the amount of caffeine present in coffee is determined. Determination of isotope ratio in caffeine present in the coffee by the Mass spectrometry requires the sample to be converted into a suitable form, usually Nitrogen or carbon dioxide.

***Distinction between Cis and Trans isomere*:** Both cis and trans isomers yield similar mass spectra but the molecular ion peak for the trans-isomer is more intense than the cis isomer. Another distinction is that the dehydration fragment for the cis-isomer is much stronger than the trans-isomer.

***Thermodynamic Studies*:** Mass spectrometry has also been found to be very useful in thermodynamic studies and can be used over a wide temperature range.

Heat of vapourisation of high temperature materials can be determined by making use of a graph in which ion intensities are plotted against temperature. Change of partial pressure with temperature can be calculated from the slope of the line in the graph.

Heat of sublimation is determined by mass spectrometry. If a subliming solid is kept in a thermostated sample reservoir at the given temperature, the solid phase and vapour phase in the reservoir are in equilibrium. Suppose a small quantity of the vapour if diffused from the reservoir into the ionization chamber. If the mass spectrum is run, there occurs a change in peak intensity which is directly proportional to the vapour pressures of the subliming substances are calculated from the peak heights in the mass spectrum at different temperatures. Then the heat of sublimation can be obtained from the slope of the plot for Pvs 1/T.

***Measurement of Ionization Potential*:** Ionizatiob potential of a molecule is defined as the amount of energy needed to form a molecular ion. If no further energy is supplied, only molecular ion is produced. Fragmentation may take place if sufficient additional energy is transferred to the molecular ion. The energy level at which fragmentation occurs is called appearance potential of the fragment ion. The appearance potential must be equal to the sum of the ionization potential and the bond dissociation energy.

***Impurity detection*:** If the molecular weights of the impurities are much larger than major components, their detection is more easy because their higher mass peaks are free from contributions by those of the major components.

Mass Spectrometry has also been useful for analyzing various plant constituents which are used chemically (or) therapeutically, along with various other technical methods like Gas chromatography. Liquid chromatography, U.V. spectroscopy and Diode Array detector methods and HPLC.

(a) A new GC-MS method for monitoring lignans was developed to study the variation in plants and elucidate the biosynthetic steps. This new GC-MS method gave a clear liganan profile of plant material. It was possible to show the large vaiation in the concentrations of deoxypodophyllotoxin, yatein and anhydropodorhizol in Antrhriscus Sylvestris. In contrast with existing GC methods for lignan analysis no derivatisation is needed. This method is also used for the detection of different classes of lignans in biosynthetically related plant species.

The essential oils of Shorea robusta heartwood and resin were isolated by hydrodistillation of their respective petroleum ether extracts. Nine and seventeen compounds representing 80.35% and 78.43% of the oil respectively were identified by GC-MS.

(b) A method to identify triterpene glycosides using reversed-phase liquid chromatography with positive atmospheric pressure chemical ionization mass spectrometry was developed. Based on the analysis of the molecular weight, fragment ions, selected ion chromatograms, a number of triterpene glycosides, including actein, 27-deoxyacetin, cimifugoside M, and cimifugoside from cimifuga racemosa were studied. A chromone, climifugin, from C foetida was also identified.

Cimifugoside M and cimifugin can specifically serve as indicators for species identification. The method can, therefore, be used to distinguish black cohosh products from among different plant species for quality control.

LC/MS was now used for analysis of chemical composition of hydroalcoholic extract of Tinnivelly Senna which is widely used as laxative in phyto medicine. This method allows the on-line identification of flavonoids, anthroquinones and the typical dianthronic sennosides.

(c) A new method using direct on-line coupling between HPLC and UV-DAD/MS was developed for the rapid detection of Aristolochic acid 1 in plant preparations. Aristolochic acid 1 was quantitatively determined by this method.

The Aristolochia genus contains nephrotoxic and carcinogenic compounds named Aristolochic acids. These nitrated products were associated with renal insufficiency and urothelial carcinoma. These toxic components were detected and quantified by using LC/UV-DAD/MS to prevent further cases of intoxication.

An online HPLC – diode array detector (DAD)-Mass spectrometry has been developed to simultaneously separate and identify 17 main constituents of chuanxiong. The dried rhizome of ligusticum chuanxiong is one of the major clinically used cardiovascular protective traditional Chinese medicines. These constituents have a reputation for facilitating blood circulation and dispersing blood stasis so this herb is commonly prescribed for the treatment of Angina pectoris cardiac arrhythmia, hypertension and stroke

CHAPTER 16

INFRARED SPECTROSCOPY

Introduction

Infrared spectroscopy is one of the most powerful analytical techniques.

- Infrared absorption spectra are due to changes in vibrational energy, accompanied by changes in rotational energy.
- Energy of a molecule = Electronic energy + Vibrational energy + Rotational energy.
- IR spectra is mainly used in structure elucidation to determine the functional groups and bonds present in a chemical substance.
- The technique is based on a chemical substance showing marked selective absorption in the infrared region.
- After absoption of IR radiations, the molecules of a chemical substance vibrate at many rates of vibration giving rise to close packed absorption bands, called an IR absorption spectrum which may extend over a wide wavelength range.
- Band positions in an infrared spectrum may be expressed in wave numbers whose unit is cm^{-1}.
- Band intensities in IR spectrum may be expressed either as transmittance (T) or absorption (A).

  Transmittance: The ratio of radiant power transmitted by a sample to the radiant power incident on the sample.

***Absorption*:** The logarithm, to the base 10, of the reciprocal of the transmittance i.e

$$A = \log_{10}\left(\frac{1}{T}\right)$$

Range of Infrared Region

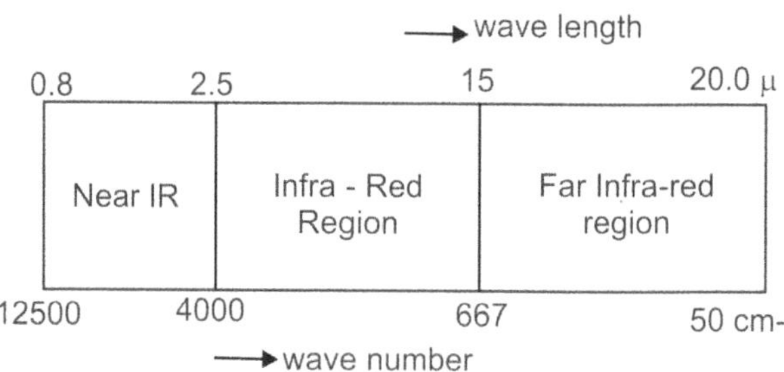

- The infrared radiation region of electromagnetic spectrum lies between the visible and microwave region.
- The regions may be divided into 4 sections:
  (a) ***The Photographic region*:** This ranges from visible 10 1.2 μ.
  (b) ***The very near infrared region*:** This is also known as overtone region and ranges from 1.2 to 2.5 μ.
  (c) ***The Near Infrared region*:** This is also known as vibration rotation region and ranges from 2.5 to 25 m.
  (d) ***The Far-Infrared region*:** This is known as the rotation region. This ranges from 25 to 300-400 μ.

S.No.	Region	Wave number (cm^{-1})	Wavelength (μ)
1.	Ordinary infrared	4000-667	2.5-15
2.	Near infrared	12,500-4,000	0.8-2.5
3.	Far infrared	667-50	15 - 200

- Another regions in infrared spectrum are
  (a) Group frequency region.
  (b) Finger print region.

Group Frequency Region

The region has a wavelength ranging from 2.5 to 8.0 μ and a wave number from 4000 – 1300 cm^{-1}. Here, the stretching and bending vibrational bands are associated with specific structural or functional groups observed frequently. Stretching frequencies are found in group frequency region.

S.No	Molecule	Frequency (cm^{-1})
C-H Stretch		
1.	$CHCl_3$	3019
2.	CH = CH	3287
C = O Stretch		
1.	CH_3COCH_3	1715
2.	CF_3COOH	1776

Finger Print Region

The region has a wavelength ranging from 8.0-2.5 μ and a wavenumber from 1300-400 cm^{-1}. Here, the vibrational modes depend solely and strongly on the rest of the molecule.

Example : The C-C stretching frequency depends largely on bonding of the carbon atoms.

Salient Features of IR Spectroscopy

There are three vital points : -

(a) Most intense peaks in the IR-spectrum are solely due to absorption peaks caused by the stretching vibrations.

(b) Molar extinction coefficient in IR-spectroscopy varies from 0-2000 cm^{-1}, and

(c) Molar extinction coefficient is directly proportional to the square of the change in the dipole moment of the molecule that the particular vibration affords.

Principle

The bonds maintain some vibrations, with some frequency, characteristic to energy portion of the molecule. This is called the natural frequency of vibration. When energy in the form of infrared radiations is applied and when, Applied infrared frequency is eaual to Natural frequency of vibration, absorption of IR radiation takes place and a peak is observed.

Every bond or portion of a molecule or functional group requires different frequency for absorption. Hence characteristic peak is observed for every functional group or part of the molecule.

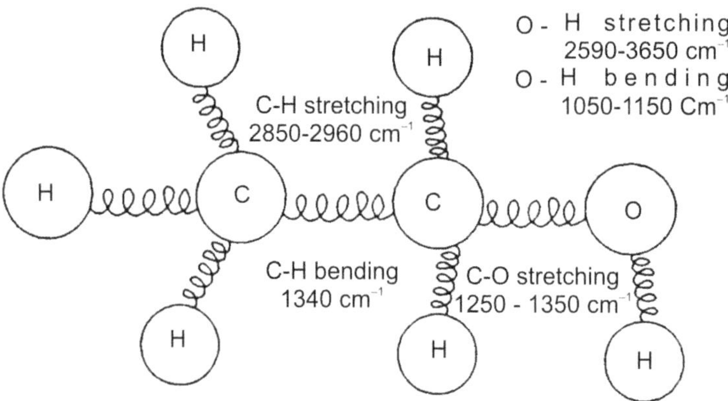

Infra red Vibrations of Ethanol

Criteria for a compound to absorb IR radiation

1. Change in dipole moment.
2. Applied IR frequency should be equal to the natural frequency of radiation. Otherwise compounds do not give IR peaks.

The Requirements for IR Absorption

(a) Correct in dipole moment.

(b) Electric dipole

(a) ***Correct wavelength of Radiation*:** A molecule absorbs radiation only when the natural frequency of vibration of some part of a molecule is the same as the frequency of the incident radiation.

After absorbing the correct wavelength of radiation, the molecule vibrateds at an increased amplitude. This occurs at the expense of the energy of the IR radiation which has been absorbed.

(b) ***Electric dipole*:** A molecule can only absorb IR radiation when its absorption causes a change in its electric dipole. A molecule is said to have electric dipole when there is a slight positive and a slight negative electric charge on its component atoms.

The symmetrical diatomic molecules, like O_2 and N_2 do not possess electric dipole, they cannot be excited by IR radiation and, they donot give rise to IR absorption spectra.

Theory

***Molecular vibrations*:** Absorption in the infrared region is due to changes in the vibrational and rotational levels, when radiations with frequency range less than 100 cm^{-1} are absorbed, molecular rotation takes place in the substance. Molecular vibrations are set in, when more energetic radiation in the region 10^4 to 10^2 cm^{-1} are passed through the sample of the substance.

In the infrared spectroscopy, the absorbed energy brings about predominant changes in the vibrational energy which depends upon:

(i) Masses of the atoms present in a molecule

(ii) Strength of the bonds, and

(iii) The arrangement of atoms within the molecule.

No two compounds except the enantiomers can have similar infrared spectra.

When Infrared light is passed through the sample, the vibrational and the rotational energies of the molecules are increased.

Two kinds of fundamental vibrations are:

(a) Stretching vibrations

(b) Bending vibrations

1. Stretching Vibrations

These are the vibrations in which the bond length is altered i.e. increased (or) decreased.

These vibrations can be sub divided into two types.

(a) Symmetrical Stretching

(b) Asymmetrical Stretching

(a) ***Symmetrical Stretching*:** In this type, the movement of the atoms with respect to a particular atom in a molecule is in the same direction. In this, two bonds increase (or) decrease in length symmetrically.

(b) ***Asymmetrical Stretching*:** In this type, one atom approaches the central atom while the other departs from it. In this, one bond length increases, the other one decreases.

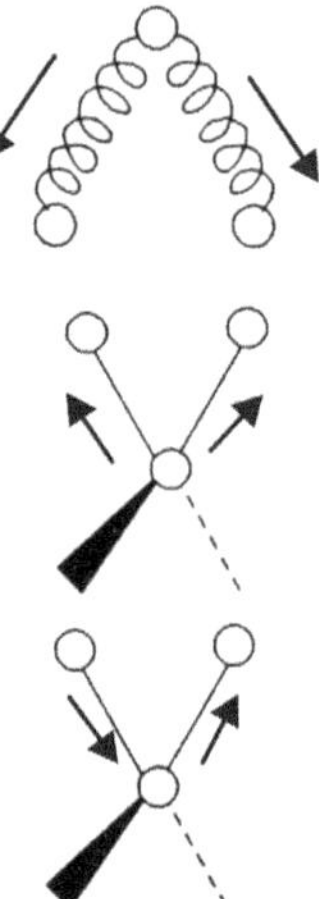

2. Bending Vibrations

In this type of vibrations, the positions of the atoms change with respect to the original bond axis.

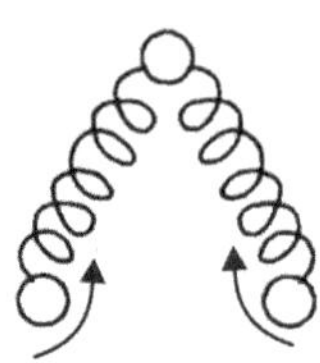

This can be divided into two types:

(a) In-plane bending

(b) Out-plane bending

(a) ***In-plane bending*****:** In these vibrations, there is change in bond angle. Bending of bonds takes place within the same plane.

This can be divided into two types :-

(i) Scissoring

(ii) Rocking

(i) Scissoring : In this, two atoms approach each other and the bond angle decreases.

(ii) ***Rocking*****:** In this type, the movement of the atoms takes place in the same direction and bond angle is maintained, but both bonds move within the plane.

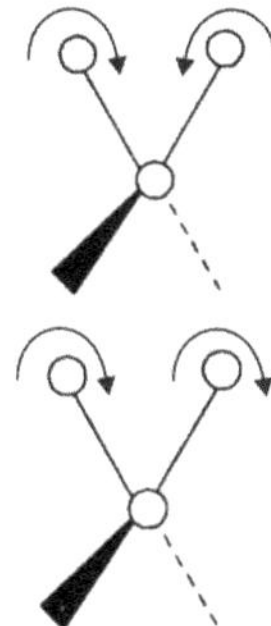

(b) *Out-plane bending*: These can be divided into two types:

(i) Wagging

(ii) Twisting

(i) ***Wagging*:** Two atoms move up and below the plane with respect to the central atom and both atoms move to one side of plane.

(ii) ***Twisting*:** In this type, one of the atoms moves up to the plane while the other moves down the plane with respect to the central atoms.

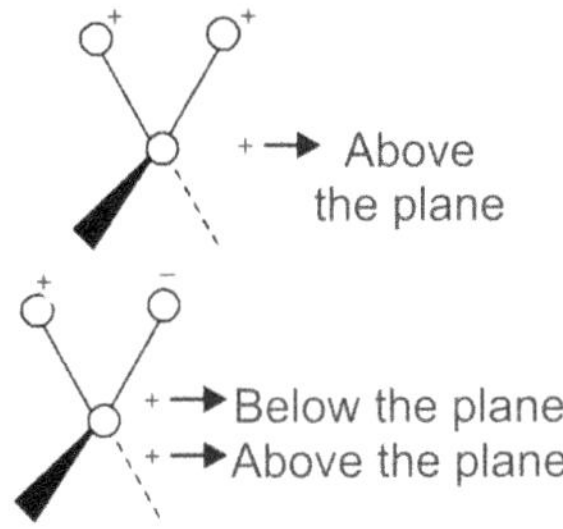

In these two vibrations, Bending vibrations require lesser energy and hence occur at higher wavelength or lower numbers than stretching vibrations.

***Vibrational frequency*:** The value of stretching vibrational frequency of a bond can be calculated by the application of Hooke's law which may be represented as :-

$$\frac{V}{c} = \overline{V} = \frac{1}{2\pi\pi}\left[\frac{k}{\frac{m_1 m_2}{m_1 + m_2}}\right]^{\frac{1}{2}}$$

$$= \frac{1}{2\pi\pi}\sqrt{\frac{K}{\mu}}$$

where μ = reduced mass

m_1, m_2 = masses of the atoms concerned in grams in a particular bond.

K = Force constant of bond

c = velocity of the radiation (2.998×1010 cm sec^{-1})

The value of vibrational frequency or wavenumber depends upon

(i) Bond Strength

(ii) Reduced Mass

If the bond strength increases or the reduced mass decreases, the value of the vibrational frequency increases.

Number of Fundamental Vibrations

The infrared light is absorbed when the oscilating dipolemoment interacts with the oscillating electric vector of an infra-red beam.

A molecule has always three translational degrees of freedom. In case of linear molecule, there are only two degrees of rotation. It is due to the rotation of such a molecule about its axis of linearity and does not bring any change in the position of the atoms while rotation about the other axes changes the position of the atoms.

For a linear molecule of '*n*' atoms

Total degrees of freedom = 3n

Translational degrees of freedom = 3

Rotational degrees of freedom = 2

∴ Vibrational degrees of freedom = 3n – 3 – 2

= 3n – 5

In case of non-linear molecule, there are three degrees of rotation. This results in a change in the position of the atoms.

For a non-linear molecule of 'n' atoms

Total degrees of freedom = 3

Translational degrees of freedom = 3

Rotational degrees of freedom = 3

∴ Vibrational degrees of freedom = 3n – 3 – 3

= 3n – 6

Factors Influencing Vibrational Frequencies

There are number of factors that influence the precise frequency of a molecular vibration, namely:

(a) Vibrational coupling
(b) Hydrigen bonding
(c) Electronic effects and
(d) Field effects

Vibrational coupling: The following four vibrations may be observed in the high – resolution spectra of compounds containing both – CH_2 and – CH_3 groups.

C – H: One stretching frequency

H – C: Two couple vibrations having different
|
H
Frequencies i.e. V_{anti} & V_{sythm} (for asymmetric and symmetric) and

H
|
H – C: Equivalent couple vibration
|
H

Example: Aldehydes (– C – H). The functional group aldehyde offers C – H str absorption band which appears as a doublet because of interaction between the two components namely : C – H str fundamental and C – H def – overtone.

Hydrogen bonding: The hydrogen bonding present in) O – H and N – H compounds give rise to a number of effects in the IP – spectra. The carbonyl group or atomatic present in the same molecule O – H or N – H group may cause similar shifts by intermolecular action.

Example: ***Amines***: Amines show two distinct bands due to N – H stretching in different environments. In condensed phase spectra, amines show bonded N – H str around 3300 cm^{-1} and in dilute solution a new band near 3600 cm^{-1} corresponding to free N – H. It may be due to the electronegativity of nitrogen being less than that of oxygen and hydrogen bonds in amines are weaker than in alcohols.

Electronic Effects: Based on the theoretical principles one may explain the frequency shifts that normally take place in molecular vibrations when the substituents are altered.

1. Conjugation effect

It is observed to lower the frequency of both C = C str and C = O str, irrespective of it is brought about by either a – b unsaturation or by an aromatic ring.

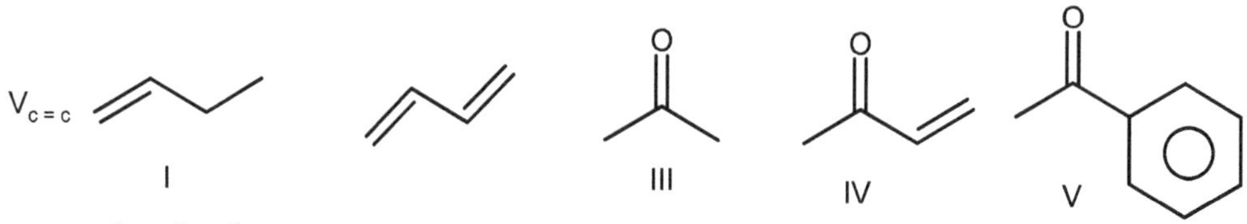

$V_{c=c}$

I α, β, saturation 1650 cm^{-1} | 1610 cm–1 | III 1720 cm^{-1} | IV 1700 cm^{-1} | V 1700 cm^{-1}

2. Mesomeric effect (or) Resonance

A molecule can be represented by two or more structures that differ only in the arrangement of electrons, i.e. by structures that have the same arrangement of atomic nuclei. There is resonance.

3. Inductive effect

The inductive effect depends upon the "intrinsic" tendency of a substituent to either release or withdraw electrons i.e. its electronegativity acting either through the molecular chain or through space. This effect usually weakens steadily with increasing distance from the substituent.

***Field effects*:** These effects can be seen when two functional groups influence each other's vibrational frequencies by a through space interaction that may be either steric or electrostatic in nature.

e.g. Ortho chlorobenzoic acid esters.

In the above example, the field effect shifts the C = O frequency in the rotational isomer (1) and not in the isomer (2). Both the isomers are found to be present together. Therefore, two C = O str absorptions are observed in the spectrum of this compound.

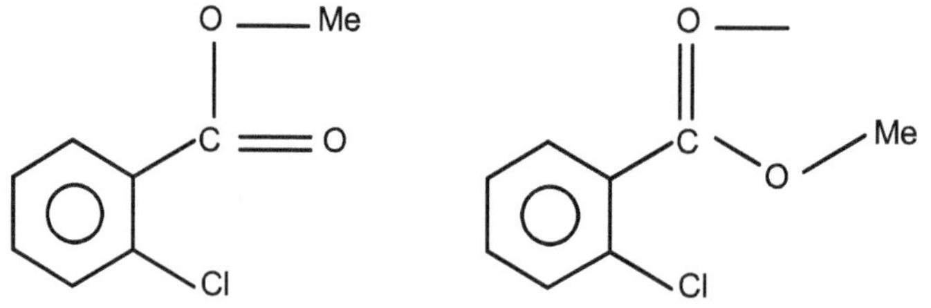

O — Me, C = O, Cl (1)

O —, C, O, Me, Cl (2)

Schematic, Automatic, Double Beam, Optical Null
IR Spectrophotometer

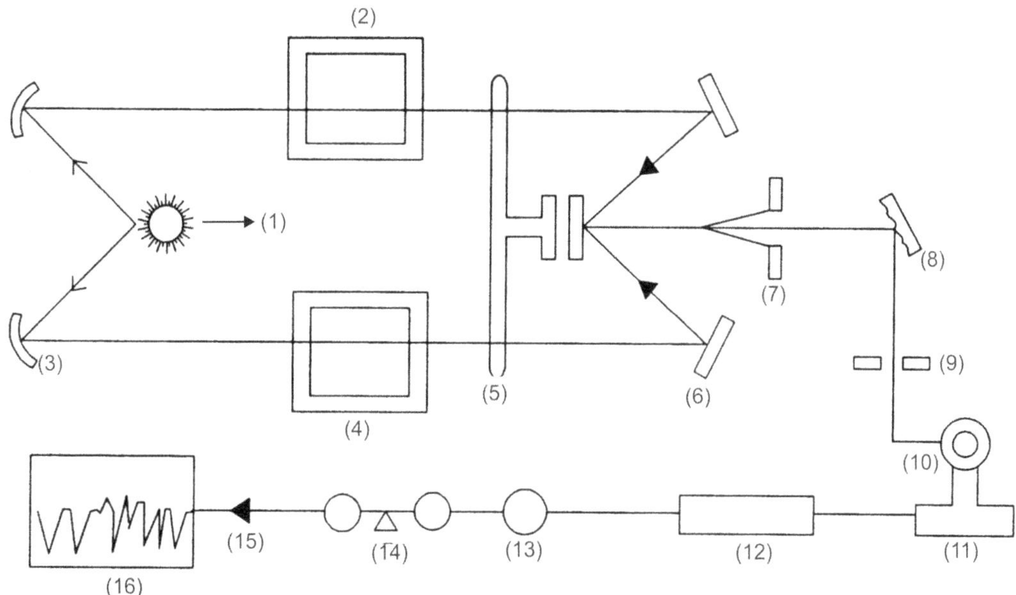

1. Source, 2. Sample Cell, 3. Collimating mirror, 4. Reference cell, 5. Chopper, 6. Reflecting mirror, 7. Entrance slit, 8. Grating, 9. Exit slit, 10. Mirror, 11. Detector, 12. Amplifier, 13. servo motor, 14. Pivot, 15. Pen, 16. Chart recorder.

Single Monochromator Infrared Spectrophotometer

The main parts of an IR spectrometer are as follows:

1. IR Radiation source
2. Monochromators
3. Sample cells and sampling of substances
4. Detectors
5. Recorder / plotter

1. Radiation Source

Infrared instruments require a source of radiant energy which provides isolating narrow frequency bands. The radiation source must emit IR radiation, which must be :

(i) Intense enough for detection

(ii) Steady

(iii) Extend over the desired wavelengths

The various sources of IR radiations are:

(a) ***Incandescent lamp***: In the near infrared instrument an ordinary incandescent lamp is used. In the far infrared, it is glass enclosed and has a low spectral emissivity.

(b) ***Nernst Glower***: It consists of a hallow rod which is about 2 mm in diameter and 30 mm in length. The glower is composed of earth exides such as Zirconia, yttria and Thoria.

Nernst glower is non-conducting at room temperature. Glower is heated to a temperature between 1000 to 1800° C. It provides maximum radiation at about 7100 cm^{-1} (1.4 μ)

Disadvantages

- It emits IR radiation over wide wavelength range.
- The intensity of radiation remains steady and constant over long periods of time.
- Nernst glower has frequent mechanical failure.

  Its energy is concentrated in the visible and near infrared region of spectrum.

(c) ***Globular source***: It is a rod of "Sintered silicon cargide" which is about 50 mm in length and 4 mm in diameter. When it is heated to a temperature between 1300 and 1700 °C, it strongly emits radiation in the IR region. It emits maximum radiation at 5200 cm^{-1}.

Advantages

- It is self starting.
- Its temperature coefficient is positive, it can be controlled with a variable transformer.
- It is more satisfactory as it works at wave lengths longer than 650 cm^{-1} (0.15 μ).

Disadvantage

It is a less intense source than the Nernst glower.

(d) ***Nichrome wire***: Coils or ribbons of Nichrome wire are used as sources in infra red spectrophotometers. The wire is raised to incandescence by resistive heating and heated to surface temperatures of 800-900 °C.

(e) ***Mercury wire***: In the far infrared region, these special high mercury arc lamps are used.

At the short wave lengths, the heated quartz emits the radiation.

At the longer wavelengths, the mercury plasma provides radiation through the quartz.

2. **Monochromators**

The radiation source emits radiation of various frequencies. The sample in IR spectroscopy absorbs only at certain frequencies, it therefore becomes necessary to select desired frequencies from the radiation source and reject the radiations of other frequencies. This selection has been achieved by means of monochromators which are mainly of two types.

(a) Prism monochromator

(b) Grating monochromator.

(a) ***Prism Monochromator*****:** Two types of substances are normally employed as monochromators. They are:

(i) ***Metal halide prism*****:** Various metal prisms such as

KBr – 12-25 μ m

CiF – 0.2-6 μ m

CeBr – 15-38 μ m

These prisms become more or less out of use now-a-days.

(ii) ***NaCl prism*** **(2-15 μ m):** Sodium chloride prisms are used for the whole of the region from 4000-6500 cm^{-1}. Because it offers low resolution at 4000-2500 cm^{-1} and its hygroscopic nature, the optics have got to be protected at 20 °C above the ambient temperature.

In this two types of monochromators are used. They are as follows:

Single Pass Monochromator

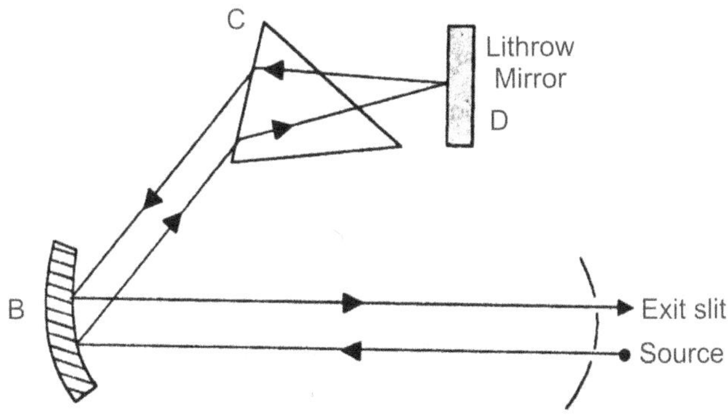

The sample is kept at or near the focus of the beam, just before the entrance slit 'A' to the monochromator. The radiation from the source after passing through the sample and entrance slit strikes the off-axis parabolic littrow mirror B which renders the radiation parallel and sends it to the prism C. The dispersed radiation after reflecting from a plane mirror D returns through the prism a second time and focuses into the exist slit of the monochromator, through which it finally passes into the detector section.

Double Pass Monochromator

In this, there occurs a total of four passes of radiation through the prism as shown (1), (2), (3) and (4). The double pass monochromator produces more resolution than the monochromator in the radiation, before it finally passes onto the detector.

(b) ***Grating monochromator*****:** Gratings are more commonly used in the design of the instruments and gives better resolution at high frequency than the prisms. They offer much better resolution at low frequency. Typical rulings are 240 lines per nm for the 1500-650 cm^{-1} region.

The grating is essentially a series of parallel straight lines cut into a plane surface. Dispersion by gratings follows the law of diffraction. It follows the following mathematical relation:

$$n\lambda = d(\sin i \pm \sin \theta)$$

where

n = order

λ = The wavelength of the radiation

d = The distance between grooves

i – The angle of incidence of beam of IR radiation

θ = angle of dispersion of light of a particular wavelength

Advantages

1. Grating can be made with materials like aluminium which are not attacked by moisture i.e. metal salt prisms are subject to etching from atmospheric moisture.
2. Grating can be used over considerable wavelength ranges.

Grating can be used in combination with a small prism which acts as an order sorter.

Magnified view of a grating monochromator

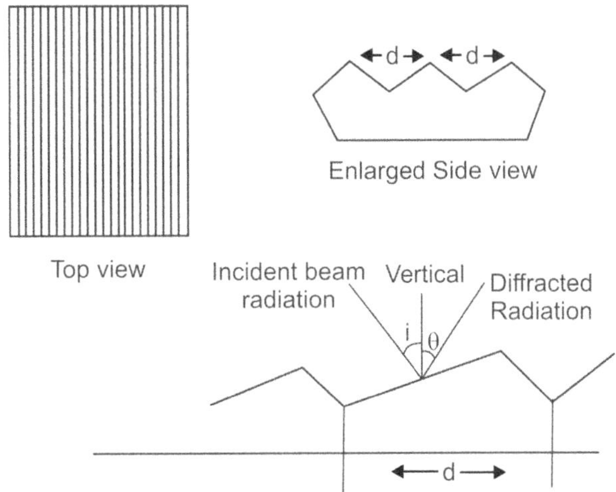

Path of IR Radiation diffracted by a grating monochromator

3. Sample cells and sampling of substances

Infra red spectroscopy is used for the characterization of solid, liquid or gas samples.

(a) Sampling of Solids

(i) Solids Run in Solution : Solids are dissolved in a non-aqueous solvent without chemical interactions.

A drop of the solid solution is placed on an alkali metal disc and the solvent allowed to evaporate leaving a thin film of the solute, or the entire solution is placed in a liquid sample cell. If the solution of solid can be prepared in a suitable solvent then the solution is run in one of the cells for liquids.

Disadvantages

This method cannot be used for all solids because suitable solvents are limited in number.

There is no single solvent which is transparent throughout the region.

(ii) ***Solid films*****:** If a solid is amorphous in nature the sample is deposited on the surface of KBr of NaCl cell by evaporation of a solution of the solid.

Advantage

This technique is useful for rapid qualitative analysis.

Disadvantage

This technique is not useful for qualitative analysis.

(iii) ***Multi technique***: In the technique, the finely ground solid sampes are mixed with Nujol (Mineral oil) to make a thick paste, which is then spread in between IR transmitting windows, this which is then spread in between IR transmitting windows. This is then mounted in a path of Infra red beam and the spectrum is run.

The solid sample in the Nujol is used in combination with hexachlorobutadiene which absorbs in the regions (630-1510, 1200-1140 and 1010-760 cm^{-1}).

Advantage

This method is good for qualitative analysis.

Disadvantages

- It has the absorption maxima at 2915, 1462, 1376 and 719 cm^{-1}.
- This method is not good for quantitative analysis.

(iv) **Pressed pellet technique :** In this technique, finely ground sample is thoroughly mixed with same weight of powderedpotassium bromide. The mixture is then passed under very high pressure in a press to form a small pellet. The resulting pellet is transparent to IR radiation and then run.

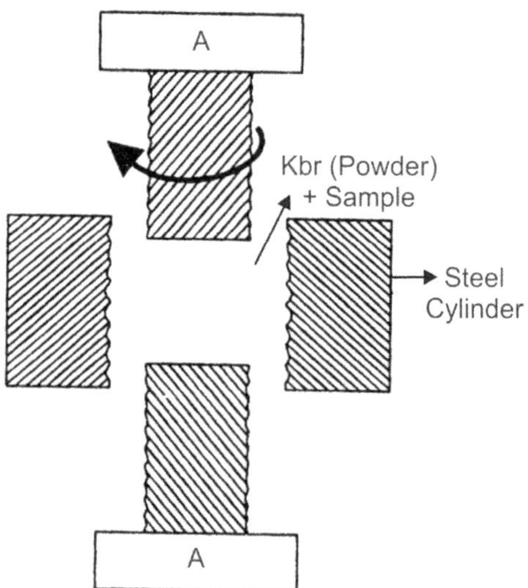

Advantages

1. KBr pellets can be stored for long period of time.
2. The concentration of sample can be adjusted in the pellets, it can be used for qualitative analysis.
3. The resolution of the spectrum in the KBr is superior to that obtained with mulls.

Disadvantages

1. It always has a band at 3450 cm^{-1}, from the OH group of moisture present in the sample.
2. Care must be needed.
3. The high pressure involved during the formation of pellets has polymorphic changes in crystallinity in the samples, which cause complications in IR spectrum.
4. Substitution by bromide may be possible in inorganic complexes.
5. This method is not successful for some polymers which are difficult to grind KBr.

(b) ***Sampling of Liquids*****:** Liquids at room temperature are usually put frequently with no preparation, into rectangular cells made or NaCl, KBr or ThBr and their IR spectra are obtained directly. The liquids represent a thin layer of 0.01-0.05 min thickness and transmittance lies between 15 and 20%.

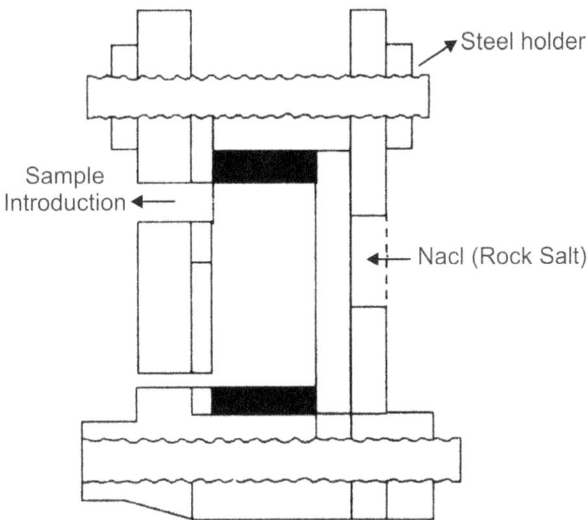

If a cell possesses good quality windows, flat and parallel, its thickness in cm can be calculated from the following equation.

$$2t = \frac{N}{W_1 - W_2}$$

where N = No. of fringes

W_1, W_2 = wave numbers

For double-beam work, "matched cells" are used. One cell will contain the sample and the other will have a solvent used in the sample. All cells should be protected from moisure because they dissolve in water.

(c) ***Sampling of Gases*****:** Gas sample cell is similar to the cell for liquid samples. To compensate for the small number of molecules of a sample that is contained in a gas, the cells are larger. They are about 10 cm long, but they may be upto 1 m long. Multiple reflections can be used to make the effective path length as long as 40m, so the constituents of the gas can be determined.

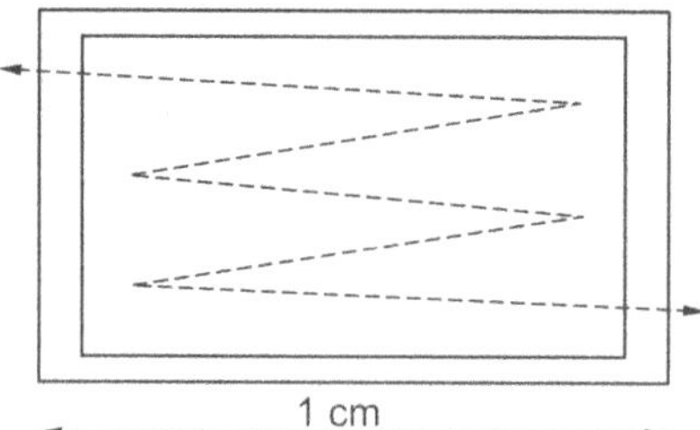

The gas must not react with the cell windows or the reflecting surfaces. Gas analysis are performed with IR but the method is not much used because of its lack of sensitivity.

Moisture must be avoided. Its strong absorption bands at $3710 cm^{-1}$ and $1625 cm^{-1}$ may interfere in the analysis.

4. Detectors

The various types of detectors used in IR spectroscopy are

(a) Bolometers

(b) Thermocouple

(c) Thermistors

(d) Golay cells

(e) Photo conductivity cell

(f) Semi conductor detectors

(g) Pyro electric detectors

(h) Fourier Transform systems

(a) ***Bolometers*****:** A bolometer is based on the fact that the electrical resistance of a metal increases 0.4% for every Celsius degree increases of temperature. A bolometer consists of a thin metal conductor. When radiation falls on this conductor its temperature changes. The metallic conductor resistance changes with temperature the degree of change in resistance is taken as a measure of the amount of radiation that has fallen on the bolometer. The response time for a bolometer is 4 m sec.

(b) ***Thermocouple***: The thermocouple detector is based on electrical current which flows with two dissimilar metal wires are connected together at both ends and a temperature differential exists between two ends. The end exposed to the Infrared radiation is called the "hot junction". In order to increase the energy gathering efficiency there is a black body. The other connection, the cold jundtion, is thermally insulated and carefully screened from stray light. The electricity flow is directly proportional to the energy differential between the two connections.

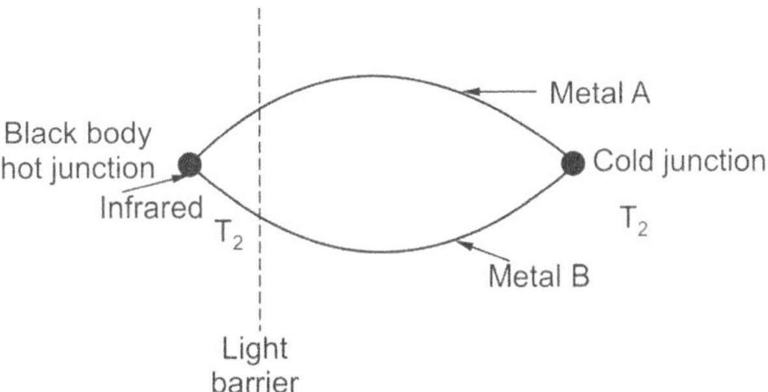

A thermocouple is made by welding together at each end of two wires of different semi conductors materials of high thermoelectric efficiency. If two welded joints are kept at different temperatures, a small electrical potential is developed between the joints. A thermocouple is closed in an evacuated steel casing with a KBr of CsI window to avoid losses of energy by convection.

In the IR spectroscopy, one welded joint (cold junction) is kept at a constant temperature and is not exposed to IR radiation, but the other welded joint (hot junction) is exposed to the IR radiation which increases the temperature of the junction. The temperature difference between the two junctions generate potential difference which depends on how much IR radiation falls on the hot junction. The response time of a thermocouple is about 60 m sec.

(c) ***Thermistors*****:** A thermistor is made of a fused mixture of metal oxides. When the temperature of the mixture increases, its electrical resistance decreases. The thermistor changes resistance by 5 per ^{o}C. Its response time is slow.

(d) ***Golay Cell*****:** It consists of a small metal cylinder which is closed by a black ended metal place at one end and by a flexible metalized diaghragm at the other. The cylinder is filled with xenon, and then it is sealed. When IR radation is allowed to fall on the black end metal plate. It heats the gas. The resulting pressure increase in the gas deforms the metalized diaghragm which separates two chambers. Light from a lamp is made to fall on the diaphragm which reflects the light onto a photo cell.

Motion of the diaphragm changes the output of cell. The signal seen by the photo tube is modulated in accordance with the power of the radiant beam incident on the gas cell.

Advantages

- It possesses the same sensitivity as a thermocouple in the mid-IR region.
- It is used when working at wave lengths greater than 15 μ.

Its reponse time is 10-2 sec, faster than that of the bolometer, thermistor or thermocouple.

Disadvantages

- Less convenient than other detectors.
- It is more expensive and bulky.

(e) ***Photo conductivity cell*:** This is a non-thermal detector or greater sensitivity. It consists of a thin layer of lead sulphide or lead telluride supported on glass and enclosed in to an evacuated glass envelope. When IR radiation if focussed on lead sulphide or lead telluride, its conductance increases and more current flows. Response time is 0.5 m sec.

Advantage

It has good speed of response and high sensitivity.

Disadvantage

When operated at room temperature it is limited to the near infrared.

The range can be broadened by drastic cooling.

(f) ***Semi Conductor detector*:** Semi conductor materials are insulators when no radiations falls on them, but which become conductors when radiation falls on them. Exposure to radiation causes a very rapid change in their electrical resistance and therefore a very rapid response to the IR signal. The basic concept is that an IR photon displaces an electron in the detector, Changing its conductivity. Recently other materials such as each telluride, indium antimonide and germanium doped with copper or mercury have been used as semiconductor detectors.

A semiconductor detector is fabricated with the semiconductor material deposited on glass in a sealed, evacuated envelope. Exposure to radiation causes a rapid range in the material's conductivity. The response time of this detector is the time required to change the semiconductor from an insulator to a conductor, which is frequently as short as 1m sec. Semi conductor detectors are very sensitive, very fast and are finding wide acceptance in the field of IR spectroscopy.

(g) ***Pyro electric detectors*:** A dielectric spacer placed in an electrostatic field becomes polarized, depending on the dielectric constant. If the field is removed, the polarization disappears, except with ferroelectric compounds, which retain a stron residual polarization. Sometimes their residual polarization is temperature sensitive, if the materials are pyro electric.

A pyro electric detector consists of a thin dielectric flake on the face of which an electro static charge appears when the temperature of the flake changes.

This happens upon exposure to IR radiation. A pyro electric flake is cut from a single crystal and is very small. It varies in size from about 0.25 to 12.0 mm^2.

The most common pyroelectric detector is tri glycerine sulphate and its response rapidly deteriorates above 45°C and is lost above the curie point (49°C).

For this reason it is usually cooled in liquid N_2. Recently deuterated TGS detectors are the choice with fourier transform IR, superseding Golay detectors. Their response is fast, so they can be used for multiplex scanning.

(h) ***Fourier transform systems*****:** If two beams of light of the same wavelength are brought together in phase, the beams reinforce each other and continue down the light path. If two beams are out of phase, destructive interference takes place. This interference is at a maximum when the two beams of light are 180° out of phase.

This system consists of four optical arms, at right angles to each other with a beam splitter at their point of intersection. Radiation passes down the first arm and is separated by a beam splitter in to two perpendicular half beams of equal intensity that pass down into other arms of the spectrometer. At the ends of these arms, the two half-beams are reflected by mirrors back to the beam splitter, where they recombine and are reflected together onto the detector.

If the initial radiations at one wavelength and in phase with itself and if the side arm paths are equal in length, then, when the two half beam are recombined, they will be in phase, reinforcing each other and the maximum signal will be obtained on the detector. If the mirror on one arm is moved up by one quarter of a wavelength, then the half beams will be one half of a wavelength out of phase in one arm is kept stationary and that in the second arm is moved slowly in the direction of the beam splitter. The net signal falling on the detector will then be a cosine wave with the usual maxima and minima when plotted against the travel of the mirror. The frequency of the cosine signal is equal to

$$f = \frac{2v}{\lambda}$$

where f = frequency

v = velocity of the moving mirror

λ = wavelength of radiation

The frequency of modulation is proportional to both the wavelength of the incident radiation and the velocity of the mirror.

Repeated bursts of radiation of all wavelengths to be considered are obtained from the source and travel down the arms of interferometer. They proceed through the sample holder before reaching the detector, where absorption by the sample can take place.

It is mechanically difficult to move the reflecting mirror at a controlled, known, steady velocity. The velocity is controlled by using a laser beam that is shown down the light path and which causes an interference pattern with itself. The cosine pattern of the interference pattern of the laser is used to regulate the velocity of the moving mirror.

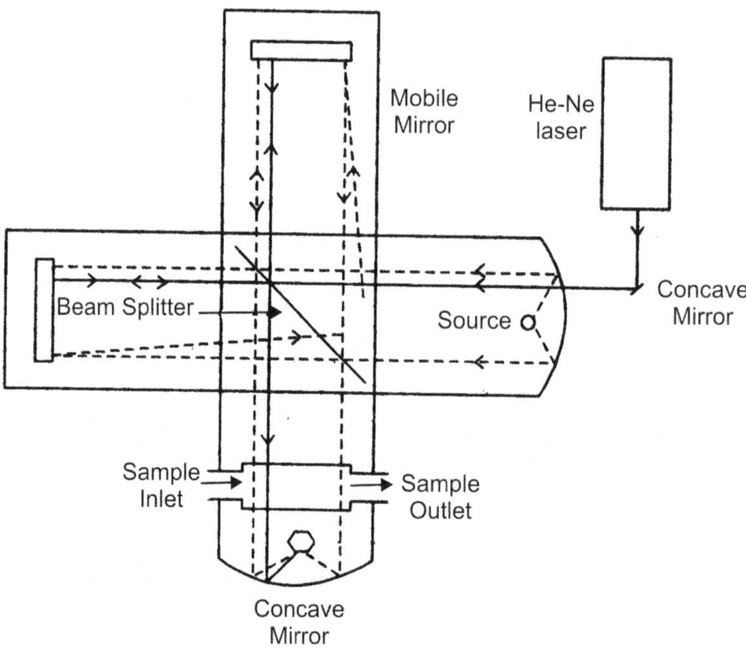

Advantages

- Only the mirror moves during an experiment.
- Use of a laser provides high frequency accuracy (to 0.01 cm^{-1})
- Stray light does not affect the detector, since all signals are modulated.

- A much larger beam may be used at all times. Data collection is easier.
- All frequencies of radiation fall on the detector simultaneously.
- Rapid scan speeds permit monitoring sample undergoing rapid change.
- The sample is not subject to the thermal effects.
- Any emission of IR radiation by the sample will not be detected.

Quantitative Analysis for Infrared Spectroscopy

There are two methods, frequently, employed for the determination of the transmittance ratio in quantitative analysis namely:

(a) Empirical Ratio Method

(b) Base-line Method

(a) *Empirical Ratio Method*: This method is employed in a situation where the absorption bands of the analyte are found to be very close to those of the main constituent or the internal standard.

The quantitative analysis of pharmaceutical substances may be achieved by empirical ratio method, either by plotting percentage transmittance against wavelength or by plotting the log-1 0/T1 against concentration.

(b) *Base-line Method*: This method involves the selection of an absorption band of an analyte which does not remain very close to the bands of other constituents present in matrix.

The value of the incident radiant energy P_0 may be achieved by drawing straight line tangent to the spectral absorption curve at the position of the analyte's absorption band. Consequently, the transmittance P is usually measured at the point of maximum absorption. Finally, the value of log P_0/P is plotted against the concentration.

The application of both empirical ratio method and base-line method helps in eliminating to a great extent the errors caused due to changes in source intensity and adjustment of the optical system.

Finger Print Region

IR spectroscopy function is to determine the identity of two compounds. In a spectrum, the number of bonding vibrations is usually more than the number of stretching vibrations, the region is usually rich in absorption bands and shoulders. It is called finger print region.

Finger-print region can be divided into 3 regions. They are :-

(i) 1500 = 1350 cm^{-1}

(ii) 1350 – 1000 cm^{-1}

(iii) Below 1000 cm^{-1}

(i) ***Region*: 1500-1350 cm^{-1}:** The appearance of a doublet near 1380 cm^{-1} and 1365 cm^{-1} shows the presence of tertiary butyl group in the compound. Out of the two strong bands for the nitro compounds, one appears in the finger print region near 1350 cm^{-1}.

(ii) ***Region*: 1350-1000 cm^{-1}:** All classes of compounds like alcohols, esters, lactones, acid anhydrides show characteristic absorptions in this region due to C – O stretching. Primary alcohols form two strong bands at 1350-1260 cm^{-1} and near 1050 cm^{-1}. Phenols absorb near 1200 cm^{-1}. Esters show two strong bands between 1380-1050cm^{-1}. Absorption in the region 1150-1070 cm^{-1} is most characteristic of other i.e. C – O stretching C – O – C group.

(iii) ***Region*: below 1000 cm^{-1}:** C = C – H deformation at 700 cm^{-1} and that at 970-960 cm^{-1} distinguishes between cis and trans alkenes. The higher value indicates that the hydrogen atoms in the alkene are trans with respect to each other.

The presence of monosubtitution and also disubstitution at ortho, meta and para positions in benzene are detected by most characteristic absorptions in the region. A band in the region 750-700 cm^{-1} shows monosubstituted benzene.

Intensity Absorption Bands

The intensity of infrared absorption bands is dependent on mainly on the magnitude of the dipole. The more the polar character of a bond, the greater the intensity of absorption. For example strongly polar bonds between carbon and oxygen gives rise to absorption bands having high intensity.

Units of Measurement

The position of the IR peak is expressed either in wave number (cm^{-1}), which represent frequency, or in microns μ which represent wavelength.

Interconversion of two units can be carried out to the following relationship.

$$\overline{\text{v}}\,(\text{cm}^{-1}) \times \lambda_{\mu} = 10^4.$$

The wavelength of the radiation in vacuum is slightly different from the wavelength in air.

$$\lambda_{\text{vacuum}} = n_{\text{air}} \times \lambda_{\text{air}}$$

where λ = wavelength

n = Refractive index

Intensity of IR bands may be recorded as a percentage of the intensity of the incident radiation or as percentage absorption.

To obtain exactly superimposable spectra (e.g. for confirmation of the identity of two samples), they should be recorded on the same instrument.

Applications

Infrared spectrum of a compound provides more information than is normally available from the electronic spectra. In this technique, all groups absorb characteristically within a definite range. The shift in the position of absorption for a particular group may change with the chages in the structure of the molecule.

Impurities in a compound can be detected from the nature of the bands which no longer remain sharp. If the spectrum contains a strong absorption band between 1900-1600 cm^{-1}, the presence of carbonyl group (C = O) in a compound is suspected. Aldehydes can be recognised from its characteristic C – H stretching, esters from C – O stretching and amides show absorptions for N – H stretching and N – H bending absorptions in addition to VC = O in the range.

Presence of conjugation with carbonyl group can be detected it shifts VC = O stretching to the lower wavenumber. The absorption values for certain groups such as C = O, O – H are also important in detecting hydrogen bonding. In case of hydrogen bonding, the wave number of absorption is shifted downwards for both the donor and acceptor group. It can also make distinction between intermolecular hydrogen bonding and intra-molecular hydrogen bonding; the absorption position due to the latter being independent of the change in concentration.

Due to different positions of abosorptions, it is also possible to know the axial and the equatorial positions of certain groups in a cyclic structure. The force constants responsible for the absorption peaks can be used to calculate bond distances and bond angles in simple cases.

Some of important families giving characteristic absorptions and the environmental effects on them are discussed below :-

A. Hydro Carbons

These compounds are made up of carbon and hydrogen only. Hydrocarbons may be saturated and unsaturated aliphatics, cyclics or aromatics.

(i) ***Alkanes and alkyl residues*:** The alkane residues are detected from C – H stretching and C – H deformation absorptions. C – H does not take part in hydrogen bonding, its apsorption position is little affected by chemical environments since most of the organic compounds possess alkanes residue. Two C – H stretching absorption bands appear just below 3000 cm^{-1}. One for symmetrical and the other for asymmetrical vibrational frequencies. The group of bands corresponding to C – H is characteristic of alkyl groups provided, it is not under some electrical influence.

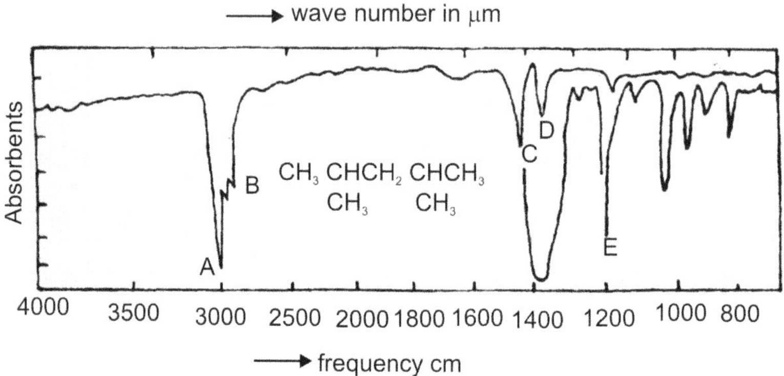

Positions of characteristic absorptions

Infra red spectrum of 2, 4 dimethyl, 1-pentane

A = 2962 cm^{-1}; C – H Str

B = 2872 cm^{-1}; C – H str in CH_3

C = 1465 cm^{-1} ; C – H def

D = 1450 cm^{-1} ; C – H def in CH_2

E = 772 cm^{-1}; CH_2 (Rocking).

Group	Type of Vibration	Region in cm
C – H	C – H str	2960-2850 (m, s)
C – C	C – H def	1485-1340 (w)
- CH_2 -	C – C str	1300-800 (w)
- CH_3	C – H def	1485-1440 (m)
- $(CH_3)_2$	C – H def	1470-1430 (m)
Germdimethyl	C – H def	~ 1380 (m)
- C $(CH_3)_3$	C – H def	~ 1365 (s)
Terbutyl	C – H def	1395-1385 (m)

For molecules containing – OCH_3, - $N(CH_3)$, O – CH_2 – O etc, C – H stretch absorption appears below 3000 cm^{-1}.

(ii) ***Alkenes*:** In alkenes (olefines), C – H str absorption band appears in the region 3100-3000 cm^{-1}. Conjugation of double bond with an aromatic ring shows C = C str near 1625 cm^{-1}.

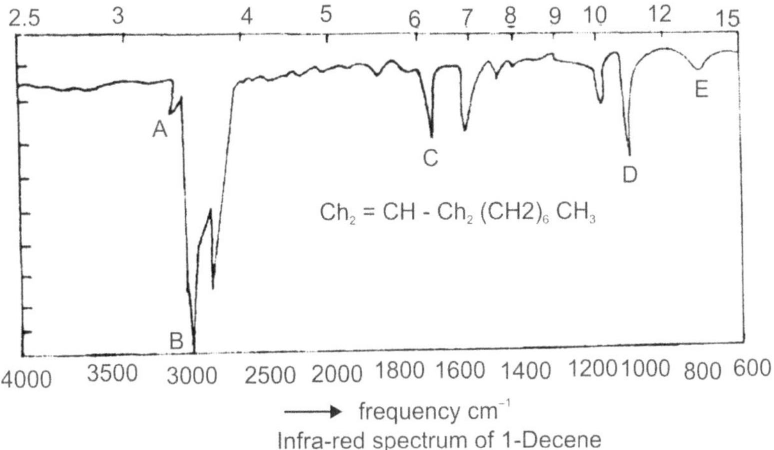

Infra-red spectrum of 1-Decene

Positions of some characteristic absorptions.

A = 3049 cm^{-1}	C - H str in olefines.
B = 2960-2850 cm^{-1}	C – H str in CH_3, CH_2
C = 1645 cm^{-1}	C = C str
D = 986 cm^{-1}	C – H def out of plane
E = 720 cm^{-1}	Methylene rocking

For trans alkenes, C – H def comes around 970 cm^{-1} and for the corresponding cis-isomer, it appears at about 700 cm^{-1}. This helps in distinguishing cis- and trans-alkenes. Conjugated dienes which form a symmetrical molecules as butadiene ($CH_2 = CH – CH = CH_2$) shows one band near 1000 cm^{-1} (C = C stretching). Similar absorptions for molecules without centre of symmetry as 1, 3 pentadiene appear in the region 1650- 1600 cm^{-1} cumulative double bonds such as C = C = C shows strong absorption band around 2000 bonds such as C = C = C shows strong absorption band around 2000-1900 cm^{-1}. For a symmetrical alkene, C = C, absorption is Raman active due to molecular symmetry.

(iii) ***Alkynes*****:** In acetylenes, a strong band for – C = C – H str appears at about 3300 cm^{-1} and a weak C = C str occur at about 2200 cm^{-1}. For mono-substituted acetylenes, C – H stretching appears at about 3300 cm^{-1}. This band is strong and narrow and can be distinguished from the hydrogen bonded O – H and N – H stretching occurring in the same region. C – H bending for acetylenes and mono-substituted acetylenes occur at 650-610 cm^{-1}.

Infra-red spectrum of 1-Hexyene.

Positions of some characteristic absorptions.

A = 3268 cm^{-1} ≡ C – H str

B = 2940-2860 cm^{-1} C – H str in CH_3, CH_2

C = 2110 cm^{-1} C ≡ C str

D = 1247 cm^{-1} ≡ C – H def (Overtone)

E = 630 cm^{-1} ≡ C – H def (Fundamental)

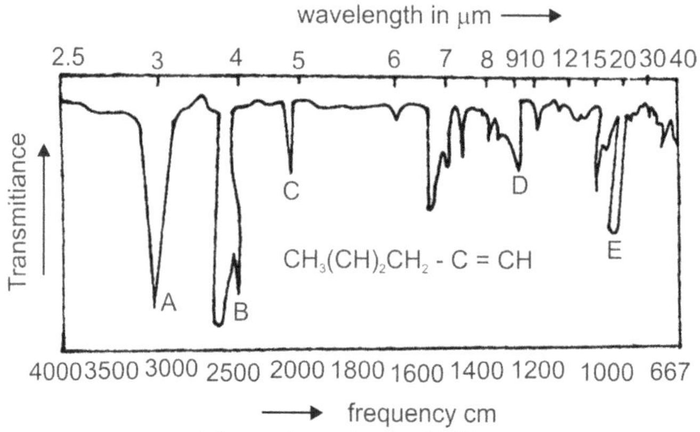

Infra-red spectrum of 1-Hexyene

(iv) ***Cyclone alkenes*****:** In cyclo alkenes, the value of C – H str increases with the increasing angle of strain in the ring. The asymmetric CH_2 stretching vibrations for cyclopropane is between 3100- 2919 cm^{-1} and that for cyclohexane is 2950 cm^{-1}. With increasing strain in the ring, C – H bending also shows an increase. For example, C – H bending in cyclopentane is at 1455 cm^{-1} while that in cyclohexane is at 1442 cm^{-1}.

Note**:** Such a spectrum (Cyclohexane) is important as a finger print and can be used for comparison.

(v) ***Aromatic hydrocarbons*****:** In aromatic hydrocarbons, a variable C – H stretching absorption occurs in the region 3050-3000 cm^{-1}; C = C str at 1650-1450 cm^{-1} and C – H def vibrations at 900 – 700 cm^{-1}. For aromatic compounds, the most characteristic C = C stretching bands are at 1600 cm^{-1}, 1580 cm^{-1}, 1500 cm^{-1} and 1450 cm^{-1} (m). If there is no absorption in this region, it is a fair proof that the compound is not aromatic. Monosubstituted benzene can be easily recognised by bands at 710-690 cm^{-1} (s) and at 770-730 cm^{-1} (s). Metasubstituted benzene usually shows two bands (i) 710-690 cm^{-1} (m) and (ii) 800-750 cm^{-1} (m) ortha and para substituted benzene show one band each at 770-735 cm^{-1} (v, s) and at 840-800 cm^{-1} (m) respectively.

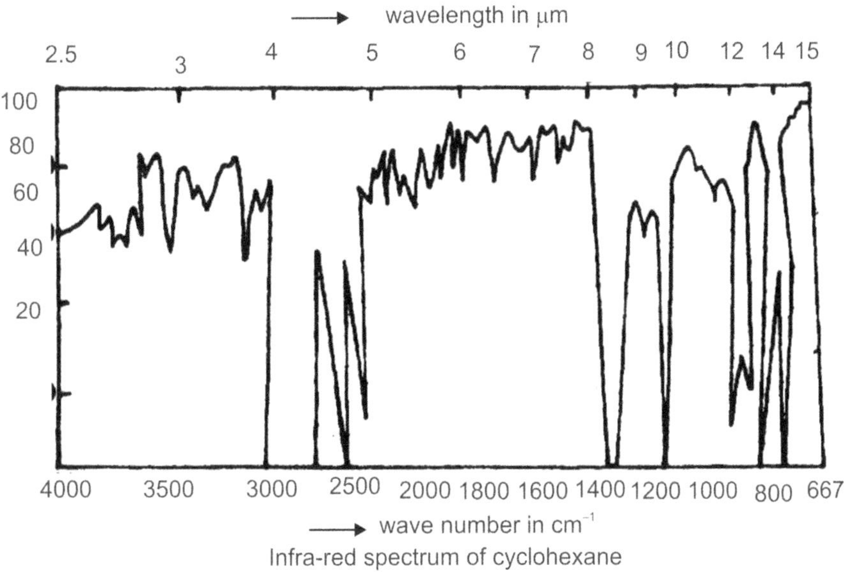

Infra-red spectrum of cyclohexane

Positions of some characteristic absorptions.

A = 3030 cm^{-1}	= C – H str in olefines aromatics
B = 2940 cm^{-1}	C – H str in methyl
C, D, E = 1624, 1510, 1450 cm^{-1};	C = C str in aromatic nuclei.
F = 1370 cm^{-1};	C – H def
G = 802 cm^{-1} ;	Para – disubstituted benzene.

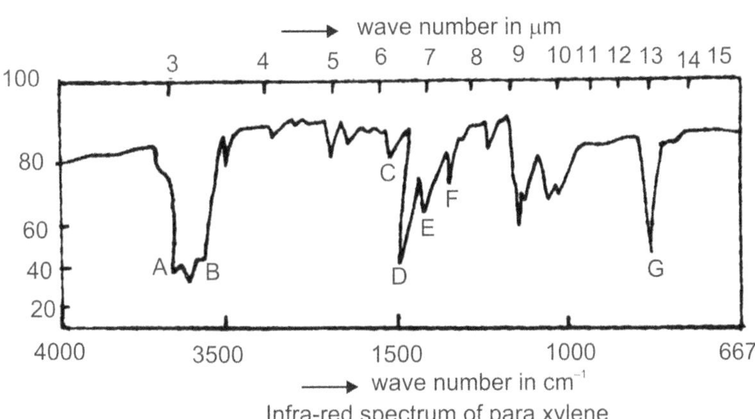

Infra-red spectrum of para xylene

Representation of C – H str and CH def vibration for – CH3, - CH2 – C – H groups.

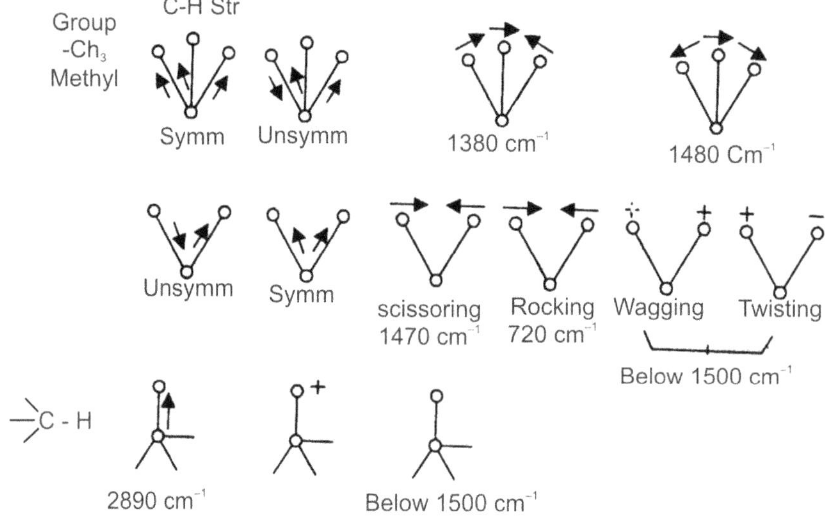

B . Halogen Compounds

In the halogen compounds, the C – H stretching shifts to higher wave number due to the – I effect of the halogen atom. Due to the I (Inductive) effect of halogen, C – H part of the molecule becomes rich in s-component and hence force constant increases. Greater the electronegativity of the halogen atom, greater is the value of C – H stretching. C – X bands show lower values of absorption frequencies as compared to C – H band due to the decreased force constant and increase in the reduced mass. C – X str (X = Cl, Br, I) absorption lies between 800-500 cm^{-1} while in case of C = F band, stretching vibrations occur in the region 1400-1000 cm^{-1} Bromides and chlorides are best detected by their mass spectra. The asymmetric C – H stretching vibrations of – CH_3 group in CH_3 occur above 3000 cm^{-1} which is also the region for aromatic and unsaturated compounds. C – H stretching shifts to higher frequencies in dihalogen and trihalogen derivatives. The detection of halogen by this technique is not reliable as most of the absorptions occur below $\pm$ 650 cm^{-1}.

C. Alcohols and Phenols

Alcohols and phenols exhibit an excellent property of hydrogen bonding. Due to this reason, O – H stretching bands for such compounds are normally recorded in dilute solutions of the sample in non-associating solvents. A variable sharp band appears in the region 3700-3500 cm^{-1}, when a spectrum of a dilute solution of alcohol in carbontetrachloride is scanned. Because of its high intensity, the O – H absorption band can be differentiated from the overtones and the combination bands of this region. Spectra for alcohols are best determined in the vapour phase. If the spectrum is taken with increased concentration of alcoholic solution, a sharp band disappears and a broad band at lower frequency appears instead. In polar solvents, O – H str appears at lower wave number due to the association of alcohol molecules with the solvent molecules.

The absorption maximum for O – H stretching depends upon concent action, nature of the solvent and temperature. The strength of the hydrogen bond is not influenced by the nature or the volume of the substituents in these positions e.g. substituent group may be methyl or the tertiary butyl.

Compared with alcohols, phenol can be classified as sterically hindered, partially hindered and normally. If Phenol is substituted in the ortho positions, it is said to be sterically hindered. The spectrum for such a compound shows a strong band corresponding to free hydroxyl group near 3640 cm^{-1}. If a single alkyl group is present in the ortho position in phenol, the absorption shows a slight downward shift. Spectra of ortho substituted phenols (capable of forming hydrogen bonds with – OH group), show a free OH band along with another band arising from intramolecularly bonded O – H group. In such a case, bonded O – H band has a lower frequency of absorption. Di and poly hydroxylic phenols with adjacent O – H groups form intra molecular hydrogen bonds. Catechol in dilute solution shows two bands at 3610 cm^{-1} (due to free O – H group) and another at 3570 cm^{-1} (due to intramolecularly bonded O – H group).

Group	Type of Vibrations	Region in cm^{-1} and intensity
Alcohols		
Free O – H group	O – H str	3700-3500 (v, sh)
Intermolecular hydrogen		
Bonded OH* (poly meric association)	O – H str	3400-3200 (v, b)
Intramolecular hydrogen bonded OH**	O – H str	3570-3470 (v, sh)
Chelate Compounds	O – H str	3000-2500 (w, b)
Primary alcohols	C – O str	(i) 1350-1260 (s) (ii) ~ 1050 (s)
Secondary alcohols	C – O str	(i) 1350-1260 (s) (ii) ~ 1100(s)
Tertiary alcohols	C – O str	(i) 1400 -1310 (s) (ii) ~ 1150 (s)
Cis-1, 2 cyclohexanediol	O – H str	(i) 3626 (free) (ii)3600 (bonded)
Phenols	C – O str	(i) ~ 1200 (s) (ii) 1410- 1300 (s)

* Absorption shifts to higher wave-number on dilution

** Not absorption shift on dilution

Infra-red spectrum of methyl cyclohexanol

D. Ethers

Ethers are derivatives of alcohols and show characteristic C – O – C bands. Since the masses of C – C and C – O are comparable, their force constants are quite close. But due to the large difference in their dipole moments, the C – O bonds are stronger as compared to C – C bonds. Ethers show only one characteristic band in the region 1300-1050 cm^{-1}. The identification of Ether in an unknown compound is difficult in presence of another oxygenated compound because many other strong bands appear in the same region. Saturated aliphatic ethers show a strong band in the region 1150-1070 cm^{-1} for asymmetric C – O – C stretching and another at 940 cm^{-1} for symmetrical stretching. The C – O – C absorption spectrum of higher members lie in the broad region 1250-1070 cm^{-1} keto ethers and esters are difficult to distinguish since both are identified for the values of C = O stretching and C – O stretching.

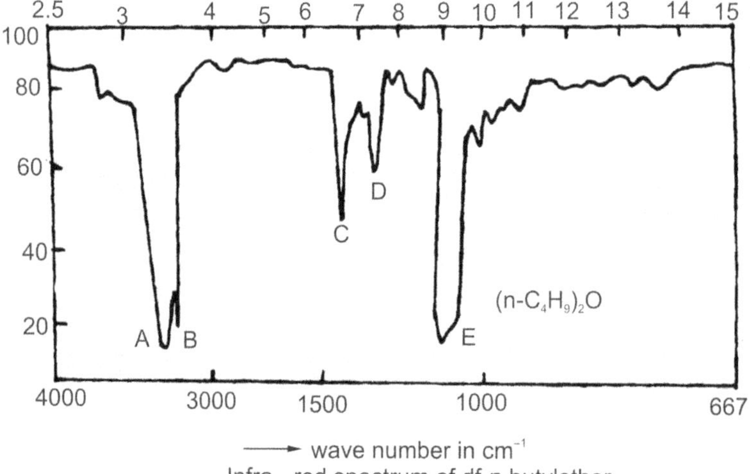

Infra - red spectrum of df-n butylether

Positons of some characteristic absorptions.

A = 2960 cm^{-1}	C – H str in methyl
B = 2880 cm^{-1}	C – H str
C = 1462 cm^{-1}	C – H def methyl methylene
D = 1372 cm^{-1}	C – H def in methyl
E = 1124 cm^{-1}	C – O str in C – O – C group.

Group	Type of Vibrations	Region in cm^{-1} and intensity
C — O — C C — O — CH_3 C — C (O)	C – O str	1150-1070 (s)
	C – H str	2850-2810 (m)
	C – O str	- 1250 (s)
		- 910 (s)
		- 800 (s)
C = C – O – C	C – O str	1070-1020 (s)
		1270-1200 (s)

E. Carbonyl Compounds

The appearance of a strong band in the spectrum between 1650-1950 cm^{-1} shows the presence of carbonyl group in the compound. It is due to C = O str and is the most representative type of vibration localised in an individual bond. After detecting the carbonyl group, the next step is to examine other peaks in the spectrum for the determination of the exact functional group, aldehyde, ketone, ester, amide, quinine etc. Greater is the number of peaks in the spectrum, easier becomes the detection. The frequency of absorption due to carbonyl group depends mainly on the force constant which in turn depends upon inductive effect, conjugative effect, field effect and steric effects.

All these effects operate simultaneously. A carbonyl compound can be written in the following two forms :-

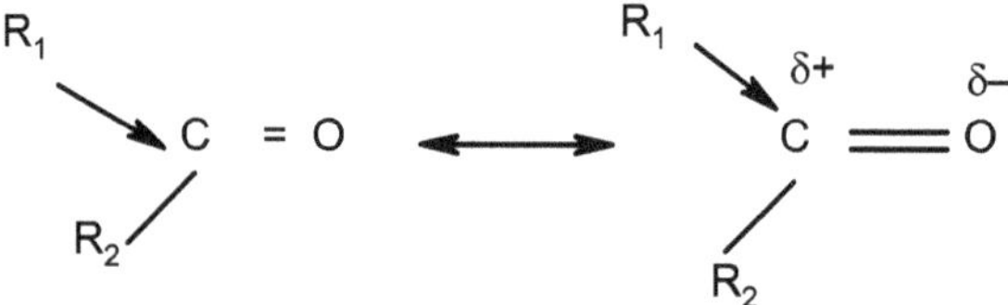

If R_1 and R_2 are electron repelling groups, the structure II is favoured, the force constant (also bond order) is lowered and absorption occurs at lower wave number. If R_1 or / and R_2 is large electron withdrawing group (s), then under its/their influence, the structure I is favoured. The force constant for structure I is more and hence absorption occurs at higher wave number. The position of absorption is also sensitive to unsaturation. C = O stretching for α, β - unsaturated ketones occurs at a lower frequency as compared to its saturated analogue. Aryl ketones show C = O stretching absorption at a lower wave number as compared to aliphaticketones. The position of C = O stretching absorption also depends upon the ring size. The wave number of absorption if raised with the decrease in the size of the ring.

(i) ***Aldehydes and ketones***: Due to larger + I effect operating in ketones as compared to that in aldehydes, the latter usually absorb at higher wave number as compared to the former. The C = O stretching absorption for formaldehyde (HCHO), acetaldehyde (CH_3CHO) and acetone (CH_3 $COCH_3$) are 1750, 1745 and 1718 cm^{-1} respectively. Aldehydes can be easily distinguished from ketones due to the presence of two weak C – H str (asymm and symm) absorption bands one near 2820 cm^{-1} and the other near 2720 cm^{-1}.

The band at higher wave number is not observed if there is another C – H str due to some other part of the molecule. Ketones exist in equilibrium with their enolic forms. The enolic form can be detected by a broad band in the bonded O – H region and the another at a very low C = O stretching frequency. Lower the value of the carbonyl frequency, greater is the enolic content in equilibrium.

In case of some electron withdrawing groups which also cause λ, β unsaturation, viz, alkenyl, alkynyl, aryl etc the conjugative effect dominates over inductive effect and the result is the net decrease in wave number of carbonyl absorption.

In the spectra of cis and trans 2-bromo-4-tertiary butyl cyclohexanone the bulky tertiary butyl group must be in the equatorial position.

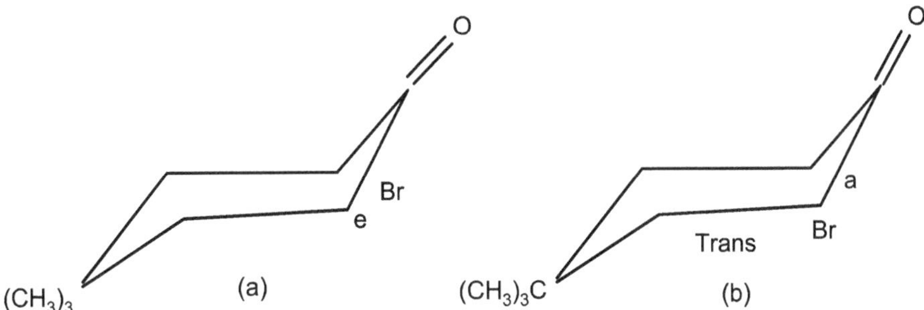

When bromine atom is equatorial, it (form a) becomes cis and VC = O absorption is raised by about 20 cm^{-1}. When bromine atom is axial (form b), the configuration is trans which does not show any VC = O shift from the normal value.

VC = O 1700 cm^{-1}, lowering is due to conjugation of C = O with the ring.

CHO

(I)

VC = O 1651 cm^{-1}, lowering is due to conjugation as well as intramelecular hydrogen bonding.

HO

CHO

(il)

VC = O 1685 cm^{-1}, lowering is due to conjugation of C = O with the ring.

$COCH_3$

(iii)

VC = O 1625 cm^{-1}, lowering is due to conjugation as well as intramolecular hydrogen bonding.

$COCH_3$ OH

(iv)

In hydroxyl aldehydes and ketones, intramolecular hydrogen bonding lowers the VC = O and VO – H absorptions. In saturated hydroxyl ketones, the intramolecular hydrogen bonds give a strong O – H band in the region 3400-3200 cm^{-1}.

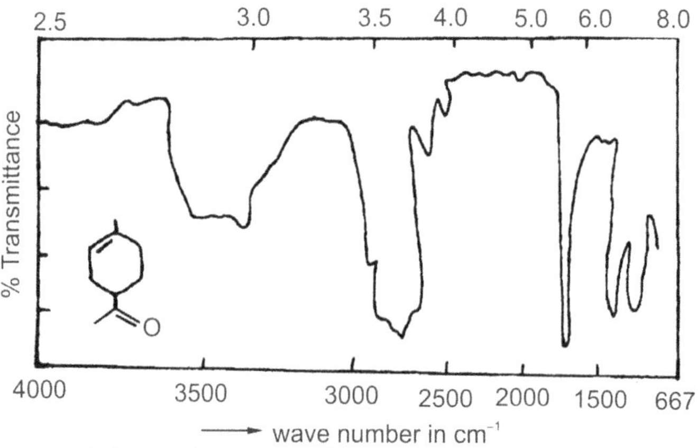

Infra - red spectrum of 1-acetyt-4-methyl cyclohexzene

β - diketones exist as a mixture of ketonic and enolic forms in equilibrium with each other. The enolic form is established by resonance.

OH ------------- O

R —— C = C R′—— C —— R ⟷ R —— C = C R′ = CR

$\overset{+}{OH}$ ---------- $\overset{-}{O}$

For enolic form, VC = O absorption band appears in the region 1640-1580 cm^{-1}, which is much lower than that for conjugated ketones. This much lowering is due to the intramolecular hydrogen bonding stabilised by resonance. Acetyl acetone absorptions in the ketones form at 1725 cm^{-1} and in the enolic form, at 1630 cm^{-1}. Quantitative studies of these forms are possible from the peak intensities.

Quinones are a special case of α, β - unsaturated ketones. For this class of compounds, characteristic frequencies of absorption due to C = O stretching and C = C stretching lie in the region 1695 to 1587 cm^{-1}. P-quinones with two carbonyl groups in the same ring absorb in the range 1680 – 1660 cm–1. Presence of electron repelling groups (+ 1 effect) lowers the frequency of absorption while the presence of electron attracting group (–1 effect) increases the force constant and hence raises the wave number of absorption.

F. Esters and Lactones

An ester can be recognised if there are two stron bands owing to C = O str and C = O string in an infrared spectrum, Ester shows the VC = O absorption at 1750-1735 cm^{-1}. The position of VC = O absorption is sensitive to ring and unsaturated due to conjugation. The presence of one more oxygen atom in esters R-COOR' compared to ketones RCOR' raises the wave number of absorption due to Z effect. The carbonyl absorption for aryl ester or α, β unsaturated esters is shifted to lower wave number. The carbonyl absorption occurs at higher wave number if the carbonyl group of an ester is present in the five membered ring.

The VC = O absorption for lactone is raised to higher wave number which the decrease in the size of the ring. β - lactones shows strong band near 1820 cm^{-1} and δ -lactone absorb at comparatively lower wave numbers. α, β unsaturation in lactones brings down the VC = O absorption. β - keto esters exist as an equilibrium mixture of keto and enol forms. The ketonic form shows C = O stretching at 1724 cm^{-1} while absorption band for hydrogen bonded C = O group (established by resources) occurs at 1650 cm^{-1}.

Positions of some characteristic absorptions:

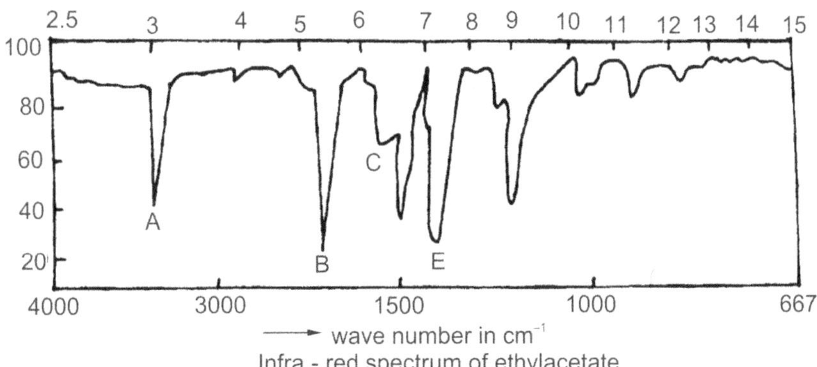

Infra - red spectrum of ethylacetate

A = 3002 cm^{-1} ;	C – H str in methyl methylene
B = 1742 cm^{-1} ;	C = O str (in esters)
C and D 1450 and 1370 cm^{-1} ;	C – H def
E = 1240 cm^{-1};	C = O str in esters.

Group	Type of Vrations	Region in Cm^{-1} and intensity
Saturated esters	C = O str	1750-1735 (s)
a – b unsaturated esters	C = O str	1730-1715 (s)
Aryl esters	C = O str	1730-1715 (s)
β - lactones	C = O str	~ 1820 (s)
δ - lactones	C = O str	1780-1760 (s)
α, β unsaturated	C = O str	1760-1740 (s)
α, β unsaturated	C = O str	1730-1715 (s)
δ - lactones		
β - ketones esters	C = O str	(i) 1725 (s) ketonic (ii) ~ 1650 (s) enolic.

G. Carboxylic Acids

Carboxylic group (- COOH) is the easiest functional group to be detected by Infra-red spectroscopy because this group is formed from C = O and O – H units. The absorption of O – H stretching appears as broad band near 3000-2500 cm^{-1}. The VC = O stretching absorption in aliphatic occurs at 1725-1700 cm^{-1}. An acid (-COOH) is formed from an aldehyde (-CHO) on replacing a hydrogen atom by an OH group. Due to the –I effect of OH group, VC = O absorption for acids should occur at higher wave number as compared to aldehydes. But actually it is not so. VC = O absorption for acids is lowered due to internal conjugation (lone pair on oxygen in conjugation with C = O) working in opposite direction, α, β - unsaturated acids or aryl acids show carbonyl absorption at a lower wave number.

Some of the acids like acetic acid, benzoic acid, exist as dimmers due to hydrogen bonding formation of bridge lowers the force constants and VC = O and VO – H absorption occur at lower wave numbers. As the hydrogen bonded structure is stabilised by resonance, the O – H stretching occurs as a broad band in the region 3000-2500 cm^{-1}. If the acid is converted into its soluble salt, then in the carboxylate anion formed, both the C = O bonds become exactly equivalent as shown below.

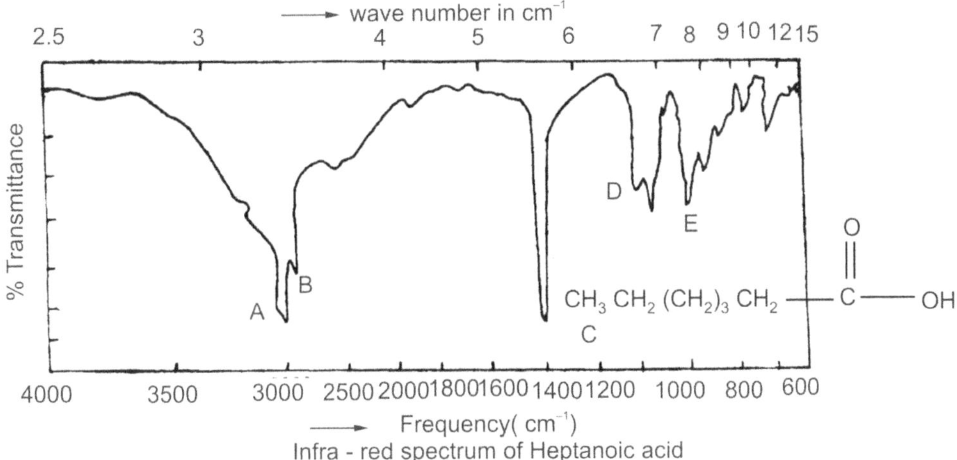

Infra - red spectrum of Heptanoic acid

Positions of some characteristic absorptions.

A = 3300-2500 cm^{-1}	Broad O – H str
B = 2950-2850 cm^{-1}	C – H str (super imposed upon O – H str)
C = 1715 cm^{-1}	C = O str Normal dimeric carboxylic acid
D = 1408 cm^{-1}	C – O – H in – plance band
E = 1280 cm^{-1}	C – O str
F = 930 cm^{-1}	O – H def (out-of-plane).

As the internal conjugation is prevalent in carboxylate anion, the force constant for C = O is less in it as compared to that in case of an acid. Hence VC = O absorption occurs at a highter wave-number for an acid as compared to that in carboxylate anion. In cis-trans isomers of an acid, small differences in VC = O observations are observed. But in case of cis/trans cinnamic acid, Maleic acid-Fumeric acid etc, VC = O absorption differences are larger.

Cis-cinnamic acid absorbs a a higher wave number. It is partially explained dut to the steric effect caused by the bulky groups on the same side of the double bond. Due to repulsive interactions, the C = O part of – COOH group goes out of the plane of the double bond. Thus, conjugation diminishes and hence VC = O absorption occurs at a highet wave number. Similar explanation can be given for malei acid (cis) which absorbs at 1705 cm^{-1} as compared to fumaric acid (trans) at 1680 cm^{-1}.

$C_6H_5 - C - H$
$\quad\quad\quad \|$
$HOOC - C - H$

Cis Cinamic acid
1705 Cm^{-1}

$C_6H_5 - C - H$
$\quad\quad\quad \|$
$H - C - H$

Trans-Cinnamic acid
1680 cm^{-1}

H. Acid Halides

In acid halides (RCOX), the presence of electronegative atom displays-I effect which increases the force constant of the carbonyl group and hence its wave number of absorption increases. In halogenated acids, -I effect is more pronounced when halogen is present in the α-position. When halogen atom is in a more remote position, the VC = O absorption returns to normal.

$BrCH_2COOH$	VC = O	730 cm^{-1} (s)
$ClCH_2COOH$		1736 cm^{-1} (s)
Cl_2 CH COOH		1751 cm^{-1} (s)
F_3C COOH		1776 cm^{-1} (s)
$BrCH_2CH_2CH_2COOH$		1725 cm^{-1} (s)

(Br is in more remote position)

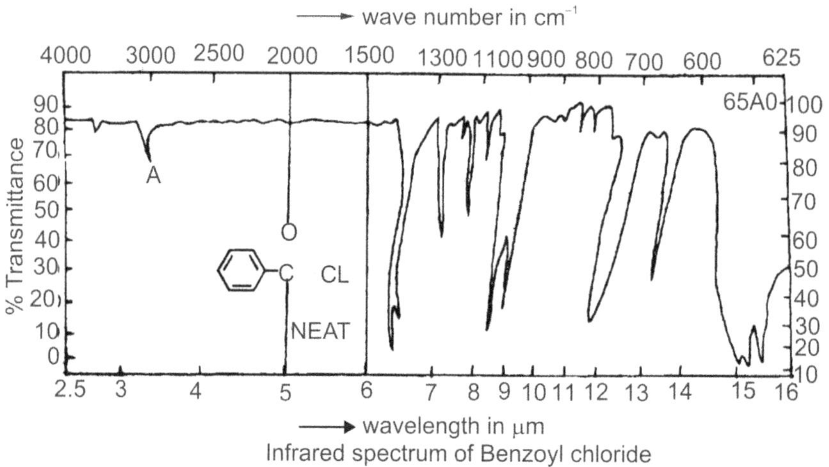

Infrared spectrum of Benzoyl chloride

Positions of some characteristic absorptions.

A = 3080 cm^{-1}	C – H str aromatic
B = 1790 cm^{-1}	C = O str (raised due to electronegative Cl atom)
C = 1745 cm^{-1}	Fermi resonance band (C = O str and overtone of 875 cm^{-1} band)

In para halobenzoic acid, –I and +E effects cancel each other (work in opposite directions) and thus, frequency of absorption returns to normal. For m-halo benzoic acid, the VC = O is higher than that for benzoic acid due to the absence of conjugation.

I. Acid Anhydrides

An acid anhydride can be easily detected due to the appearance of two frequency bands in the region 1850-1750 cm^{-1}. The doublet appears because of the coupled vibrations of two C = O groups. The high frequency band is assigned to symmetrical vibrations and lower frequency band to asymmetric vibrations. The splitting of the band is due to Fermi Resonance. In acyclic anhydrides of saturated carboxylic acids, the two bands appear at (i) 1850-1800 cm^{-1} and (ii) 1790-1740 cm^{-1}. The absorption at higher wave number is more intense. In the α, β unsaturated anhydrides, the higher absorption band shifts downward by 20-40 cm^{-1} while the second band due to asymmetric vibrations maintain its position. Symmetric vibrations towards lower frequencies takes place in aromatic anhydrides. In cyclic anhydrides, both the bands shift towards higher frequencies.

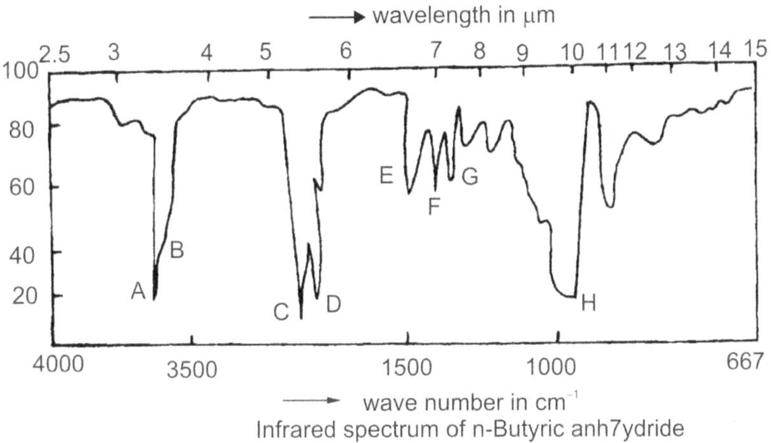

Infrared spectrum of n-Butyric anh7ydride

Positions of some characteristic absorptions.

A = 2980 cm^{-1}	C – H str in methyl
B = 2890 cm^{-1}	C – H str
C and D = 1820 and 1748 cm^{-1}	C = O str in acyclic anhydrides
E, F, G = 1460, 1406, 1380 cm^{-1}	C – H def in methyl
1035 cm^{-1}	C – O str in acyclic anhydrides

Amides

The presence of nitrogen atom has – I effect but a lone pair of electrons present on nitrogen atom are involved in conjugation which tend to decreases C = O force constant. This effect is more pronounced in amides due to greater mobility of electron pair on nitrogen atom (less electronegative) and hence, its greater participation in conjugation. The VC = O absorption in amides takes place at lower wave number. In addition to the

VC = O absorption, amides can be recognised by N – H stretching and N – H def bands. Primary amides in dilute solutions show two bands (N – H str) near 3400 cm^{-1} and 3500 cm^{-1}. These two bands arise due to symmetrical and asymmetrical N – H stretching. Secondary amides give only one band while tertiary amides which donot show any band in the region 3500-3100 cm^{-1}. In tertiary amides which donot contain N-H group, VC = O absorption does not show any marked shift due to dilution. Since hydrogen bonding is absent in tertiary amides, it spectra in the solid and in solution forms are almost the same.

K.Lactams

Cyclic amides of the amino acids are called lactams. The VC = O absorptions in lactams depend upon the ring size. The VC = O absorption is higher in γ - lactams due to the greater ring strain as compared to that in δ – lactams due to the greater ring strain as compared to that in δ – lactams. The value of VC = O absorption is raised further in β-lactams. β - lactams in dilute solution absorb at 1760 – 1730 cm^{-1} whereas γ – and δ - lactams. The value of VC = O absorption is raised further in β-lactams. β – lactams in dilute solution absorb at 1760-1730 cm^{-1} whereas γ – and δ - lactams absorb at: 1700 cm^{-1} and : 1680 cm^{-1} respectively.

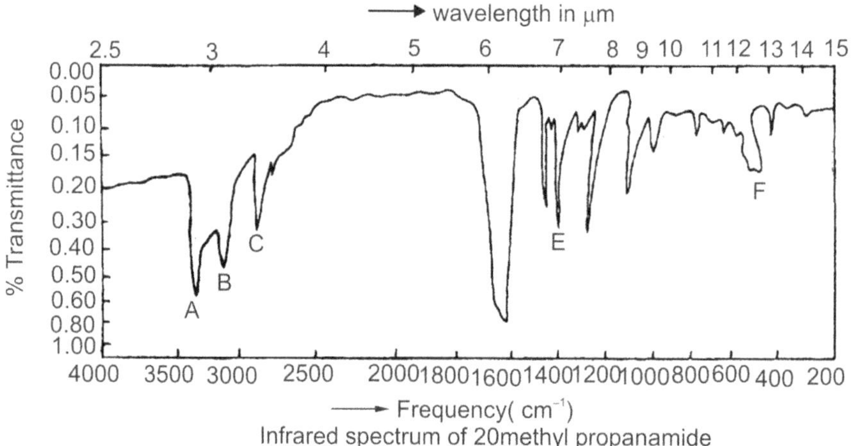

Infrared spectrum of 20methyl propanamide

Positions of same characteristic absorptions.

A = 3350 cm^{-1}	N – H str coupled, primary amides Hydrogen bonded-symmetric
B = 3170 cm^{-1}	N – H str symmetric
C = 2960 cm^{-}1	C – H str alphatic
D = 1640 cm^{-1}	C = O str amide
E = 1425 cm^{-1}	C – N str
F = 700 – 600 cm^{-1}	N – H def (out of plane band)

β - lactams have been extensively studied in connection with the structure of penicillin. In penicillin, the VC = O absorption occurs at 1760 cm^{-1}.

In cyclic amides the VC = O absorptions are very sensitive to ring size and α, β – unsaturation. The VC = O absorption is raised with the decrease in the size of the ring whil α, β – unsaturation brings down the wave number of absorption.

L. Amino Acids

All Aminoacids exist as Zwitter ions at the isoelectric points due to the internal neutralisation of the acidic and the basic group in the molecule.

$$NH_2CH_2COOH \rightleftharpoons NH_3^+ CH_2COO^-$$

Due to the insolubility of amino acids in common solvents, infra-red spectrum of aminoacids are usually taken in the solid state. In the aqueous solution or in the solid state, its presence can be detected by the absorption of $^+NH_3$ and COO^- groups. Amino acids in the form of zwitter ions donot show N – H stretching at 3200 cm^{-1} but show a broad band between 3130 cm^{-1} and 3030 cm^{-1} assigned to asymmetric stretching of $^+NH_3$ group. Absorption depends upon the structure of amino acids. Hydrochlorides of Amino acids containing $+NH_3$ group absorb between 3145 and 3050 cm^{-1}. In zwitter ions, two vibrational modes of the carbohydrate ion are readily identified between 1600-1410 cm^{-1}. The asymmetric vibrational band at 1600-1560 cm^{-1} is broad and strong. In hydrochlorides of amino acids, the VC = O absorptions are shifted to higher frequencies. In the hydrochloride of α – amino acid C = O stetching occurs at 1754-1724 cm^{-1}. This higher frequency absorption is due to the – I effect of $^+NH^3$ group. When $^+NH_3$ group is present in the more remote position e.g. in δ amino valeric acid, VC = O stretching returns to 1710 cm^{-1}. N – H deformation bands occur near 1600 cm^{-1}.

M. Amines

Amines are the alkyl derivatives of ammonia. These can be recognised by absorption due to N – H str in the region 3500-3300 cm^{-1}. The position of absorption depends upon the degree of hydrogen bonding. Primary amines show two sharp bands; secondary amines give only one band while tertiary amines do not absorb in the said N – H str region. N – H and O – H groups have common properties and their absorptions due to these groups have common properties and their absorptions due to these groups are superimposed making their identification difficult. Since nitrogen atom is less electronegative then oxygen atom, the N – H ... N hyderogen bonds are weaker as compared to O – H.. O bonds and hence frequency shifts due to hydrogen bonding in amines are smaller. VN – H absorptions occur at lower frequencies compared to VO-H frequencies. The dilute solution of primary amine in an inert solvent gives two sharp bands due to asymmetric and symmetric stretching vibrations between 3500-3300 cm^{-1}.

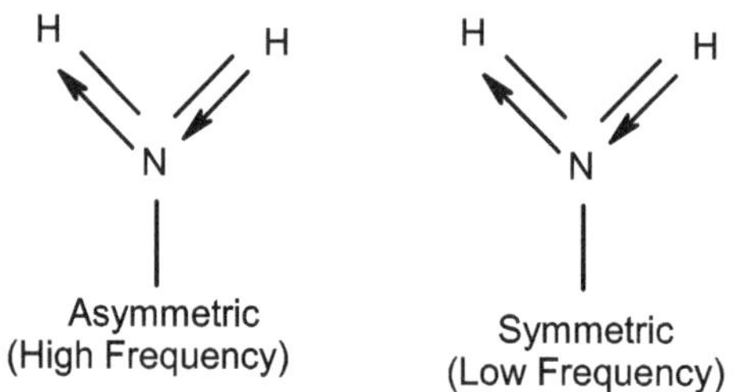

Positions of some characteristic absorptions:

A and B 3450 and 3390 cm^{-1} ;	N – H str in primary amines.
C 3226 cm^{-1} ;	N – H str (hydrogen bonded)
D 3030 cm^{-1} ;	C – H str in olefines/aromatics.
E, F and G 1620, ~ 1602, 1499 cm^{-1} ;	C = C str in aromatic nuclei
H and I 1360, 1275 cm^{-1} ;	C – N str in primary aromatic amines
J and K 754 and 696 cm–1 ;	characteristic of monosubstituted benzene.

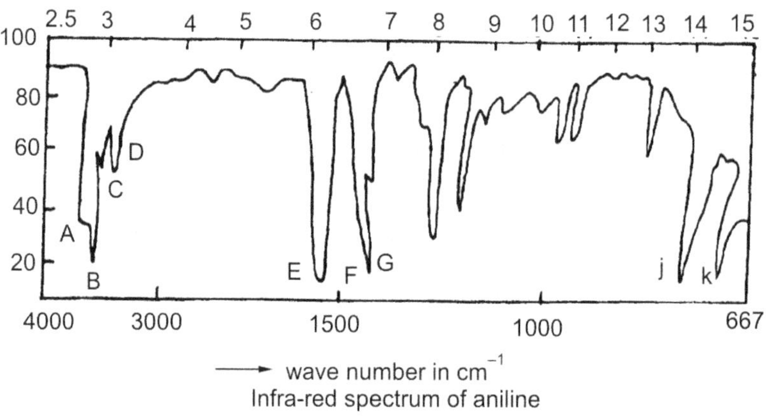

Infra-red spectrum of aniline

VN – H stretching absorptions for aromatic amines are comparatively higher than those of aliphatic amines. For aromatic amines, lower VN – H absorption values are expected due to –I and +E effects. In phenols, similar electronic effects (–I and +E) produce a decrease in the force constant and thus, phenols absorb at a lower frequency as compared to alcohols but it is not so in amines since electronic effect is shielded by hybridisation effect. In aliphatic amines, the nitrogen atom has pyramidal configuration (almost sp^3) and force constant is influenced by the adjacent atoms or groups in the same way as in alcohols. In aromatic amines, the nitrogen atom is partially rehybridised towards sp^2 due to conjugation. This increases the S-character in N – H bond and thus, due to the formation of a stronger bond, the VC = O absorption rises.

Aliphatic Amines are more sensitive to hydrogen bonding than aromatic amines because they are more stronger bases. The VN – H absorption is usually broad unless spectrum is scanned in dilute solutions. It has been noted that in aliphatic and aromatic amines, the VNH_2 symmetric absorption band is more intense than the asymmetric band. The N – H stretching band depends upon the state of the amines. Samples in the solid form show N – H stretching at lower wave number due to greater degree of hydrogen bonding. The amines, the shift due to hydrogen bonding does not exceed 100 cm^{-1}. The N – H bending vibration for primary amines occur at higher wave number as compared to secondary amines. The N – H def, vibrations for amino salts appear as strong bands at 1600-1575 cm^{-1} and also near 1500 cm^{-1}. The C – N vibrations for aliphatic amines appears as weak bands at ~ 1410 cm^{-1} and also at 1220-1020 cm^{-1}.

N. Nitro Compounds

The electron diffraction method and X-ray analysis have shown that the two oxygen atoms are equidistant from the nitrogen atom (1.22A°) and also π electrons are equally distributed between the two N – O bonds by isovalent conjugation. The uniform p electron distribution in the nitro group can be expressed as follows.

The vibrational behaviour of the nitro group also supports this structure. The presence of nitrogroup in a compound is characterised by the presence of two strong bands in its infra-red spectrum which arises from the symmetrical and a symmetrical stretching modes which occur in the regin (i) 1620-1535 cm^{-1} and (iii) 1375-1275 cm^{-1}. Bands arising from deformation modes are difficult to distinguish from other bands occurring in the low frequency region. Primary derivatives ($RCH_2 – NO_2$) absorb at higher frequency as compared to secondary (R_2CHNO_2). Tertiary nitro compounds ($R_3C.NO_2$) absorb at lower frequency.

Aromatic compounds show two strong bands (i) 1570-1500 cm^{-1} and (ii) 1370-1300 cm^{-1}. Nitrites (- O – N = O) can be readily recognised from the two strong bands in the regions(i) 1680-1650 cm^{-1} and (ii) 1625-1605 cm^{-1}.

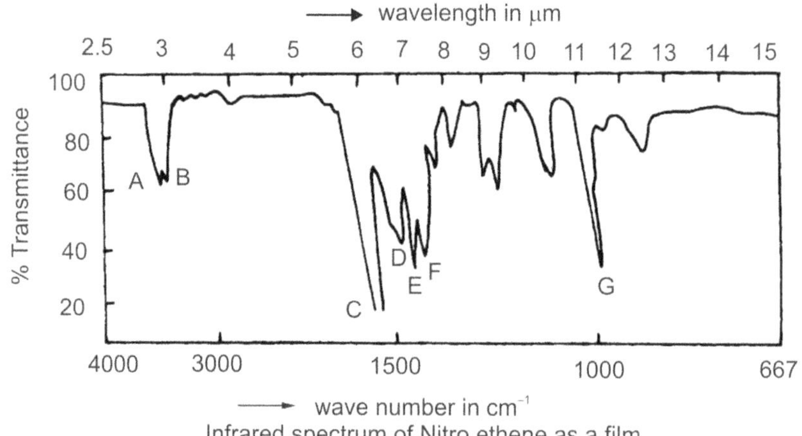

Infrared spectrum of Nitro ethene as a film

Positions of some characteristic absorptions.

A and B 3003 and 2940 cm^{-1} ;	C – H str in CH_3
C and F 1562 and 1394 cm^{-1} ;	characteristic of nitro group
O = 1440 cm^{-1}	C – H def in methyl
F = 1362 cm^{-1}	C – H def
G = 875 cm^{-1}	C – N str

O. Nitriles and Related Compounds

Nitriles are the functional derivatives of the carboxylic acids containing C ≡N group. Various equivalent structures of cyanides can be written as

The electronegative nitrogen atom makes the carbon atom more positive the polar – CN group has – I effect on the adjacent bond the Infra-red spectra of various cyanides (nitriles) have shown coredominant forms with a triple bond between carbon and nitrogen atoms. Thus, the infrared absorption occurs in the triple bond region between 2280-2200 cm^{-1}. The shift in VC ≡ N stretching abosorption depends upon the electronic effect of atoms of groups attached to C ≡ N group.

In aliphatic nitriles, the intensity of VC ≡ N stretching band is low.

$CH_3 - C \equiv N$	2280 cm^{-1}
$CH_3 - CH_2 \equiv N$	2257 cm^{-1}

The decrease in the wave number of absorption is due to + 1 effect of the alkyl group (s) attached to C ≡ N group. In α, β- unsaturated nitriles, conjugation of electrons of the double bond with C ≡ N group lowers the force constant and hence the wave number of absorption is lowered.

Conjugative effect dominates and VC ≡ N stretching which occurs at a lower wave number if a group exerting –I and +E effects is attached with the C ≡ N group.

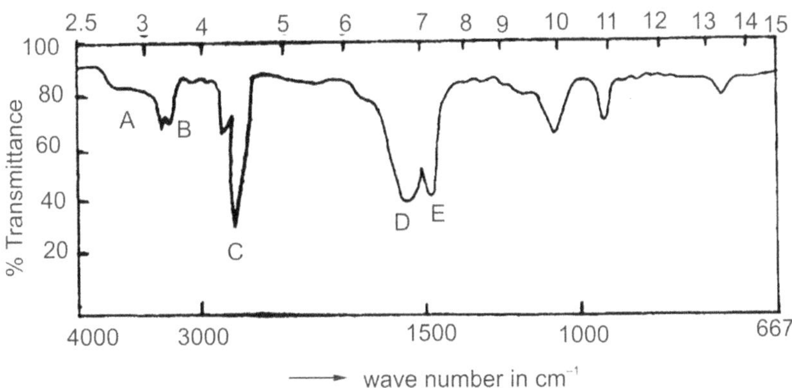

Positions of some characteristic absorptions

A = 3002 cm^{-1}	C – H str in CH_3
B = 2940 cm^{-1}	C – H str
D = 1440 cm^{-1}	C – H def in CH_3
E = 1370 cm^{-1}	C – H def
C = 2256 cm^{-1}	C ≡ N str in alkyl cyanides

P. Hetero Aromatic Compounds

Hetero aromatics such as pyridine, furan, thiophene etc show C – H str bands in the region 3077-3000 cm^{-1}. Compounds containing N – H group shows N – H str absorption in the region 3500-3220 cm^{-1}. In this region of absorption, the exact positon depends upon the degree of hydrogen bonding and hence upon the physical state of the sample or the polarity of the solvent. Pyrole and Indolein dilute solution in non-polar solvents show a sharp band near 3945 cm^{-1}.

Ring stretching vibrations occur in the general region between 1600-1300 cm^{-1}. The absorption involves stretching and contraction of all the bonds in the ring and interation between these stretching modes, pyridine shows four absorption bands in this absorption. In this respect, it closely resembles a mono-substituted benzene.

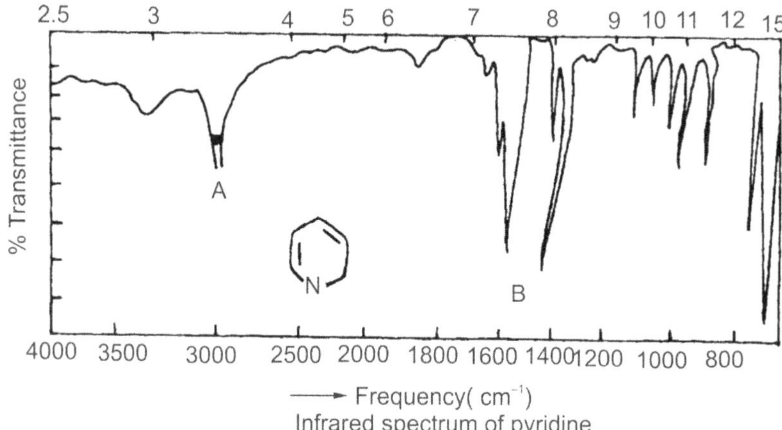

Infrared spectrum of pyridine

Positions of some characteristic absorptions.

A = 3080 – 3010 cm^{-1}	C – H str aromatic
B = 1600 – 1430 cm^{-1}	C = C and C = N str (in Ring)
C = 748, 703 cm^{-1}	C – H def out of plane

Important Tips for Interpreting an Infrared Spectrum

Following are some useful tips for interpreting an infrared spectrum:

(i) Always place more reliance upon the negative evidence. The absence of a band in a particular region is a sure indication of the absence of group(s) absorbing in that region. For example if there is not absorption in the region 1900-1600 cm^{-1}, the carbonyl group (C = O) must be absent in the compound.

(ii) Always start from the higher frequency end of the spectrum. Mostly stretching vibrations occur in the region above 1500 cm^{-1} and are most informative. The region 1500-1000 cm^{-1} may be used for confirming esters, alcohols, ethers etc.

(iii) To distinguish between inter molecular and intra molecular hydrogen bonding, the spectra of the sample are scanned at two different concentrations. Various solvents may be used to study association effects.

(iv) For easy detection of the various groups present in the compound, the infrared region (14000 to 667 cm^{-1}) may be visualised as consisting of the following portions:

(a) 3600-3200 cm^{-1}: The appearance of the bands in this region shows the presence of – OH – NH_2 NH group in the compound. The position, intensity and the breadth of the bands tell the group is free, intra molecularly bonded or exhibit inter molecular hydrogen bonding. ≡C – H str also shows a medium band near 3300 cm^{-1}.

(b) 3200-3300 cm^{-1}: Absorptions due to = C – H str and Ar – H stretching occur in this region. The sharp bands of weak to medium intensities are observed.

(c) 3000-2500 cm^{-1}: The absorptions due to C – H stretching from methyl or methylene groups occur in this region. The asymmetric C – H stretching occur at slightly higher wave number as compared to that of symmetric C – H str. A very broad band between 3000-2500 cm^{-1} is most characteristic of acids (- COOH group). Two weak bands, one at 2720 cm^{-1} and the other near 2820 cm^{-1} are most characteristics of C – H stretching in aldehydes. The higher frequency band is observed.

(d) 2300-2100 cm^{-1}: This is the region in which alkynes, cyanides, cyanates, isocyanates, absorb. The bands observed are weak and variable – C ≡ C stretching occurs between 2140-2100 cm^{-1}. –C ≡ N stretching shows a variable band between 2260-2200 cm^{-1}. Isocyanates show a strong band between 2280-2250 cm^{-1}.

(e) 1900-1650 cm^{-1}: Strong bands due to C = O stretching occur in this region.

Anhydrides show two strong bands in the region 1850-1740 cm^{-1}. Esters, aldehydes, ketones, lactones, carboxylic acids, amides show strong bands due to C = O stretching in this region. Imides are also recognised by two strong bands (doublet) in the region around 1700 cm^{-1}. Following points regarding C = O stretching may be helpful.

(i) $\alpha - \beta$ – unsaturation lowers the frequency of absorption by 15-40 cm^{-1}. But in Amides, a small absorption shift towards lower frequency is observed.

(ii) Increase in the ring strain in case of cyclic ketones raises VC = O absorption.

(iii) Hydrogen bonding to the carbonyl compounds lowers VC = O absorption by 40 – 60 cm^{-1}.

(f) 1600-1000 cm^{-1}: This region is very important for identifying nitro compounds and also confirming the presence of ethers, esters, primary, secondary and tertiary alcohols. The appearance of strong bands due to C – O stretching at 1300-1050 indicates.

(i) an ester provided C = O stretching is observed in the region 1750-1735 cm^{-1} and

(ii) an alcohol if O – H stretching free and/or bonded occurs between 3600-3200 cm^{-1}. Ethers show a strong band in the region 1150-1070 cm^{-1} due to C – O stretching in – C – O – C -. This region also helps to identify C – H str in aromatic compounds. For aromatic rings, medium bands around 1600 cm^{-1}, 1580 cm^{-1} and 1500 cm^{-1} are observed.

(g) **Below 1000 cm^{-1}:** This region is very useful in identifying the type of substitution on the aromatic ring.

(i) a strong band at 770-730 cm^{-1} (s) shows monosubstitution.

(ii) ortho and para disubstituted compounds show one band each. The latter absorbs at a higher wave number.

(iii) Meta-disubstituted compounds are usually recognised by two medium bands in the region 850-710 cm^{-1}.

CHAPTER 17

NUCLEAR MAGNETIC RESONANCE SPECTROSCOPY

Introduction

When a substance is subjected simultaneously to two magnetic fields one stationary and the other varying at some radio frequency, at a particular combinations of fields, energy is absorbed by the sample and the absorption can be observed as a change in the signal developed by a radio frequency detector and amplifier.

This energy absorption can be related to the magnetic dipolar nature of spinning nuclei. This technique is known as NMR (Nuclear magnetic resonance).

In general, the study of radio frequency radiation by Nuclei is called NMR. This method was first developed by E.M. Purcell and Fell Bloch in 1946.

This spectroscopy is more superior than I.R. & U.V. spectroscopy, but the cost of instrument is very high.

The spectra given by all forms of spectroscopy may be described by these important factor.

1. Frequency of spectral lines or bands.
2. Intensity of spectral lines or bands.
3. Shape of spectral lines or bands.

These parameters depend on the molecular parameters of the system.

In case of NMR, these molecular parameters are found to be

1. Shielding constant of nuclei.
2. Coupling constant of nuclei.
3. Life time of energy level.

All these parameters are of fundamental importance in NMR spectroscopy.

Nuclear Spin

Nuclei of atoms are composed of protons and neutrons. These particles also have the property to spin on their own axis and each of them possess angular momentum $\frac{1}{2}(h/2\pi)$ in accordance with quantum theory. The net resultant of the angular momentum of all nuclear particles is called nuclear spin. For a nucleus having nuclear spin quantum number I, there are (2I + 1) spin states.

Number of protons	Number of neutrons	Spin Quantum number I
odd	odd or eveny	$\frac{1}{2}, \frac{3}{2}, \frac{5}{2}$
even	even	0
even	odd	1, 2, 3

(a) There are three broad principles for the Nuclear spin. (*a*) If the sum of protons and neutrons is even, I is zero integral. If the spins of all the particles are paired, there will be no net spin and the nuclear spin quantum number I will be zero.

e.g. ^{12}C, ^{16}O, ^{18}O, $^{38}\delta$ have even number of neutrons and even number of protons and will show zero spin. Consequently, there will be no magnetic moment.

(b) If the sum of the protons and neutrons is odd, it is half integral $\left[\frac{1}{2}, \frac{3}{2}, \frac{5}{2} \text{ etc}\right]$.

e.g. ^{1}H, ^{19}C, ^{13}C have $I = \frac{1}{2}$ and a uniform charge distribution ^{35}Cl, $I = \frac{3}{2}$.

(c) If both protons and neutrons are even numbered I is zero. 12C, 16O fall in this category and give no NMR signal.

In fact magnetic properties and odd mass number

1. Odd atomic number and odd mass number

e.g. H^1, $_7H^{15}$, $_9D^{19}$

2. Odd atomic number and even mass number

e.g. H^1, $_7N^{14}$ etc.

3. Even atomic number and odd mass number

   e.g. $_{3}C^{13}$

NMR Phenomenon

These are five different aspects that essentially govern the NMR Phenomenon namely:

1. The spinning nucleus.
2. The effect of an external magnetic field.
3. The precessional motion.
4. The precessional frequency.
5. The energy Transitions.

1. The Spinning Nucleus

The nucleus of the hydrogen atom i.e. the proton just behaves as if it is a small spinning bar magnet. It does so because it evidently possesses an electrical charge as well as a mechanical spin. Consequently, a spinning charged body will generate a magnetic field and hence the nucleus of hydrogen atom is not an exception.

2. The Effect of an External Magnetic Field

As a "compass needle" possesses an inherent tendency to align itself with the earth's magnetic field, the proton not only responds to the influence of an external magnetic field but also tends to align itself with the field. Restrictions, as applicable to nuclei, the proton can only have the two orientations with regard to an external magnetic field.

(i) When proton is aligned with the field [lower energy state].

(ii) When proton is opposed to the field [higher energy state].

3. The Precessional Motion

The proton appears as "spinning magnetic" and not only it aligns itself with or apposite to an external field, but also may move in a characteristic manner under the influence of the external magnet.

The energy of reorientation of magnetic dipole ΔE, may be expressed as

$$\Delta E = hv$$

Where h = Plank's constant

v = frequency of radiation.

4. The Precessional Frequency

The spinning frequency of the nucleus does not change at all whereas the speed of precession does. Therefore, the precessional frequency is directly proportional to the strength of the external field.

5. The Energy Transitions

Whenever a proton is precessing in the aligned orientations it can absorb energy and pass into the orientation and subsequently it can lose this extra energy and relax back into the aligned state. It is called energy transitions. The transition from one energy state to the other is called flipping of the proton. The transition between the two energy states can be brought about by the absorption of a quantum of electromagnetic radiation in the radio wave region with energy *hv*.

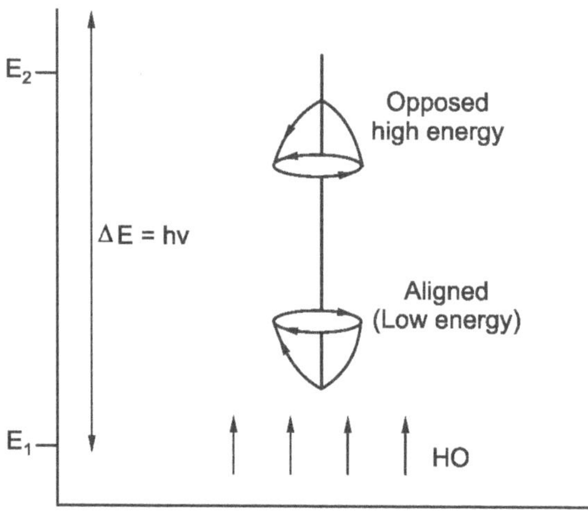

The energy required to bring about the transition ($\Delta E = hv$) or flip the proton depends upon the strength of the external field. Stronger the field, greater will be the tendency of the nuclear magnet to remain lined up with it and higher will be the frequency of the radiation needed to flip the proton to the higher energy state.

$$v = \frac{\gamma H_o}{2\pi}$$

v = frequency in cycles per sec or Hz.

H_o = strength of the magnetic field in gauss.

γ = Nuclear constant or Gyromagnetic ratio and is equal to 26750 for the proton.

Resonance

In NMR experiment, a strong homogeneous magnetic field is applied, causing the nuclei to precess. Radiation of energy comparable to ΔE is then imposed with a radio frequency source. When the applied frequency from the radio frequency source becomes equal to the angular frequency of precession, the two are said to be in resonance. As a result of this resonance, some nuclei are excited from the low energy state $\left[m = \frac{+1}{2}\right]$ to the high energy state $\left[m = \frac{-1}{2}\right]$ by the absorption of energy ΔE from the source at a frequency equal to the precessional frequency. The transition from one energy state to the other is known as flipping of the proton.

Principle

Any proton with odd mass number spins on its own axis. By the application of an external magnetic field (H_o), the nucleus spins on its own axis and a magnetic moment is created, resulting in a precessional orbit, with a frequency called as precessional frequency. This state is called as ground state or parallel orientation. In this state, the magnetic field caused by the pin of nuclei is aligned with the externally applied magnetic field.

When applied energy is in the form of radio frequency and when applied energy is equal to precessional frequency, absorption of energy occurs and a NMR signal is recorded.

Relaxation Process in NMR

Relaxation is the process of transition from excited state to ground state (or) relaxation process involve some non-radiative transitions by which a nucleus in an upper transition state to the lower spin state. Two kinds of relaxation peocesses are

1. Space lattice relaxation (or) longitudinal relaxation process.
2. Spin spin relaxation (or) Transverse relaxation process.

1. Spin Lattice Relaxation

It involves the transfer of energy from the nucleus in its higher energy state to the molecular lattice. Spin-lattice relaxation time T_1 which is a measure of the average lifetime of the nuclei in the higher energy state. The energy is transferred to the components of the lattice as the additional translational, vibrational and rotational energy. The total energy of the system remains the same. T_1 is strongly affected by the mobility of the lattice. In crystalline solids and viscous liquids, mobilities are low, T_1 is large. As the mobility of the lattice is (at higher temperature) the vibrational and rotational frequencies increase.

2. Spin-Spin Relaxation

It is due to the mutual exchange of spins by two precessing nuclei which are in close proximity to each other. It is also known as transfer relaxation time T_2. In this, nuclei exchange spins with neighbouring nuclei by interaction of their magnetic moments. Although no spin energy is lost by this mechanism, T_2 values are generally so small for crystalline solids or viscous liquids (as low as 10^{-4}).

When two neighbouring nuclei of the same kind have identical precession rates, but are in different magnetic quantum states, the magnetic fields of each can interact to cause and interchange of states, a nucleus in the lower spin state is excited while the excited nucleus relaxes to the lower energy state. No net change in the relative spin state population and no ↓ in saturation results. But the average lifetime of a particular excited nucleus is shortened.

Number of Signals

1. The number of signals in the NMR spectrum tell the number of different sets of equivalent protons in a molecule. The position of the signal gives information about what kind of protons they are i.e. they are either aliphatic or aromatic 1° or 2° or 3° or adjacent to halogen or other atom or group etc. Different kinds of protons have different electronic environments. Each signal corresponds to a set of equivalent protons. It may be noted the magnetically equivalent protons are chemically equivalent protons.

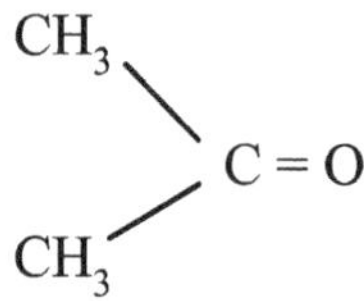

e.g. 1. Acetone all the six protons are in exactly similar environment. Therefore only one signal is observed.

2. Some compounds showing more than one signal because the protons are not in exactly one environment.

e.g. $CH_3 - OH$ — 2 nmr signals; $CH_3 - CH_2 - NH_2$ — 3 nmr signals

3. Chemically equivalent protons must also be stereo chemically equivalent i.e. a particular set of protons are said to be chemically equivalent only if they remain exactly similar environment.

e.g. 2 chloro propane $CH_3 - C\ (Cl) = CH_2$ it shows 3 signals.

Instrumentation

There are thus two types of NMR spectrometers, the single coil spectrometers, in which absorption is measured and the two coil instruments in which resonant radiation is measured.

Spectrometers may be further divided into absorption or induction types. The absorption spectrometer makes use of a bridge circuit to detect the absorption of radio frequency energy from a coil surrounding the sample.

In Induction Spectrometers, two coils at right angles are used and energy is absorbed from the transmeter coils to orient the nuclei. This orientation process induces a voltage in the receiver coils.

NMR Spectrometers have also been classified as wide line or low resolution instruments and high resolution instruments.

- An effective quantitative analysis is possible. Quantitative measurements are also possible through integration of the areas beneath the peaks.
- Such type of experiments can be performed by making use of an instrument called wide line or low resolution NMR spectrometer. It is also used for quantitative element analysis and for the physical environment of a nucleus.
- The high resolution instruments are capable of resolving the fine structure that is associated with the absorption peak for given nucleus. By making use of chemical environment of the nucleus it is then possible to determine the nature of this fine structure.
- A high resolution spectrometer can evidence two distinct types of structures in NMR absorption due to proton resonance, known respectively as the chemical shift and spin spin coupling.

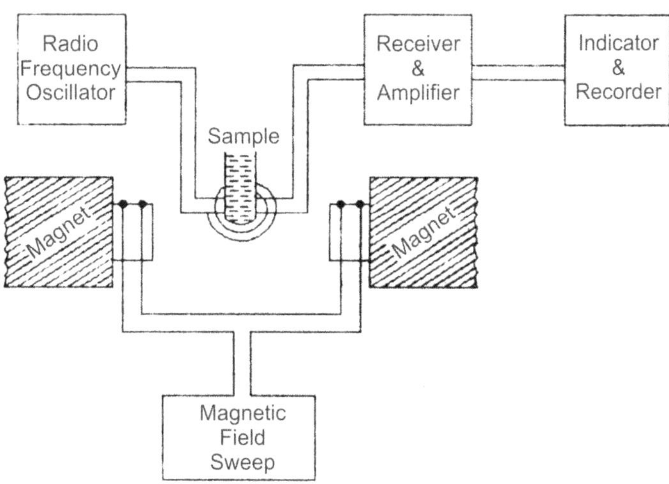

A brief description of the important components:

1. **The Magnet**

   It is used to supply the principal part of the field H. The important feature of the magnet is that it should give homogeneous magnetic field i.e. the strength and direction of the magnetic field should not change from point to point. The strength of the field should be very high i.e. at least 20,000 gauss, because the chemical shifts are proportional to the field strength. Two factors are important in the design of magnets (i) homogeneity or uniformity of the field (ii) The constancy of the field, strength and maximum obtainable strength of the field.

   Permanent magnets can provide fields which are sufficiently constant provided that these are thermostated very carefully.

   Conventional electromagnets are less suitable but the desired stability can be produced by producting anicillary stabilising devices.

   Permanent and conventional electromagnets are generally used in spectrometers operating up to 100 MHz to 230 MHz.

2. **The Magnetic Field Sweep**

   An alteration over a small range in the applied field may be made by making use of a pair of coils [Helmholtz coils] located parallel to the magnet face. These coils superimpose on the main field of the magnet, the additional field, required to bring the total to the resonance condition by varying a direct current through the coils, the effective field can be changed by a few hundred milligauss without any loss in field homogenicity. The field strength is changed automatically and linearly with time and this change is synchronized with the linear device or a chart-recorder.

3. **Sweep Generator**

   In order for a nucleus to resonate, the precession frequency should be equal with that of applied frequency or R_f radiation. If the applied magnetic field H_0 is kept constant and the precession frequency is fixed in order to bring about resonance. The frequency of R_f field should be changed so that it becomes equal to the resonance frequency (frequency sweep method) if the R_f radiation is kept constant, the resonance frequency of the nucleus must be changed by varying H_0 (field sweep method).

   Generally the field sweep method is regarded as better because it is easier to vary H_0 than R_f radiation.

4. The Sample Hoder

Ausual NMR sample cell consists of a 7.5 cm to 0.3 in diameter. The sample holder should be chemically inert, durable and transparent to R_f radiation. Generally the glass tubes are sturdy, practicable and cheap. The sample must be in the liquid or solution state for high resolution spectra.

5. The Sample Probe

It is a device that holds the sample tube in a fixed position in the field and it is also provided with an driven turbine for rotating the sample tube along its longitudinal axis at several hundred RPM. This rotation minimises the effects of inhomogeneities in the field and as a consequence sharper lines and better resolution are obtained.

The design of probe depends upon the type of instrument, probe may be single coil or a turn coil system. Single coil serves as transmitter as well as receiver coils. In turn coil, the two coils are orthogonal to each other.

6. Radio Frequency Generator

To generate it, radio frequency oscillator is used. A fixed oscillator having a capacity of exactly 60 MHz normally used. For high resolution work, about one part in 10^8 can be used. The maximum interaction of the R_f radiation with the sample, the coil of oscillator is wound around the sample container. The oscillator irradiates the sample with R_f radiation. The coil is wound perpendicular to the applied magnetic field. The applied R_f field should not change the effective magnetic field in the process of irradiation.

7. Radio Frequency Receiver

When the radio frequency radiation is passed through the magnetised sample, two phenomena, namely, absorption and dispersion, may occur. The line shapes are the interpretation of absorption spectrum and it is easier as compared to dispersion spectrum.

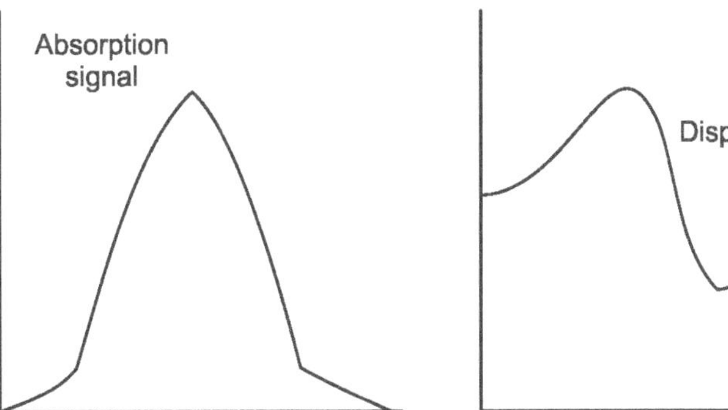

The detector should be capable of separating absorption signal from dispersion signal and from that of the R_f oscillator. There are two main methods of detection. These are as follows:

(i) The first method uses a radio frequency bridge. Its network balances out the transmitter signal and allows the absorption and dispersion signals to appear as an out of emf across the bridge. In this method the coil used for surrounding the samples serves as both a transmitter as well as a receiver coil.

(ii) The second method employs a separate receiver coil. This method is some times called the crossed coil or nuclear induction method. If the two coils are fixed at right angles to each other as well as to the direction of static magnetic field, they will not be effectively coupled. In this way, the transmitter signal is separated from the absorption and dispersion signals.

The separation of absorption and dispersion signals is achieved by knowing the fact that they differ in phase by an angle of 90°. The general method in practice is to use a phase sensitive detector.

8. The Signal Detector and Recording System

The coil has been used to direct the radio frequency signal produced by the resonating nuclei. The electrical signal generated into the coil must be amplified before it can be recorded.

***Technique and Principle*:** A radio frequency oscillator which is adjusted to generate a certain preset or definite frequency v which passes through a coil located between the magnetic poles surrounding the sample, is a receiver coil. The receiver coil is used to pickup the broadcast signal. These signals are carried to a receiver and amplifier and then to a cathode ray oscillograph recorder. The strength of the magnetic field can be varied with the help of a suitable device known as magnetic field sweep. The frequency of the magnetic field is gradually varied in such a manner that the frequency emitted by the nuclei of the sample is equal to the radio frequency of the oscillator. Under these conditions, the same will be in resonance with the applied frequency. As a result, absorption occurs, and stops again when H is raised further. The result is then a trace, where the peaks represent the values of H at which the sample is in resonance with the applied frequency. A signal from the receiver is plotted versus magnetic field strength. Such plots are called NMR spectrum.

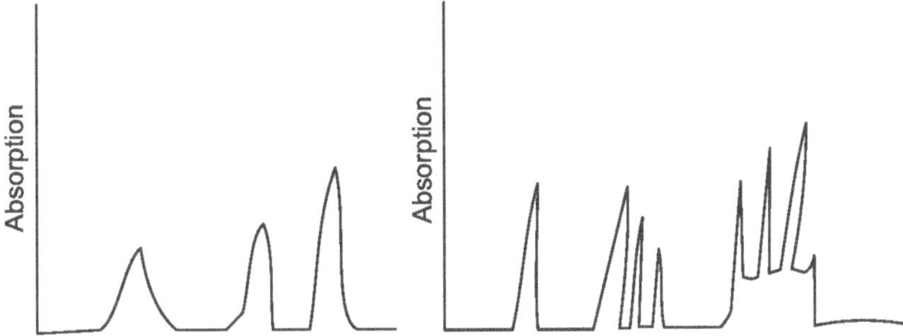

Chemical Shift (origin of the chemical shift): The chemical shift is caused by small magnetic fields that are generated by electrons as they circulate around nuclei.

These fields usually oppose the applied field. Although the chemical shift is measured as a field or frequency, it is the ratio of the necessary change in field to the applied field or the necessary change in the frequency to the standard frequency and hence it is dimensionless constant usually denoted by δ expressed in parts per million (PPM)

$$\delta PPM = \frac{H_S - H_R}{H_R} \times 10^6 \text{ or } \frac{V_s - V_r}{V} \times 10^6 \text{ PPM}$$

where H_S and H_R refer field at resonance of sample and the reference substance such as H_2O.

If the induced field opposes the applied field, then proton is said to be shielded. But if the induced field reinforces the applied field, the proton feels a higher field strength and thus such a proton is said to be deshielded.

Shielding shifts the absorption upfield and deshielding shifts the absorption down field to get an effective field strength necessary for absorption. Such shifts in the positions of nmr absorptions which arise due to the shielding or deshielding of protons by electrons are called chemical shifts.

For measuring chemical shifts of various protons in molecule the signal for tetramethul silane (TMS is taken as a reference). In addition, TMS is chemically inert, relatively volatile (BP 27° C) and soluble in most organic solvents. As TMS is not soluble in aqueous solutions, it is not suitable for aqueous solutions. For water soluble substances, DDS [2, 2 dimethyl 2 silapentane-5-sulphonate] may be used as a reference.

The chemical shift is caused mainly due to different nuclei in a molecule experiencing different magnetic fields as a result of the 2° magnetic fields associated with the molecules.

Shielding and Deshielding Effects

In a molecule Hydrogen nuclei is surrounded by the electronic charge which shields the nucleus from the influence of the applied field. To overcome the shielding effect and to bring the protons to resonance, greater external field is required. Greater the electron density around the proton, greater will be induced secondary magnetic field will cause proton absorption. The extent of shielding is represented in terms of shielding parameter α, when absorption occurs the field H felt by the proton is represented as

$$H = H_0 (1 - \alpha) \quad .....(1)$$

Where H_0 is the applied field strength. The field felt by the proton does not correspond to the applied field. Greater the value α, greater will be the value of applied strength which has to be applied to get the effective field required for absorption and vice versa.

Also

$$V = \frac{\gamma H}{2\pi} \quad .....(2)$$

From 1 and 2

$$V = \frac{\gamma H_0 (1 - \alpha)}{2\pi}$$

From this relation, it is clear that the protons, with different electronic environments or with different shielding parameters, can be brought in to resonance in two ways:

(i) The strength of the external field is kept steady and the radio frequency is constantly varied.

(ii) The radio-frequency is kept steady and the strength of the applied field is constantly varied.

At constant radio-frequency shielding shifts the absorption upfield in the molecules where there is a spherical distribution of electrons around the proton. It is called "Positive Shielding".

If the 2° field produced by the circulating electrons reinforces the applied field, the position of resonance moves down field. This is known as "negative shielding". There are two types of shielding phenomenon.

The field experienced by a nucleus may be modified by fields due to induced circulation of electrons localised on that nucleus. This is known as local shielding.

Low-range Shielding

In aromatic compounds the 2° fields set up the induced circulation of π electrons often influence the field experienced by nuclei not directly associated with the π electrons.

Due to this additional shielding and deshielding, effects may be included within the molecule.

Factors Influencing Chemical Shift

Following are the factors which influence the chemical shift

(a) Inductive effect

(b) Vander Waal's deshielding

(c) Anisotropic effects

(d) Hydrogen bonding

(e) Concentration, solvent and temperature

(a) ***Inductive Effect***: A proton is said to be deshielded, if it is attached with an electronegative atom or group. Greater the electronegativity of the atom, greater is the deshielding caused to the proton. If the deshielding is more for a proton, then its δ value will also be more.

e.g. $\overset{b}{C}H_3\ \overset{a}{C}H_2\ F$, $\overset{b}{C}H_3 - \overset{a}{C}H_2 Cl$ 2 signals are expected from each one. As the distance from the electronegative atom increases, the deshielding effect due to it diminishes. Protons 'b' are comparatively less deshielding and hence will resonate at comparatively lower value of δ.

(b) *Vander Waal's Deshielding*: In over crowded molecules it is possible that some proton may be occupying sterically hindered position. Electron cloud of a bulky group (hindering group) will tend to repel the electron cloud surrounding the proton. Thus such a proton will be deshielding and will resonate at slightly higher value of δ than expected in the absence of this effect.

(c) *Anisotropic Effects (space effect)*: The deshielding effect on proton attached to C = C is higher than that can be accounted by the inductive effect alone. Aldehydic and aromatic protons are much more deshielded. Consider an alkene, it is so orientated that the plane of the double bond is at right angles to the applied field. Induced circulation of π electrons generates induced magnetic field. Induced circulation of π electrons generates induced magnetic field which is diamagnetic around carbon atom and paramagnetic in the region of the alkene protons. Thus the protons will feel greater field strength and hence resonance occurs at lower applied field.

(d) *Hydrogen Bonding*: The hydrogen bonded proton being attached to a highly electronegative atom will have smaller electron density around it. Being less shielded the field felt by such a proton will be more and hence resonance will occur down field. The down field shift depends upon the strength of hydrogen

bonding can be easily distinguished as the latter does not show any shift in absorption due to the change in concentration.

(e) *Concentration, Solvent and Temperature Effect*: In CCl_4 and $COCl_3$ chemical shift of proton attached to carbon is independent of concentration and temperature while protons of COH, – NH_2, – SH groups exhibit a substantial concentration and temperature effect due to hydrogen bonding.

Intra molecular hydrogen bonding is less affected than Intermolecular bonding by concentration change. Both types of hydrogen bonding are affected by temperature variations.

Solvents Used

A substance free if proton should be used as a solvent i.e. which does not give absorption of its own in NMR spectrum.

The solvent should be capable of dissolving at least 10% of the substance under investigation.

Following solvents are commonly used in NMR spectroscopy:

1. Carbon tetrachloride (CCl_4)
2. Carbon disulphide (CS_2)
3. Deuterated chloroform ($COCl_3$)
4. Deuterated water (D_2O)
5. Deuterated methanol, dimethyl sulphide, acetic acid.
6. Hexa chloro acetone $(CCl_3)_2$ C = O etc.

Solvents should have the following properties:

1. Chemical inertness
2. Magnetic isotropy (magnetically neutral)
3. Volatality (to facilitate sample recovery)
4. Absence of Hydrogen atoms.
5. Easily available and inexpensive.

Peak Area and Proton Counting

In an nmr spectrum, various peaks represent equivalent sets of protons. The size or the area of each peak tells the number of protons in each set present in the compound under investigation. The are under an nmr signal is directly proportional to the number of protons giving rise to signal. For flipping over of a proton, a quantum of energy is absorbed in the same effective magnetic field. Greater the number of protons that flip over at a particular frequency, greater will be the energy absorbed and greater is the area under the absorption on peak squares under each peak are simply counted and from this, the ratio between various kinds of protons out. These ratios are then converted into whole numbers. These whole numbers tell various nmr signals e.g. toluene.

(i) Five proton signal (down field due to deshielding).

(ii) Three proton signal (up-field)

Note: When drawing small squares in the nmr spectrum of a compound like the squares in a graph paper, the number of squares under each signal are carefully counted and then the said ration is found out.

Splitting of Signals

Each signal in an nmr spectrum represents one set of protons in a molecule. It is found that in certain molecules, a single peak is not observed, but instead, a multiplet is observed.

e.g. Consider a molecule "ethyl bromide". This molecule has two kinds of protons and thus two signals are expected in nmr spectrum. It has been observed that for each kind of protons, we do not get singlets but a group of peaks are observed. For 'a' kind of protons, a triplet, a group of three peaks is observed and a quarter is noticed for 'b' kind of protons.

e.g. Consider a molecule "ethyl bromide". This molecule has two kinds of protons and thus two signals are expected in nmr spectrum. It has been observed that for each kind of protons, we do not get singlets but a group of peaks are observed. For 'a' kind of protons, a triplet, a group of three peaks is observed and a quarter is noticed for 'b' kind of protons.

$\overset{b}{C}H_3\ \overset{a}{C}H_2\ Br$

Signals and their absorption positions.

1. A three proton triplet 8.35 τ
2. A two proton quarter 6.6τ
3. A two proton doublet 6.05 τ
4. A one proton triplet 4.2 τ

Spin-Spin Coupling

Spin: Spin is a fundamental property of nature like electrical chare of mass.

Two or more particles with spins having opposite signs can pair uo to eliminate the observable manifestations of spin.

Nuclei can interact with each other to cause mutual splitting of the sharp resonance lines into multiplets, called "spin-spin" coupling.

These multiplets arise because magnetic moments of nuclei interact with each other through the strongly magnetic electrons in the intervening bonds. The strength of the coupling is denoted by 'J' expressed in hertz.

e.g. Consider molecule ethylbromide (CH_3CH_2Br). The spin of two protons ($-CH_2-$) can couple with the adjacent methyl group ($-CH_3-$) in 3 different ways relative to the external field as follows:

1. ↑ ↑ (Reinforcing)
2. ↓ ↑ ↑ ↓ (Not effecting)
3. ↓ ↓ (Opposing)

external field ↑

Thus, a triplet of peaks results with the intensity ratio of 1 : 2: 1 which corresponds to the distribution ration of alignment.

Note: Spin-spin coupling takes place between non equivalent neighbouring protons. Non equivalent protons are those which have different chemical shifts.

NMR Absorption by Other Nuclei

The nucleus of an isotope whose spin quantum number I is less than O shows absorption in the nmr spectroscopy. The nmr spectroscopy studied for the absorption of most abundant natural isotope of hydrogen, H^1 is called proton magnetic resonance (PMR) spectroscopy. The numerical value of I is related to the mass number and the atomic number of the concerned isotope. Such nuclei are said to be magnetic and assume only a discrete set of orientations.

Ex:

Isotope	Spin quantum number I
H^1	1/2
H^2	1
B^{10}	3
C^{13}	1/2
N^{14}	1
F^{19}	1/2
P^{31}	1/2
Cl^{35}	3/2
Br^{79}	3/2
I^{127}	5/2

The nuclei of some isotopes like C^{12}, O^{16} etc. for which I = O are non magnetic and hence cannot cause such orientations. Thus such nuclei are not capable of causing absorption in the nmr spectroscopy.

The spin quantum number 'I' indicates the number of orientations that a nucleus may assume in a magnetic field. For nmr, spectroscopy other nuclei, no modification compared with H^1 nmr spectrometer is needed except for the appropriate radio frequency source. Out of the halogens (F, Cl, B, I) protons can couple only with fluorine atom present on the same (or) on the adjacent carbon atom. It is due to a very large electric quadrupole moment of the halogen atoms (Cl, Br, I) effectively cause spin decoupling of adjacent protons. Fluorine resonances are well separated and donot appear in the normal range from 0-10ppm. Moreover the values of coupling constants in the absorption for the fluorine nuclei are very high as compared to those observed in H^1 nmr signals.

e.g. Geminal F – F coupling ranges from 40-370 cps while vicinal F – F couplings have values of J between 0-40 cps.

NMR spectrum of other nuclei provide structural information just as PMR.

Generally very broad bands are observed compared with proton spectrum. Double resonance technique can be used to remove broadening of absorption.

Calculating the Ratio in the Heights of Signals

It has been noticed that due to spin-spin coupling, each signal is split up into a multiplet. The ration in the heights of lines in a multiplet can be easily calculated.

e.g. Ethyl alcohol CH_3 CH_2 OH

In this, due to deshielding effect of oxygen atom, the signal for OH proton will be down field. Next signal comes for methylene (– CH_2 –) which appears as a quartet while a signal for methyl protons appears as a triplet and will be up field. The mutual coupling between – OH and – CH_2 – does not take place. It is due to the fact that the proton oxygen atom is rapidly exchanging, i.e. it does not stay in the same environment long enough for its coupling with – CH_2 – protons to be detected and hence – OH proton is seen as a singlet.

Thus in ethyl alcohol

1. Singlet 1 H (for hydroxyl proton)

   [1+ = 1 peak height 1 unit]

2. Triplet3 H

   Intensity 1 : 2 : 1

   1 unit = ¾ = 0.75

   Thus peak heights will be in the ratio 0.75 : 1.5 : 0.75

3. Quartet 2H

   Intensity 1 : 3 : 3 : 1

   1 unit = 2/8 = 0.25

The peak heights will be in the ration of 0.25 : 0.75 : 0.75 : 0.25.

Chemical Exchange (Proton Exchange Reactions)

In a molecule, if a proton shuttles between two magnetic environments at a rate which is much faster in comparison with nmr transition times, then the resonance observed for that proton will be simply that of the average effective field in the two environments.

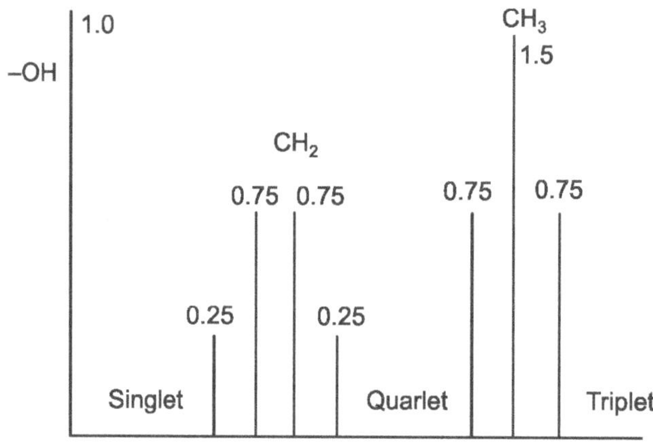

We see only one signal in nmr spectrum of acetic acid in water at an average position according to the following formula;

$$N_a S_a + N_b S_b$$

where N_a = mole fraction of the proton 'a'

N_b = mole fraction of the proton 'b'

S_a = chemical shift of unexchanged proton 'a'

S_b = chemical shift of unexchanged proton 'b'

The phenomenon of chemical exchange can be explained by considering the nmr spectrum of anhydrous ethanol and also the spectrum of ethanol containing small quantities of water. In the case of pure anhydrous ethanol $\overset{a}{C}H_3\ \overset{b}{C}H_2 - \overset{c}{O}H$, three signals are observed.

1. A triplet for $-CH_3$ protons at 8.82 τ due to coupling with CH_2 – protons.
2. A multiplet consisting of eight lines for – CH_2 – protons at 6.38 τ. The – CH_2 – protons are under the influence of two kinds of protons in different chemical environments. Thus the multiplet consists of (n + 1) (n + 1) = (3 + 1) (1 + 1) = 8 lines.
3. A triplet for – OH proton at 4.72 τ. The OH proton appears as a triplet because of coupling to – CH_2 – protons.

If we scan the spectrum of ethyl alcohol containing water, the OH signal appears as a singlet and its coupling with adjacent – CH_2 – does not take place. The proton exchange becomes faster as the water content in increased. The exchange of OH protons among ethanol molecules in presence of water or at high temperature or in acidic medium is normally so rapid that a particular proton does not reside on a particular oxygen atom long enough for the nuclear coupling to be observed.

$$ROH^* + HOH \equiv R-OH + HOH^*$$

Rapid chemical exchange causes spin decoupling, because the spin values get averaged. The proton exchange does not occur.

1. If the sample is pure.
2. If the sample is recorded at a low temp. (or)
3. If the sample is dissolved in a highly polar solvent like dimethyl sulphoxide.

Low temperature and solution of the polar sample in a highly polar solvent are some of the factors which reduce the chemical exchange and hence, coupling of – OH proton with the neighbouring proton does take place. Proton exchange also occurs rapidly in some other compounds in which hydrogen is attached with nitrogen, sulphur and oxygen and hence no coupling is observed between the protons of these functional groups with the protons on the adjacent carbon atoms.

Note: A proton undergoing chemical exchange does not show spin-spin coupling.

Coupling Constant (J)

The distance between the centres of the two adjacent peaks in a multiplet is usually constant and is called the "coupling constant". It is denoted by latter 'J'. It is a direct measure of the spin coupling of the protons and is known as the "spin-spin coupling constant. It is expressed in "cycles per second" cps, the units of frequency.

The "J" value is in between 1 and 20 Hz. It is independent upon the magnetic field.

If we work the spectrum of a particular compound at different radio-frequencies, the separation of signals due to different chemical shifts change.

From the value of coupling constant one can distinguish between the two singlets and one doublet and also a quarter from two doublets. It can be determined by simply recording the spectrum at two different radio frequencies. If the separation between the lines does not change, that signal indicates the doublet, and the separation of the lines increases with increasing frequency will be two singlets.

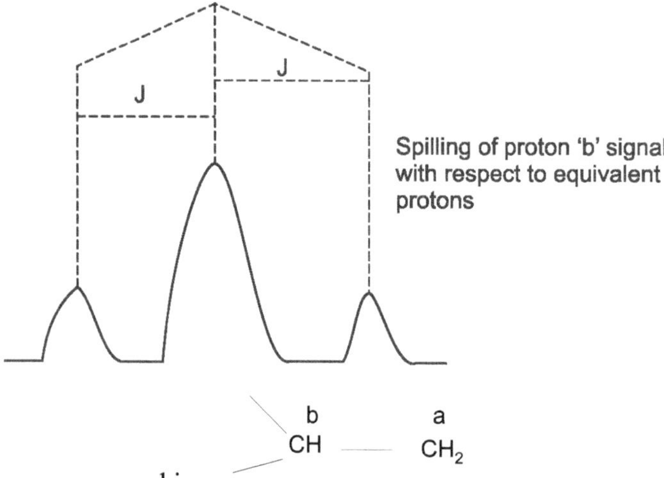

e.g. consider a compound i.e.

In this two signals are expected in nmr, under the influence of two equivalent protons a and b, the distance between any two adjacent peaks in a multiplet will be exactly the same. This is triplet formed due to spin-spin coupling.

Hence it is useful in characterising the relative orientations of interacting protons.

Few examples of 'H' coupling constants (J) are given below :-

C-C linkage **Value of J**

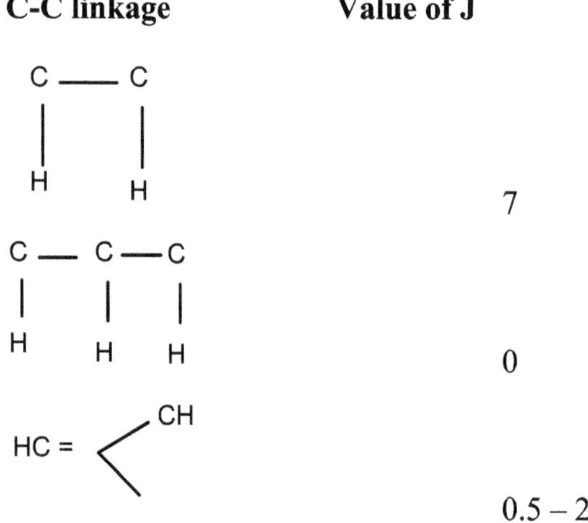

C = C<(H)(H)	0 – 3
C = C<(H)(H)	4 – 10
H–C = C–H (cis)	6-14
H–C = C–H (trans)	11-20

Restricted Rotation

The isomers which arise due to rotation about single bond are called conformational isomers (or) conformers. The presence of conformations in a solution can not be detected by nmr spectroscopy. But at temps much below room temp., the rate of inter conversion of rotational isomers is usually restricted (or) diminished and results in nmr absorption. This is the "restricted rotation".

The presence of double bond (a sigma and a π bond) in a compound restricts rotations and results in the formation of cis and tran isomers. Cis and trans isomers are the distinct compounds with different properties and different nmr spectra.

In a compound, where a double bond may originate in its equivalent resonating structure, the rate of rotation about the given bond becomes intermediate between free rotation about unhindered single bond in one structure and hindered rotation about the double bond in the structure.

e.g. N – N dimethyl formamide at room temperature.

The nmr spectrum for such a compound usually consists of a super imposition of spectra resulting from two (or) more rotational isomers present at equilibrium.

Amides, oximes, nitroso amines show restricted rotation.

Important Tips for Interpreting an NMR spectrum

(a) Following points regarding the value of chemical shift may be useful :

1. The value of methyl, methylene and methane protons have the order,

Methyl > Methylene > Methine.

2. Tau value depends upon the nature of the substitution on the carbon atom bearing the proton. Greater the electronegativity of the substituent, lower is the value of Tau.
3. The value of tau depends upon the type of the hydrid orbital holding the proton, $Sp^3 > Sp > Sp^2$.
4. The Tau value for aromatic protons is always less that 4 ppm. The value depends upon the degree and the nature of substitution.
5. Tau values for the aldehydic protons are generally lower i.e., 0.8 ppm lower.
6. Tau value of protons in a cyclic compound is always higher than that of any other proton.

(b) The number of signals in nmr spectrum tells the number of sets of the protons in different chemical environments.

(c) It also tells the number of equivalent protons causing the splitting of a signal.

Some Important NMR Spectra

1. All protons in an organic molecule, at a given radio frequency, may give NMR signals at different applied field strengths.
2. The number of signals or peaks signifies how many different kinds of protons are present in the molecule.
3. The positions of the signals tell us about the electronic environment of the different types of protons present.
4. The intensities of signals tell us about the different kinds of protons present.
5. The splitting of a signal into several peaks tell us the number of protons in the adjacent positions.
6. Whether the protons in a given compound are equivalent or not, can be determined by mentally replacing the each proton by another atom. If the replacement results in one product, the protons are equivalent. If replacement gives isomers, the protons are not equivalent.

Double Resonance Techniques

Double resonance experiments include a sample that is simultaneously irradiated with two or more signals of different radio frequency among these methods.

Spin-spin decoupling, nuclear overhauser effect, spin tickling, internuclear double resonance.

Spin Spin de coupling or indoor or Double resonance: Simultaneous use of two radio frequency sources, in addition to the normal nmr instrument, a second tunable radio frequency source is needed to irradiate H_a at the necessary frequency and the recording of the spectrum is done in the same way. It is called double resonance or double irradiation. Since the multiplet collapses to singlet in the process, it is also called spin decoupling.

It is a powerful tool for simplifying a spectra. In a complex molecule if several of the coupling constants have nearly the same values or if the long range coupling present or if complex absorption gives multiplets then it becomes very difficult to determine structure.

A proton spin couples with neighbouring proton because it has sufficient life time in a given state. If life time of a spin is reduced i.e., if the exchange between spin states of nuclei is speeded up then little information about the neighbouring neclei will be obtained.

In case of such compounds where H_a and H_b are in different

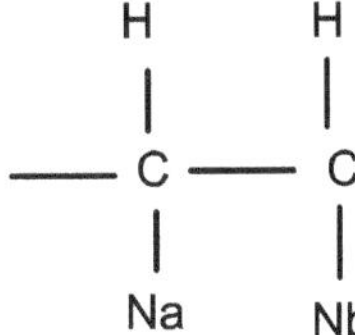

Environments therefore two doublets are different field strengths are observed. If H_a is irradiated with strong correct radio frequency so that the rate of its transition between the two energy becomes larger than the life time of this nucleus in any one spin state will be too short to resolve coupling with H_b. In such a case H_b proton will have one time average view of H_a and hence H_a will come to resonance only once and H_b will appear as a singlet and not doublet. Time dt is needed to resolve the two lines of a doublet which is related to J thus, formation of a doublet is possible if each spin state of H_a has a life time greater than dt due to double irradiation life time becomes still less and thus coupling is not possible. So it results in a singlet by spin-spin decoupling.

Nuclear overhauser Effect

Magnetic nuclei also interact through space but it does not lead to coupling. The interaction is seen when one of the nuclei is irradiated at its resonance frequency. Then the other is detected as a more intense or weak signal than usual or normal signal, this is known as Nuclear overhauser effect. This effect is seen over short distance (2-4 A) between two nuclei.

The interaction is dependent upon the relation of the observed nucleus by the irradiated nucleus. The NOE effect shows molecular geometry. It tells us whether the two protons are in close proximity with in the molecule or not. Line intensities observed in the normal spectrum may be the same as in the decoupled spectrum.

NMR Spectrum at more than one Radio-Frequency

- The chemical shift positions for the various sets of protons are field dependant.
- If we work the spectra of a particular compound at different radio-frequencies, the value of coupling constant remains same whatever the applied field. Scanning at different radio-frequencies tell clearly a particular signal is multiplet or a few singlets.

  e.g. A doublet is observed and is being suspected as two singlets. For this, the spectrum of the same compound is rerun at a higher radio frequency. Now the signal will appear at a different field strength, but if the distance between the two peaks remains same, then it is necessarily a doublet.
- If the distance between the two peaks increase at a higher radio-frequency, there are two singlets.
- The two signals in the NMR spectrum overlap and the analysis becomes difficult. The multipliets can be pulled apart by scanning same compound at a higher radio frequency.

Deuterium Exchange Reactions

Few drops of deuterium oxide are added in the sample, the D_2O exchanges with the labile protons such as – OH – NH – SH and also with the reactive methylene protons flanked by the carbonyl groups. The mechanism involves same process as is seen in proton exchange reactions.

When little D_2O is added to ROH, then due to rapid exchange, ROH becomes ROD

$$ROH + D_2O \rightleftharpoons R - OD + H - OD$$

The signal for OH proton normally observed in ROH will be missing in the NMR, the signal for proton in H – OD will appear.

D_2O is added to RCOOH, due to rapid exchange becomes RCOOD.

$$RCOOH + D_2O \rightleftharpoons RCOOD + H - OD$$

RCOOH signal disappears, H – OD signal appears.

This technique which is employed for detecting the presence of OH, NH groups etc, is called deuteration for these two spectra are

1. One with the sample dissolved in a solvent other that D_2O.
2. Second spectrum with sample dissolved in the same solvent and containing a few drops of D_2O. On comparing the two spectra, if the peak areas are seen to diminish then the sample contain – OH, -NH, -SH group in which deuterium exchange is possible.

^{13}C NMR Spectroscopy

^{13}C nmr to a strategically much advanced stage where it gives a clear edge over[1] H-NMR in terms of not only its versatility but also its wide application in analysis.

^{13}C NMR refers to recording another NMR spectrum but of C_{13} atoms rather than the hydrogen atoms. In actual practice, these spectra are recorded in such a manner that each chemically distinct carbon gives rise to single peak, without any coupling or fine structure.

Hence simply a count of the peaks can be used to see how many carbons are actually present in the molecule. But this particular technique is not reliable for a molecule that exhibits symmetry, because this would ultimately reduce the number of peaks.

F^{19} NMR

It is naturally occurring isotope. It has I = ½ Except frequency source, no major modification in the instrument is needed. Chemical shifts are commonly measured with $COCl_3$ as standard. The range of chemical shift covered by fluorine containing compound is 0-200 ppm compared to 0-10 ppm in case of proton magnetic resonance. Moreover, signals corresponding to fluorine resonances are well separated on spectrum. The values of coupling constants in such compounds have higher values.

NMR of Carbocations

There are certain carbocations which are sufficiently stable under definite conditions and their proton magnetic spectra can be easily studies e.g. alkyl fluorides in liquid sulphur dioxide with Lewis acid.

Applications

1. Identification Testing

The versatility and ability of NMR to distinctly differentiate nuclei in various intramolecular environments has placed it as the most reliable and dependable technique for carrying out the identification testing of a host of pure drugs.

2. Identification of Structural Isomers

The distinction between the following isomers can be easily made from their nmr spectra.

In the isomer these signals are observed where as we see only two signals in the spectrum for ‘b’ which is a clear distinction between the above isomers, the three signals for isomer ‘a’ in order of decreasing tau values are

1. A three proton triplet (CH_3 –)

   A two proton sextet (–CH_2–) and

   A two proton triplet (–CH_2Cl)

   For isomer (b) two signals have their multiplicities as (1) doublet (6 H) upfield and

2. Sextet (H^+) down field

   Similarly position isomers like propranol and propranalol 2 can also be determined.

3. **Detection of Aromaticity**

   Protons attached to the benzoyl, polynuclear and heteroyclic compounds whose π electrons follow Huckel’s rule $(4n + 2)_n$ electrons where n = 1, 2, 3 whose number) are extremely dishielded due to circulating sextet (ring current) of π electrons. As a result of this, the signal for the aromatic protons appear at a very low field than that observed even for benzene. From this, the aromatic character of the compound under investigation can be predicted.

   The primary applications of NMR spectroscopy are in the field of structure determination and delineration. Integration of the NMR spectrum furnishes information that can be used for quantitative determination of one or more compounds present in a mixture.

4. **Structural Diagnosis by NMR**

   1. The chemical shift indicates the type of hydrogen atoms present e.g. methylene, methyl, olefins etc.
   2. The spin-spin splitting or multiplicity reveals about the possible arrangement of groups in the molecule.
   3. From the area of peaks, the number of hydrogen nuclei present in each group can be determined.

      e.g. The relative areas of methyl (CH_3) and methylene (CH_2) peaks in $CH_3 – CH_2$ CH_3 would be 6 : 2 in butane 6 : 4.

5. Quantitative Analysis

NMR spectroscopy has been used to determine the molar ratio of the components in a mixture. Equilibrium mixtures can be analysed when the proton signals of the components are well separated. In the NMR spectrum of pure ethanol a triplet is formed for the OH proton but when water is added in alcohol, then due to proton exchange, the triplet collapses to a singlet. The position of this singlet depends upon the water content in alcohol. From the values of the chemical shift, the ratio of water and alcohol can be estimated by comparing with the known results.

6. Ketoenol Tautomerism

The NMR spectrisciot us very useful in studying ketoenol tautomerism. In the case of acetyl acetone, the following exists :-

The NME spectrum of acetyl acetone the peaks are assigned to –OH, = CH – and – C H_3 group of enol form, and to the – CH_2 and – CH_3 groups of keto.

7. Hydrogen Bonding

The NMR can be used to study the hydrogen bonding in metal chelates as well as in organic compounds. Proton signal is shifted towards low field in the case of hydrogen bonding. This reveals that hydrogen bond formation results in the decrease in the electron shielding of the proton.

In these an upfield shift of the signal occurs, this may be ascribed to the breaking of intermolecular hydrogen bonds. This can be seen in the case of ethanol on increasing temperature or on diluting the ethanol with carbon tetrachloride.

- The electrostatic effect of the donor atom or group, this is dominated in strong hydrogen bonds.
- The diamagnetic anisotropy of the donor atom or group, this is dominant in the case of weak hydrogen bonds.
- Changes in long-range shielding of the acceptor group, appears in the case of intermolecular hydrogen bonding.

8. Elemental Analysis

NMR spectroscopy can be used for the determination of the total concentration of a given kind of magnetic nucleus in a sample of an accurate quantitative determination of total hydrogen in organic mixture is possible.

9. Exchange Effects

The width of an absorption band in NMR spectrum depends upon the physical state of the sample and also upon the type of the nycleus, in a particular environment. In the case of liquids the width of absorption band in their NMR spectra is very small i.e., of the order of 2-2 Hz. However in some liquids, broad bands are observed in their NMR spectra which can normally be accounted for in terms of exchange effects.

10. Distinction Between Cis-Trans Isomers

The cis and trans isomers of a compound can be easily distinguished as the concerned protons have different values of the chemical shifts as well as the coupling constants.

H_A C = C H_B (Cis) ⟷ H_A C = C H_B (Trans)

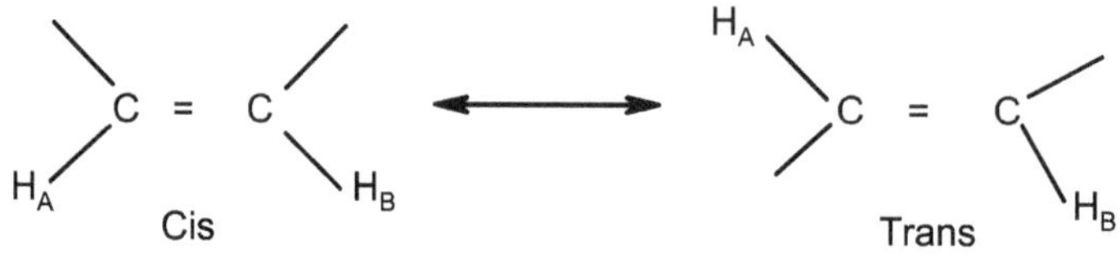

Similarly, the various concentrations of a compound, the axial and equatorial positions of the proton or group carrying a proton can be distinguished from their different values of the coupling constants.

11. Detection of Electronegative Atom or Group

It is known that the presence of an electronegative atom or group in the neighbourhood of the proton causes deshielding and the signal is shifted down field. Greater the electronegativity of the adjacent atom, smaller is the tau value of absorption for the concerned proton. Fluorine causes more downward shift as compared to oxygen which in turn causes more downward shift as compared to nitrogen and so on.

12. Study of Isotopes Other than Proton

Several nuclei in addition to the proton which have magnetic moments can thus be studied by the magnetic resonance technique, such as fluorine, phosphorous. Phosphorus^{-31} with spin number $\frac{1}{2}$ also gives sharp nmr peaks with chemical shifts extending over a range of 100 PPM. The resonance frequency of ^{31}P at 14000 guass is 24.3 MHZ.

13. Intermolecular Exchange Reaction

In high resolution spectrum of ethyl alcohol, it should be kept in mind that spin spin interaction between the hydroxyl group proton and the CH_2 group is to be taken into consideration if such a spectrum arises in the presence of acid or base.

If the nucleus undergoes exchange between two chemically and hence magnetically different sites, the resonance of the nucleus in these two sites will be broadened if the frequency of exchange is of comparable magnitude to the difference in chemical shifts.

14. Detection of some Double Bond Character Due to Resonance

In some compounds the molecule acquires a little double bond character due to resonance. Due to this, two signals can be expected for apparently equivalent protons. It is due to the hindered rotation which changes the geometry of the molecules.

e.g. NN dimethyl formamide

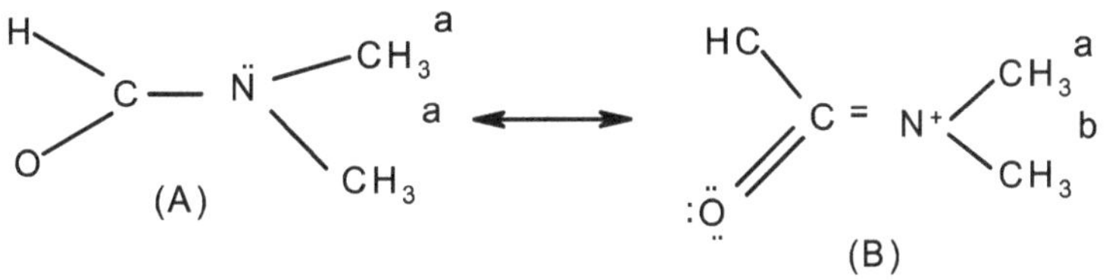

(A) H–C(=O)–N̈($\overset{a}{CH_3}$)($\overset{a}{CH_3}$) ⟷ (B) HC(=Ö:)=N⁺($\overset{a}{CH_3}$)($\overset{b}{CH_3}$)

For (a) two signals should be expected with peak areas 6 : 1 as the two methyls are exactly equivalent.

In (b) the presence of double bond restricts rotation and now the two methyl groups remain no longer equivalent (geometrical isomers). For this, two signals appear for two methyl groups.

15. Determination of Activation Energy

The activation energy ΔE can be calculated by using the Arrhenius equation

$$GK = \text{In } A - \frac{\Delta E}{RT}$$

A → constant

ΔE → activation energy

K is the rate of rotation and $K = \frac{1}{2}\pi$

Limitations of NMR spectroscopy

1. NMR having lack of sensitivity.

   The maximum sample size is about 0.1 ml having maximum concentration of about 1%.
2. In some compounds, two different types of hydrogen atoms resonate at similar resonance frequencies. This results in an overlap of spectra and makes such spectra difficult to interpret.
3. While characterizing the organic compounds, no information about molecular weight is given but the relative number of different protons present are only known.
4. In most of the cases only liquids can be studied by NMR spectroscopy. Although polymers when pre heated with various solvents, frequently become fluids which can be treated as liquids.

CHAPTER 18

WATER ANALYSIS

Introduction

Water is the most common solvent used in the general chemistry laboratory and is present in nearly all reaction mixtures studied in the typical teaching lab. We tend to take water for granted unless we are investigating physical properties which are conveniently demonstrated with it. The versatility of water in the laboratory only hints at its importance in the larger world.

Exobiologists remind us of the literally "vital" importance of water as they search for other planetary bodies which sport liquid water. Water is essential for life "as we know it" whether one considers the high water content of even the simplest organisms, the speed with which chemical reactions occur in aqueous solution or the ability of water to facilitate ion formation and ion transport.

Water is required for photosynthesis :

$$6\,CO_{2(g)} + 6\,H_2O_{(1)} \rightarrow C_6H_{12}\,O_{6(aq)} + 6O_{2(g)}$$

The production of simple sugars which are used to build up more complex structures is one obvious results of this important process but the oxygen produced as a by-product should not be overlooked. Animal life depeneds on it. A large part of the photosynthetic oxygen is produced by plant life in the oceans. The careless discharge of waste material (some of it toxic) into the oceans thus representa a real threat not only to marine life but to land animals as well (including humans). Wastes may consume the dissolved oxygen in the sea water (or fresh water bodies) enabling the growth of toxic anaerobic bacteria and preventing fish from obtaining adequate oxygen.

Approximately 4 mg/L or four parts of dissolved oxygen per million parts of water (4 ppm) is the minimum required for life processes in water. The equilibrium concentration of dissolved oxygen in open water, is normally higher than that, 9.2 ppm at 20°C, but the rate of dissolving is dependent on the surface area accessible to the atmosphere and is slow unless the water is deliberately aerated (something done routinely at water treatment plants). In public drinking water the dissolved oxygen level is typically maintained in the range of 8 – 10 ppm through aeration either during the transit of the water from its original source (lakes, streams, reservoirs, etc.) or during the treatment process as disinfectants are added. In modern laboratories, the dissolved oxygen content is typically measured with a selective electrode. After calibration the electrode provides a direct reading of the dissolved O_2 in either ppm or mg/L.

There is also a classic chemical determination for dissolved oxygen in water known as Winkler's Method. The water sample is first treated with excess manganese (II) sulphate solution and then with an alkaline solution of potassium iodide. The following reactions are important :

$$Mn^{2+}(aq) + OH^-(aq) \rightarrow Mn(OH)_2(s) \text{ (not balanced)}$$

$$Mn(OH)_2(s) + O_2(aq) + H_2O \rightarrow Mn(OH)_3(s) \text{ (not balanced)}$$

The $Mn(OH)_2$ initially formed, reacts with the dissolved oxygen (boxed). The process is a heterogeneous reaction, involving the combination of a gas with a colloidal solid.

The amount of $Mn(OH)_3$ formed is determined by reaction with iodide ion, which is inert in basic solution, but in acidic solution reacts with $Mn(OH)_3$ to form Mn^{2+} and iodine (excess $Mn(OH)_2$ is redissolved in the acid) :

$$Mn(OH)_{2(s)} + H^+(aq) \rightarrow Mn^{2+}{}_{(aq)} + H_2O \text{ (not balanced)}$$

$$Mn(OH)_3 + I^-{}_{(aq)} + H^+{}_{(aq)} \rightarrow Mn^{2+}{}_{(aq)} + I_{2(aq)} + H_2O \text{ (not balanced)}$$

The iodine formed may be titrated against standard thiosulphate solution, using starch as an indicator :

$$I_2(aq) + S_2O_3^{2-}(aq) \rightarrow I^-(aq) + S_4O_6^{2-}(aq)$$

(not balanced)

From the stoichiometries of the various equations, the amount of dissolved oxygen can be readily calculated.

Natural water supplies in contact with air also absorb carbon dioxide, producing the weak acid carbonic acid in solution. This acid, found only in aqueous solution, interacts with water to form hydrated protons and hydrogen carbonate anions :

$$CO_{2(g)} + H_2O \rightleftharpoons H_2CO_3(aq)$$

$$H_2CO_{3(aq)} + H_2O_{(1)} \rightleftharpoons H_3O^+{}_{(aq)} + HCO_3{}_{(aq)}\ K_a = 4.3 \times 10^{-7}$$

Most natural water sources are therefore slightly acidic (typical drinking water : pH 6.0-8.5]. To sustain life, water must remain fairly close to neutral in character. You have seen in other experiments that it takes only a small amount of acid or alkali to alter the pH of unbuffered water. The concern over airborne acidic pollutants and acidic effluents from manufacturing plants is therefore justified. We may not live in a lake or in the rivers but our health is inevitably tied into the larger web of life.

You will test the pH of your water sample by a universal indicator paper, i.e., a paer designed to produce different colours for different pH values throughout the range 1-14.

In addition to the dissolved gases natural waters pick up due to their exposure to the atmosphere, other materials – mostly ions-accumulate in water either because they are leached out from the watercourse itself or because they are added (intentionally or unintentionally) by humans. Chloride ion is a good example. Water flowing over rocky stream beds will dissolve chloride ion and carry it along. Nominal levels of chloride (not chlorine) are not harmful and actually have physiological use. The hydrochloric acid in our stomachs must be synthesized by the body and the chloride has to come from somewhere!

Many manufacturing processes also use either hydrochloric acid or various chloride compounds, and without sufficient treatment effluents from factories can significantly raise the chloride concentration in surrounding water supplies. A much smaller amount of chloride ion is a byproduct of the purification processes used on many domestic drinking water supplies. The most obvious evidence for this is the cloudy white appearance of tap water when used to rinse beakers that held silver nitrite or lead nitrate solutions. Silver and lead chloride are fairly insoluble and even the small amount of chloride present in tap water will cause precipitates to form (typical public drinking water contains about 40 mg/LofCl-).

This suggests a technique for determining the amount of chloride ion present in a water sample. Standard solutions of chloride ion can be prepared and excess silver nitrate added to them. The degree of choudiness is a measure of the amount of chloride ion. This may seem imprecise but there are instrumental techniques (nephelometry or turbidimetry) based on this simple idea which use the amount of scattered light to determine the concentration of a substance. There is also a classic titration technique which uses chromate ion and silver nitrate as the titrant.

You have seen from earlier work that the concentration of ions in solution will affect the electric potential of a galvanic cell. This is the principle upon which pH electrodes (and many other ion-selective electrodes) operate. It is possible to construct a simple silver – sensitive electrode and use it to determine the chloride content in a water sample. The electrode consists of a $CuCu^{2+}$ half cell and a silver wire.

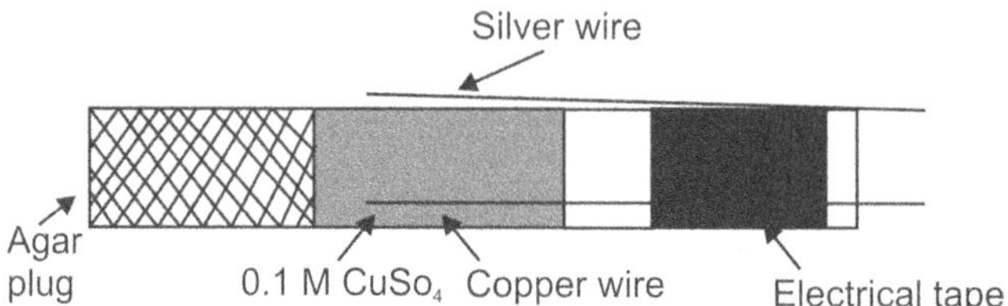

The half-cell is immersed in a water sample so that the silver wire is exposed to the water. When silver nitrate solution is added to the water sample from a burette, the silver ion concentration in the water changes slowly at first because much of the silver is immediately precipitated by any chloride ion present. This results in a gradual increase in the potential of the complete cell in which this reaction occurs :

$$2\ Ag^{+}\ (aq) + CU(s)\ 2\ Ag(s) + Cu^{2+}\ (aq)$$

This is exactly the behaviour we would predict with Le Chatelier's principle or the Nernst equation. Titrations performed in this manner, by following the voltage change in a galvanic cell, are called potentionmetric titrations.

As additional silver nitrate is added, the amount of free chloride in the mixture becomes very small until there is essentially none. Now added silver ions are not removed as AgCl and the concentration of silver rises more rapidly. This corresponds to a more rapid increase in the potential of the cell. A plot of voltage vs. mL of $AgNO_3$ in fact yields a typical s-curve and the equivalence point can be determined graphically from a derivative plot. At the equivalence point, the moles of Ag^{+} added are equal to the moles of Cl^{-} present in the sample.

Natural water supplies contain varying amounts of dissolved cations reflecting the nature of the ground over which the water has passed or is stored. Small amount of Na+ and K^{+} are common and of little concern. Both are important in biochemical processes. Less benign in some situations are Ca^{2+}, Mg^{2+} and Fe^{3+} ions because of their tendency to precipitate as insoluble salts, particularly carbonates, phosphates, and hydroxides. Deposits of these materials cause damage in domestic water heaters and pipes ($CaCO_3$ is actually less soluble in hot water). They also contribute to "scale" formation on plumbing fixtures and shower doors.

Magnesium and calcium, in particular, present additional problems because they combine with the anionic component of some soaps and detergents to form insoluble precipitates the familiar scum in the sink or washing machine. Soaps are sodium or potassium salts of aliphatic fatty acids. The binary salts are soluble, but the ternary calcium or magnesium salts are not.

Water with a high concentration of Mg^{2+} and Ca^{2+} is referred to as "hard" water, and the degree of hardness is linked to the concentrations of these two cations (typical public drinking water : 60-150 mg $CaCO_3$/L). Water with a low concentration or these ions is referred to as being "soft". Domestic water is "softenes" by exchanging sodium ions for the calcium and magnesium ions.

The hardness of a water sample can be determined by titration of the alkaline earth cations with ethylene diaminetetracetic acid (EDTA), a complexing agent. The acid itself is practically insoluble in water so it is typical to use the disodium salt of EDTA ("Na_2H_2Y").

As a complexing agent EDTA has the potential to bind at 6 sites (we say it is hexadentate – i.e., six-toothed) and its capacity to do so is somewhat determined by pH. In strongly basic solution (PH 10), the remaining two protons on the "H_2Y^{2-}" form are displaced and the Y^{4-} ion complexes 1 : 1 with magnesium and/or calcium ions.

The titration is monitored by using another complesing agent, eriochrome black T (EBT), as an indicator. EBT will also form 1 : 1 complexes with calcium and magnesium ions. But EBT-Mg complexes are more stable than EDTA-Mg complexes, whereas EBT-Ca complexes are less stable than EDTA-Ca complexes, whereas EBT-Ca complexes are less stable than EDTA-Ca complexes. In addition, the EBT-Mg complex is a wine-red colour while everything else is either colourless or blue (uncomplexed EBT is blue as well).

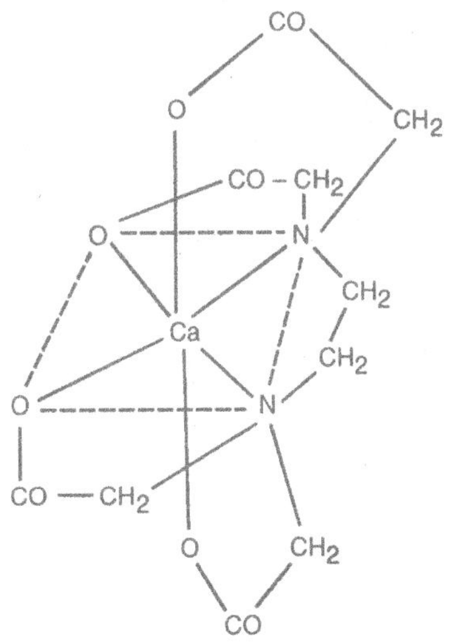

The accurate determination of total hardness (i.e., Mg + Ca) using EDTA/EBT depends on sharpening the transition from the wine-red color of the EBT-Mg complex to the blue colour of uncomplexed EBT. To ensure a sufficient amount of magnesium for this purpose, a very small amount is added to the EDTA titrant just in case the water sample itself has none (or very little).

When EBT is added to the pH 10 buffered water sample the wine-red colour of the EBT-Mg complex is evident. During the titration EDTA complexes any calcium ions in the sample and continues to do so in preference to magnesium ions (which are bound to the EBT) until all the calcium ions are complexed. At that point excess EDTA added will abstract magnesium ions from the EBT-Mg complex. As the complex comes apart the wine-red colour gives way to the blue of uncomplexed EBT. This is the end-point of the titration. The colour change can be difficult to judge without prior experience and for that reason you sill standardize the EDTA solution with a known concentration of Ca^{2+} before analyzing the actual water sample.

You will need about 250 ml of water for this experiment. Bring some from home or your favourite local supply. A bottle will be provided for this purpose.

Collect your sample in such a way as to minimize the amount of air contact. If you have a faucet aerator, remove it first before filling the bottle, and then let the water come out only in a slow stream, not a gusher. If you have a domestic water softening unit, be sure to collect water from a tap not connected to it (e.g. an outdoor hose connection.)

The Experiment

There are four parts to this experiment:

- determining the pH of the water sample
- determining the dissolved oxygen content of the water sample
- determining the Cl^- concentration of the water sample
- determining the total hardness of the water sample

The following non-locker materials will be provided:

- pH indicator paper
- 25 mL Erienmeyer flask w/stopper
- 2.6 M $MnSO_4$
- 0.90 M KI/12.5 M NaOH mixture
- concentrated H_2SO_4 (fume hood)
- 0.00050 M $Na_2S_2O_3$
- Starch indicator

- 200 mL Berzelius-style beaker w/black paper shield
- Approx. 0.004 M AgNO3 (record exact concentration)
- 0.10 M $CuSO_4$
- Pre-cut glass tubes, electrode wire pairs, electrical tape, etc.
- CBL voltage probe
- 0.10 g $CaCO_3$/L standard solution
- EBT indicator
- EDTA solution
- Four 125 mL Erienmeyer flasks
- pH10NH_3/NH_4Cl buffer (fume hood)

The chemicals

Manganese (II) sulphate is a pale red/pink powder which is slightly efflorescent. It is soluble in 1 part cold water. It has been used in dyeing, for red glazes on porcelain, in fertilizers and feeds.

Potassium iodide is a white solid, slightly deliquescent, and prone to oxidation in air. It is used in the manufacture of photographic emulsions, and in table salt and some drinking water to help prevent iodine deficiency disease.

Sodium hydroxide is commonly known as lye or caustic soda. It is a very hygroscopic white solid (absorbs water from the air rapidly) and also absorbs CO_2. It is very corrosive to vegetable and animal matter and aluminium metal especially in the presence of moisture. Dissolving NaOH in water generates considerable heat.

Besides its use in the laboratory, sodium hydroxide is used in commercial drain cleaner preparations, to treat cellulose in the manufacture of rayon and cellophane and in the manufacture of some soaps. It is corrosive to all tissues and can be detected on skin by the "slimly" feeling associated with bases. It should be rinsed off thoroughtly upon contact. It can damage delicate eye tissues and cause blindness.

Sulphuric acid is a clear, colorless, oily liquid in concentrated form (98%). It is highly corrosive and has a high affinity for water, abstracting it from wood. Paper, sugar, etc., leaving a carbon residue behind. Dilution of concentrated sulphuric acid generates a tremendous amount of heat. Here in the lab your instructor prepares the dilute sulphuric acid you use by puring the concentrated acid slowly over ICE while stirring! Even so, the resulting solution is very warm. As with all acid dilutions, acid is added to water, not the reverse, since the heat generated can boil the water at the point of contact and cause spattering.

Sulphuric acid is used to make fertilizers, explosives, dyes, parchment paper, and glue. It is used, in concentrated form, in automobile batteries as the electrolyte. It is coorosive to all body tissues and contact with eyes may result in total blindness. Ingestion may cause death. Frequent skin contact with dilute solutions may cause dermatitis.

Sodium thiosulfate (photographer's "hypo") is most commonly obtained as a pentahydrate in colorless, odourless crystals of granules. It melts at 48°C and has a tendency to form supersaturated solutions. The compound dissolves silover halides and many other salts of silver. It is used as a fixer in photography, for extraction of silver from ores, as a mordant in dyeing and printing textiles and in the manufacture of leather. The compound has relatively low toxicity. Large doses orally cause purging.

Silver nitrate forms colorless, transparent crystals. It is stable and not darkened by light in pure air but darkens in the presence of organic matter and H_2S. It decomposes at low red heat into metallic silver. It is used in photography and the manufacture of mirrors, silver plating, indelible inks, hair dyes, etching ivory and as an important reagent in analytical chemistry.

It has been used as a topical antiseptic in a 0.1 to 10% solution. However, it is caustic and irritating to skin. Silver nitrate stains skin and clothing. These stains will wear off skin in a few days to a week but clothing is generally ruined. Swallowing silver nitrate can cause severe gatroenteritis that may end fatally.

Copper(II) sulphate is available in both anhydrous form (pale blue to white), and the more common pentahydrate blue crystals (blue vitriol). It slowly effloresces in air, losing 2 waters at 30°C, 2 more at 110°C and becoming anhydrous at 250°C. It is very soluble in water and methanol. The pentahydrate is used as an agricultural fungicide and bactericide as well as an herbicide (readily available at your local hardware store to kill roots in sewer pipes). It has may other uses in the dye, tanning, plating and photography industries. Copper is a trace nutrient but is toxic when ingested in sufficient quantities.

Calcium carbonate is found in limestone, marble and chalk deposits but the commercial substance is manufactured chemically. It is a white, odourless, tasteless powder, practically insoluble in water. The compound is used in the manufacture of paint, rubber, plastics, paper, and in foods and pharmaceuticals. The solution used in this experiment was prepared to dissolving a sample of the solid in dilute HC1 and diluting to volume.

Eriochrome Black T, $C_{20}H_{12}N_3NaO_7S$, or C.I. Mordant Black 11, 3-hydroxy – 4-(1-hydroxy – 2 – naphthyl) azo] – 7- nitro – 1 – naphthalenesulfonic acid sodium salt, is a brownish – black powder with a slight metallic sheen. It is soluble in hot water. Indicator solutions are prepared according to a variety of recipes. Solutions have limited shelf-life. It can be used to dye wool and in analytical chemistry as a metal ion indicator in the determination of total water hardness with EDTA as a titrant.

Erichrome Black T

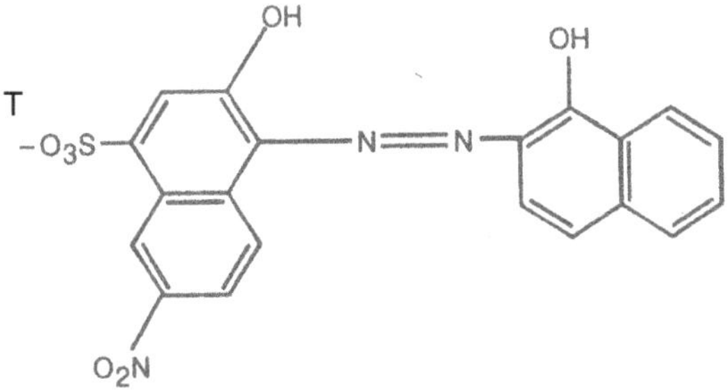

Na_2EDTA, $C_{10}H_{14}N_2Na_2O_8$, or ethylenediamminetetra acetic acid disodium salt, is very slightly soluble in water and exhibits the characteristics of a weak acid, including displacing CO_2 from carbonates and reacting with metals to form hydrogen. It is used as a sequestering agent, in particular as a chelating agent which combines with calcium, etc.

EDTA

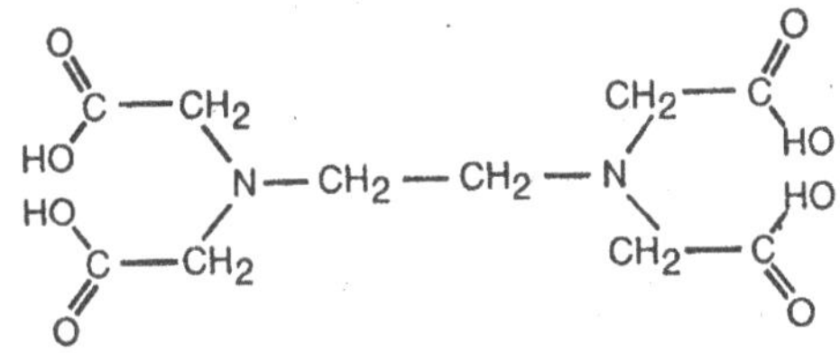

Starch (soluble starch, amyloidextrin) is a white, odourless, tasteless powder which is soluble in water when heated. It is frequently used in the lab as an indicator for iodometric analysis since it forms an intense blue-to-black complex with I_2 but not with I.

Ammonium chloride (once commonly known as "sal ammoniac") is a white crystalline or granular solid with a cooling, saline taste. It sublimes without melting, is very soluble in water and dissolves with signigicant cooling. It is used as a soldering flux, in ordinary dry cells and for slowing the melting of snow on ski slopes.

Ammonia gas can be manufactured from industrial gases associated with the processing of "coke", a spongy form of carbon obtained from processing coal and essential in steel-making. In the Haber-Bosch process nitrogen and hydrogen from these industrial gas mixtures are combined at high temperature and pressure in the presence of a catalyst to form ammonia. The gas and its aqueous solutions are colorless with a very pungent odour (lower limit of human perception : 0.04 g/m^3). Mixtures of ammonia gas and air can explode when ignited under favourable conditions. At room temperature ammonia is soluble to the extent of 31% in water, only 16% in methanol. It is used in the manufacture of nitric acid, explosives, fertilizers and in regrigeration. In anhydrous liquid form it is a good solvent for many elements and compounds, notably the alkali metals which yield blue solutions when dissolved in liquid ammonia.

Inhalation of the concentrated vapour causes swelling in the respiratory tract, spasma and asphyxia.

Technique Discussion

Checking the acidity of your water sample is the simplest procedure and might as well be done first before there is any chance of trace contamination. Remember that indicator paper is NEVER dipped into a solution (dyes leach out....). A clean stirring rod is dipped into the solution and then touched to a piece of indicator paper.

A 25 ml sample of the water is used for the dissolved oxygen determination. After the water is transferred into the 25 ml Erlenmeyer flask, 20 drops of $MnSO_4$ and 20 drops of the KI/NaOH solution (caution : use different beral pipettes for these ! They react !) are used to “fix” the dissolved oxygen so that no additional oxygen which might be inadvertently introduced during handling, stirring, pouring, etc. will react in the titration. The solution should be stoppered and inverted a few times to mix thoroughly.

The $Mn(OH)_3$ precipitate is then dissolved with 10-20 drops of concentrated H_2SO_4 (fume hood). Stopper and invert to mix. If all of the precipitate does not dissolve, a few additional drops of acid may be added, followed by further mixing. Large excesses of acid should be avoided but all of the precipitate must be dissolved. Precipitates which stand for long periods of time seem to be more difficult to dissolve.

10 mL of the acidified mixture is then placed in a 100 mL beaker and titrated to a starch endpoint with 0.00050 M $Na_2S_2O_3$ solution. As with all iodometric/starch titrations, some of the iodine should be discharged before adding the starch. The solution should be pale yellow before sufficient starch is added to give a definite blue colour. At the endpoint the sample should look like plain water. Because the decrease in blue colour is gradual it may help to place a beaker of water next to the titration beaker in order to judge when the endpoint has been reached. Repeat in order to judge when the endpoint has been reached. Repeat the titration with a second 10 ml sample only if problems are encountered with the first sample.

To construct the electrode for the chloride determination, obtain a short length of glass tubing plugged at one end with agar, and a copper/silver wire pair. Clean the wires with a steel wool pad. The bare copper wire is inserted into the glass tube and the silver wire remains outside (you can fasten the silver wire to the glass tube with a small rubber band if you like). Insert the wire as far into the tube as it will go and secure it with a piece of electrical tape. The wire should be touching the agar.

When you are ready to use the electrode, place enough 0.1 M $CuSO_4$ inside the glass tube to immerse the bare copper wire.

50 mL of the water sample is added to a tall 200 mL beaker wrapped with black paper. Place the electrode in the water. Keep the water from entering the top of the tube and diluting the copper solution and be sure the plugged end is not sitting on the bottom of the beaker. Be sure the silver wire is actually in the water before you start. Attach the wire leads to the CBL voltage probe, matching the colors of the leads with the small pieces of colored insulation on the wire ends. This ensures that the silver is connected to the + terminal. Set up the calculator to measure VOLTAGE VS, USER X (volume) and use the Graphical option, Y_{max} and Y_{min} can be 0.4 and 0.09, respectively, X_{max} and X_{min} should be 50 and 0.

Standard 0.004 M $AgNO_3$ solution (note exact concentration on bottle) is added slowly from a burette while monitoring the voltage. Chloride ion contents vary. Time can be saved by taking an initial voltage reading of your sample (once you enter the actual data-collection part of the program the CBL displays the voltage from the electrode continuously until you take a reading). It is not necessary to begin recording data until the voltage is around 0.09 volts. If your cell gives less than this, add silver nitrate from the burette in a slow stream(while stirring) until the cell voltage approaches 0.09 V. At that point record the volume of $AgNO_3$ added and the voltage. If the initial voltage is higher than 0.09 notify the instructor before continuing.

$AgNO_3$ is added in 0.5 ml increments once the minimum voltage is obtained, recording the voltage after each addition. There should be a gradual increase, then a marked increase, and then a gradual flattening out, just as in an acid/base titration but perhaps not so dramatic. Data should be taken at least 2 mL past the endpoint.

The EDTA solution for the water hardness determination must be standardized before the actual water sample can be titrated. The colour change at the endpoint is often difficult to judge. Until the endpoint is near there is practically no change in the solution. It then becomes a sort of indigo colour. At this point, you should halt and allow the solution to mix before completing (there may be additional change on mixing). The final colour at the endpoint is blue with no trace of purple. You might want to save your first titration for a reference.

The standardization should be done in triplicate using 10 mL of the CaCO3 solution in a clean, dry 125 mL Erlenmeyer flask. 5 drops of EBT indicator and 2 mL of the buffer are added (CAUTION : **the buffer contains a high concentration of ammonia).** The burette for delivering the EDTa must be rinsed with a small amount of EDTA (discard) before using. EDTA is an excellent ion scavenger and any concentration of the EDTA and give spurious results. The CaCO3 samples should be titrated to the colour of the "colour standard" mixture.

A 10 mL volume should be sufficient for the water sample titration. 5 drops of EBT and 2 mL of buffer are also required. A duplicate titration is recommended, but not required.

The Report

Your initial calculations should include:

1. The moles thiosulfate used in dissolved 02 titration (may be mean or single value).
2. The equivalent moles of I2, $Mn(OH)_3$, and O_2.
3. The mass of 02 in mg
4. The total dissolved oxygen content expressed as parts per million by mass (mg.L)
5. The volume of EDTA solution needed to titrate 1 mg $CaCO_3$ (the standard solution is 0.10 mg $CaCO_3$/mL)
6. The hardness of the water expressed as mg$CaCO_3$/L (may be mean or a single value).
7. A graph of your potentiometric titration data (voltage or E vs. mg$AgNO_3$)
8. A table of DE, DV, DE/DV and V (average mL AgNO3) for our titration (near the endpoint region only)
9. A graph of $\Delta E/\Delta V$. and V (first derivative plot)
10. The Cl^- concentration for your water sample expressed in mg/L.

You conclusion to this experiment should include the balanced equations needed to complete the calculations and a summary table for all the test done. There should be a brief discussion of any results that seem abnormal. Be sure to include the source of your water sample.

CHAPTER 19

VALIDATION

Introduction

According to the US food and drug administration (FDA).

Validation is establishing documented evidence which provides a high degree of assurance that a specific process (such as the manufacture of pharmaceutical dosage forms) will consistently produce a product meeting its predetermined specifications and quality characteristics.

According to the FDA, assurance of product quality is derived from careful (and systematic) attention to a number of (important) factors including:

Selection of quality (components) and materials

Adequate product and process design and

(statistical) control of the process through In-process and end product testing.

According to the FDA's Current Good Manufacturing Practices (CGMPs) control procedures shall be established to monitor output and to validate performance of the manufacturing processes that may be responsible for causing variability in the characteristics of In-process material and the drug product. Such control procedures shall include:

1. Tablet or capsule weight variation
2. Disintegration time
3. Adequacy of mixing to ensure uniformity and homogeneity.
4. Dissolution time and rate.

5. Clarity, completeness or pH of the solution.

- Items 1 and 3 are associated with variability in the manufacturing process.
- Items 2 and 4 are influenced by the selection of the ingredients in the product formulation.
- The first four items are directly related to the manufacture and validation of solid dosage forms.

Definition

Validation is a documented programme which provides a high degree of assurance that a specific process will consistently produce a product meeting its pre-determined specifications and quality attributes.

It is simply assessment of validity or action of providing effectiveness.

According to European Community for medicinal products

"Validation is action of proving, in accordance with the principles of Good manufacturing practices, that any procedures, process, equipment, material, activity or system actually leads to expected results."

Importance of Validation

1. Quality safety and effectiveness must be designed and built into the product.
2. Quality can not be inspected or tested in the finished product.
3. Each step of the manufacturing process must be controlled to maximise the probability that the finished product meets all quality and design specifications.

The Concept of Validation

Validation is a relatively new concept in pharmaceutical manufacturing evolved in 1980's.

- Validation is establishing documented evidence which provides a high degree of assurance that a specific process will consistently produce a product (or) service meeting its pre-determined specifications and quality characteristics.
- Validation is the action of proving that any procedure, process, equipment, method, material (or) activity actually leads to the expected results and produce a quality product.
- The concept of validation has expended to a wide range of activities from cleaning methods, Analytical methods to equipments, facilities and process for the manufacturing of drug substances and drug products.

The purpose of validation of any equipment (or) process is achieved by means of validation protocol, which details the tests to be carried out. The frequency of testing and the results expected i.e. the acceptance criteria.

- The validation of facilities, equipment and services is called 'qualification'.

  An operational qualification (OQ) documents specific dynamic attributes of a facility or equipment to prove that it operates as expected through out its opening range.

- An installation qualification (IQ) documents specific static attributes of a facility (or) equipment like U.V. Spectrophotometer to prove that the instillation of the unit has been correctly performed.

Methods of Validation

1. Prospective validation
2. Retrospective validation
3. Concurrent validation
4. Revalidation.

Validation has several methods. If validation programme is designed and implemented before the equipment of facility comes on stream i.e. before starting the production, then this constitutes prospective validation.

- Some times, however, systems or processes are in place that have not been previously validated but are functioning well and consistently producing good products.

- Already in production, validation of such facilities (or) process is called retrospective validation.

  It is activated by the review of historical manufacturing and testing data..

- Prospective and retrospective validation may be combined advantageously in sequence to provide a higher level of assurance that is given by the pre-marketing prospective validation alone.

  Concurrent validation is a newer term that is applied either to ongoing prospective validation or to the ongoing review and evaluation of historical data associated with retrospective validation.

- Revalidation is the act of repeating all (or) a portion of the validation as a result of any modification to the process (or) facility that may lead to changes in quality (or) reproducibility of the product.

  Revalidation also refers to the regular, planned repetition of validation steps for equipment or process, where performance may change with time.

Process Validation

- Critical processes should be validated prospectively (or) restrospetively.

  When any new master formula or method or preparation is adopted, it should be taken to demonstrate its suitability for routine processing. The defined process using the materials and equipment specified should be shown to yield a product consistently of the received quality.
- Significant amendments to the manufacturing process including any change in equipment or material that may effect product quality or reproducibility of the process should be validated.

Equipments of Validation

- Credibility of instrumentation depends on the use of quality machineries and proper maintenance.
- Dependability of instrumentation depends on the
  (i) The extensive testing to cover varied working condition.
  (ii) Continuous reliability of functioning of equipment can only be assured through a strictly applied validation programme to maintain accuracy and general performance.
- The equipments should be designed or selected in which product specifications are consistently achieved.
- This should be done with the participitation of all appropriate groups that are concerned with assuring a quality product.

  e.g. Engineerng design, production operation and quality assurance.

The validation of facilities, equipments and services is commonly called 'Qualification'.

Qualification is usually divided into two elements.

(i) Installation qualification (IQ)

(ii) Operational qualification (OQ)

(i) ***Installation qualification*:** Installation qualification studies establish confidence that the process equipment and ancillary systems.

- Which are capable of consistently operating within the established limits and tolerance.

This phase of validation includes:

- Examination of equipment design
- Determination of calibration
- Maintenance requirements

- Adjustment requirements
- Identification of critical elements that could affect the product etc.
- Information obtained from above mentioned studies should be used to establish written procedures for :-
- calibration
- maintenance
- Product manufacturing and control of equipments.

(ii) Operational Qualification

- The purpose of the operational qualification is to provide rigorous testing to demonstrate the effectiveness and reproducibility of the process.

This phase of qualification includes:

- Visual checking of equipment
- Checking the functioning of switches and indicator lights.
- Cleaning procedures
- Actions resulting from installation qualification
- Requalification (time scales and triggering factors) and
- Testing of processes specific for the equipment.

Validation Master Plan

- The qualification programme is co-ordinated by means of a written general plan called 'Validation master plan'.
- The administration of qualification programme is normally done by means of a validation committee comprising of representatives of the various disciplines involved with the programme.
- These representatives may be from departments such as:
  - production
  - Quality assurance
  - Research and development
  - Engineering and maintenance
- This committee defines, approves and issues written protocols and revises the data obtained against the acceptance criteria.
- Validation master plan reinforces the commitment of the company to GMP and should provide a clear overview of the validation programme including schedules and responsibilities.

- It is also a convenient guide to the validation committee and for those performing the qualifications.
- Validation master plan is maintained as live document to which new addition may be included from time to time.
- Tests and challenge conditions should include actual production and 'worst case' conditions of equipment operation.
- In evaluating an entire system, it may be necessary to study the interaction of several process elements to determine cumulative effect on th product attributes.
- The test and challenged conditions may be repeated for suitable number of items to assure reliable and meaningful results. If any derivations from specifications are found, it should be corrected and the validation procedures should be repeated to assure the process adequacy.

Regulatory Background

- Validation is best viewed as an important and integral part of GMP validation became a regulatory requirement in 1978 in order to force the industry to control their processes, so that process outcome would be pre-ordinated.
- As stated by Ted Beyers of FDA, "FDA except the industry to build quality into the product, not test quality into the product.
- FDA requires the validation to be completed even at the time of applying for approval.
- Any piece of equipment, facility to process operated under current GMP should be validated.

The requirements for process validation is contained in 21 CFR published by FDA.

"There shall be written procedures for production and process control designed to ensure that the drug products have the identity, strength, quality and purity they purport or are represented to possess".

Section 210.110, sampling and testing of in process materials and drug products states:

"In control procedures shall be established to monitor the output and validate the performance of those manufacturing processes that may be responsible for causing variability in the characteristics of Inprocess material and the drug products".

Section 211.165, testing and release and distribution says:

"The accuracy, sensitivity, specificity and reproducibility of test methods employed by the firm shall be established and documented".

A general status requirements for process validation is contained in the medical device CGmp regulations. Section 820.110 (b) (1) states:

"Where deviations from device specifications could occur as a result of the manufacturing process itself, there shall be written procedures describing any processing controls necessary to assume conformance of specifications".

Benefits of Validation

- Process consistently under control requires less process support, will have less down time, fewer batch failure and may operate more efficiently with greater output.
- In addition, timely and appropriate validation will transmit a commitment to product quality, which may facilitate pre-approval inspections and expedite granting of marketing authorisations.
- The quality should not be simply related or equated to "Compliance to specifications" rather it should be linked to "route to compliance".

Hence, a quality drug product can be manufactured and packed using qualified equipment in qualified facilities by a validated process.

Validation of Analytical Methods

- Analytical methods play a vital role in:
  - (i) New drug development
  - (ii) Pre-formulation studies
  - (iii) Stability studies
  - (iv) Quality control testing and in quality assurance programmes
- Analytical testing of a pharmaceutical product is necessary to ensure its stability, safety and efficiency.
- The need of analytical methods to give reliable results adequate for intended purpose.
- Analytical methods available to serve the above purpose are summarized in Table 1.
- For the selection of an analytical method, it is needed to establish:
  - (i) First what is to be measured and how accurately it should be measured.
  - (ii) It is also necessary to define precisely both the conditions in which the method is to be used and the purpose for which it is intended.
- The selection method must be simple, specific, accurate, precise, economical and convenient.
- The method should be validated during the development and use.

Analytical Validation

- Analytical validation refers to the evaluation and proving that an analytical method serves the intended purpose.
- Analytical validation ensures that the selected analytical method will give reproducible and reliable results, adequate for intended purpose.

Table 1 Analytical methods and the physical property

Analytical method	Physical property employed
1. Gravimetry	Mass (or) weight
2. Volumetry	Volume (of a liquid or gas)
3. Physical methods	Specific gravity (or) density, Surface tension, viscosity
4. Conductometry	Electrical conductivity
5. Potentiometry	Electrical potential
6. Amperometry and coulometry	Electrical current
7. Polarography	Current-voltage characteristics
8. Thermal Analysis	Transmission temp. (M.P. and B.P.)
9. Enthalpy method	Heat of reaction
10. Spectrophotometry	Absorption of radiations
11. (U.V, visible, IR, X-ray atomic absorptions, NMR, ESR)	
12. Flame photometry, 13. Flourimetry, X-ray emission 14. Spectroscopy	Emission of radiation
15. Turbidimetry, Nephelometry and Raman Spectroscopy	Scattering of radiations
16. Polarimetry and ORD	Rotation of radiation
17. Refractometry and Interferometry	Refraction of radiation
18. X RD (X-ray diffraction method	Diffraction of radiation
19. Mass spectroscopy	Mass to charge ratio
20. Radio chemical method	Radio activity

Main Objectives of Analytical Procedures

- The procedure is suitable for its intended purposes. Due to their complex nature, Analytical procedures for biological and biotechnological products in some cases may be approached differently.

  Well-characterized reference materials, with documentated purity, should be used through out the validation study. The degree of purity necessary depends on the intended use.

- In practice, it is usually possible to design the experimental work, so that the appropriate validation characteristics can be considered simultaneously to provide a sound, over-all knowledge of the capabilities of the analytical procedure. For instance :

Specificity, linearity, range, accuracy and precision.

1. Specificity

- An investigation of specificity should be conducted during the validation of identification tests, the determination of impurities and the array.
- It depends upon the intended objectives of the analytical procedure.

  It is not always possible to demonstrate that an analytical procedure is specific for a particular analyte (complete discrimination).

- In this case, a combination of two or more analytical procedures is recommended to achieve the necessary level of discrimination.

1.1 Identification

- The suitable identification tests should be able to discriminate between compounds of closely related structures, which are likely to be present.
- The discrimination of a procedure may be confirmed by obtaining positive results (perhaps by comparison with a known reference material) from samples containg the analyte, coupled with negative results from samples which do not contain the analyte.
- In addition the identification test may be applied to materials structurally similar to or closely related to the analyte to confirm that a positive response is not obtained.
- The choice of such potentially intergering materials should be based on sound scientific judgement with a consideration of the interference that could occur.

1.2 Assay and impurity Test (S)

For chromatographic procedures, representative chromatograms should be used to demonstrate specificity and individual components should be appropriately labelled. Similar considerations should be given to other separation techniques.

- Critical separations in chromatography should be investigated at an appropriate level. For critical separations, specificity can be demonstrated by resolution of the two components which are closest to each other.
- In cases where a non-specific assay is used, other supporting analytical procedures should be used to demonstrate over all specificity.

e.g. where a titration is adopted to assay the active substance for release, the combustion of the assay and a suitable test for impurities can be used. The approach is similar for both assay and impurity tests.

1.2.1 Discrimination of Analytes where impurities are available :

For the assay, this should involve demonstration of the discrimination of the analyte in the presence of impurities and/or excipients.

Practically this can be done by spiking pure substances (active substance or product) with appropriate levels of impurities and / or recipients and demonstrating that the assay result is unaffected by the presence of these materials. (by comparison with the assay result obtained on unspiked samples)

For the impurity test, the discrimination may be established by spiling active substance or product with appropriate levels of impurities and demonstrating the separation of these impurities individually and/or from other components in the sample matrix.

1.2.2 Discrimination of the analyte where impurities are not available

If impurity or degradation product standards are unavailable, specificity may be demonstrated by comparing the test results of samples containing impurities or degradation products to a second well-characterized procedure.

e.g. pharmacopoeial method or other validated analytical procedure (independent procedure). This should include samples stored under relevant stress conditions : light, heat, humidity, acid/base hydrolysis and oxidation.

- For the assay, the two results should be compared.
- For the impurity test, the impurity profiles should be compared.

  Peak purity test may be useful to show that the analyte chromatographic peak is not attributed to more than one component (e.g. diode array, mass spectrometry).

2. Linearity

- A linear relationship should be evaluated across the range of the analytical procedure.
- It may be demonstrated directly on the active substance (by dilution of a standard stock solution) and/or on separate weighing of synthetic mixtures of the product components. Using the proposed procedure linearity should be evaluated by visual inspection of a plot of signals as a function of analyte concentration or content. If there is a linear relationship, test results should be evaluated by appropriate statistical methods.

  For e.g. : By calculation of a regression line by the method of least squares. In some cases, to obtain linearity between assays and sample concentrations, the test data may need to be subjected to a mathematical transformation prior to the regression analysis. Data from the regression line itself may be helpful to provide mathematical estimates of the degree of linearity.
- The correlation coefficient, Y-intercept, slope of the regression line and residual sum of squares should be described by an appropriate function of the concentration (amount of an analyte in a sample.
- For the establishment of linearity, a minimum of 5 concentrations is recommended. Other approaches should be justified.

3. Range

The specified range is normally derived from linearity studies and depends on the intended application of the procedure.

- It is established by confirming that the analytical procedures provides an acceptable degree of linearity, accuracy and precision when applied to samples containing amounts of analyte within or at the extremes of the specified range of analytical procedures.

The following minimum specified ranges should be considered:

- For the assay of an active substance or a finished product normally from 80 to 120 percent of the test concentration.
- For content uniformity, covering a minimum of 70 to 130 percent of the test concentration, unless a wider more appropriate range, based on the nature of the dosage form (e.g. : metered dose inhaler) : is justified.
- For dissolution testing : + 20% over the specified range :

  e.g. : If the specifications for a controlled released product cover a region from 20%, after 1 hour, upto 90% after 24 hours, the validated range would be 0-110% of the label claim.
- For the determination of an impurity : From the reporting level of an impurity to 120% of the specification : For impurities known to be unusually potent or

to produce tonic or unexpected pharmacological effects, the detection/quantitation limit should be commensurated with the level at which the impurities must be controlled.

Note: For validation of impurity, test procedures carried out during development, it may be necessary to consider the range around a suggested (probable) limit.

If assay and purity are performed together as one test and only a 100% standard is used, linearity should cover the range from the reporting level of the impurities 1 to 120% of the assay specification.

4. Accuracy

Accuracy should be established across the specified range of the analytical procedure.

4.1 Assay

4.1.1 ***Active substance***: Several methods of determining accuracy are available.

(a) application of an analytical procedure to an analyte of known purity (e.g. : reference material).

(b) comparison of the results of the proposed analytical procedure with those of a second well characterized procedure, the accuracy of which is stated and/or defined (independent procedure, sec 1.22).

(c) accuracy may be inferred once precision, linearity and specificity have been established.

4.1.2 ***Medical Product*** **:** Several methods for determining accuracy are available:

(a) application of the analytical procedure to synthetic mixtures of the product components to which known quantities of the substance to be analysed have been added.

(b) in cases where it is impossible to obtain samples of all product components, it may be acceptable either to add known quantities of the analyte to the product or to compare the result obtained from a second, well characterized procedure, the accuracy of which is stated and/or defined (independent procedure)

(c) accuracy may be inferred once precision, linearity and specificity have been established.

4.2 Impurities (Qunatitation)

Accuracy should be assessed on samples (substance/product) spiked with known amount of impurities.

In cases where it is impossible to obtain samples of certain impurities and/or degradation products, it is considered acceptable to compare results obtained by an independent procedure. The response factor of the drug substance can be used.

It should be clar how the individual or total impurities are to be determined e.g. weight/weight or area percent, in all cases with respect to the major analyte.

4.3 Recommended Data

Accuracy should be assessed using a minimum of a determinations over a minimum of 3 concentration levels covering the specified range (e.g. 3 concentrations/3 replicates each of the total analytical procedure)

Accuracy should be reported as percent recovery by the assay of known added amount of analyte in the sample or as the difference between the mean and the accepted true value together with the confidence intervals.

5. Precision

Validation of tests for assay and for quantitative determination of impurities includes an investigation of precision.

5.1 Repeatability

Repeatability should be assessed using:

(a) a minimum of determinations covering the specified range for the procedure (e.g. : 3 concentrations/3replicates each).

(b) a minimum of 6 determinations at 100% of the test concentration.

5.2 Intermediate Precision

The extent to which intermediate precision should be established depends on the circumstances under which the procedure is intended to be used. The applicat should establish the effects of random events on the precision of the analytical procedure.

Typical variations to be studied include day, analysis, equipment, etc.

It is not considered necessary to study those effects individually, The use of an experimental design (matrix is encouraged).

5.3 Reproducibility

Reproducibility is assessed by means of an inter-laboratory trial, reproducibility should be considered in case of the standardisation of an analytical procedure, for instance, for inclusion of procedures on pharmacopecias. This data is not part of the marketing authorisation dossier.

5.4 Recommended data

The standard deviation, relative standard deviation (coefficient of variation) and confidence interval should be reported for such type of precision investigated.

6. Detection Limit

Several approaches for determining the defection limit are possible, depending on whether the procedure is a non-instrumental or instrumental. Approaches other than those listed below may be acceptable.

6.1 Based on Visual Evaluation

Visual Evaluation may be used for non-instrumental methods but may also be used with instrumental methods.

The defection limit is determined by th analysis of samples with concentrations of analyte and by establishing the minimum level at which the analyte can be reliably defected.

6.2 Based on Signal-to Noise

This approach can only be applied to analytical procedures which exhibit baseline noise.

Determination of the signal-to-noise ratio is performed by comparing measured signals form samples with known low concentrations of analyte with those of blank samples and establishing the minimum concentration at which the analyte can be reliably defected.

A signal-to-noise ratio between 3 or 2 : 1 is generally considered acceptable for estimating the defection limit.

6.3 Based on the Standard Deviation of the Response and the Slope

The slope S may be estimated from the calibrating curve of the analyte. The estimate of may be carried out on a variety of ways.

6.3.1 Based on the Standard Deviation of the Blank

Measurement of the magnitude of analytical background response is performed by analysing an appropriate number of blank samples and calculating the standard deviation of these responses.

6.3.2 Based on the Calibration Curve

A specific calibration curve should be studied using samples containing an analyte on the range of DL.

The residual standard deviation of a regression line or true standard.

Standard deviation of y-intercepts of regression lines may be used as the standard deviation.

6.4 Recommended Data

The detection limit and the method used for determining the detection limit should be presented.

- If DL is determined based on Visual Evaluation or based on signal to noise ratio, the presentation of the relevant chromatograms is considered acceptable for justification.
- In cases where an estimated value for the detection limit is obtained by Calculation or Extrapolation, this estimate may subsequently be validated by the independent analysis of a suitable number of samples known to be near or prepared at the detection limit.

7. Quantitative Limit

- Several approaches for determining the quantitation limit are possible, depending on whether the procedure is a non-instrumental or instrumental.

Approaches other than those listed below may be acceptable.

7.1 Based on Visual Evaluation

- Visual evaluation may be used for non-instrumental methods but may also be used with instrumental methods.
- The quantitative limit is generally determined by the analysis of samples with known concentrations of analyte and by establishing the minimum level at which the analyte can be quantified with acceptable accuracy and precision.

7.2 Based on Signal-to-Noise approach

This approach can only be applied to analytical procedures that exhibit baseline noise.

- Determination of the signal-to-noise ratio is performed by comparing measured signals from samples with known low concentrations of analyte with those of blank samples and by establishing the minimum concentration at which the analyte can be reliably quantified.
- A typical signal-to-noise ratio is 10 : 1.

7.3 Based on the Standard Deviation of the Response and the Slope

The slope S may be estimated from the calibration curve of the analyte. The estimate may be carried out in a variety of ways including.

7.3.1 Based on Standard Deviation of the Blank

Measurement of the magnitude of analytical background response is performed by analysing an appropriate number of blank samples and calculating the standard deviation of these responses.

7.3.2 Based on the Calibration Curve

A specific calibration curve should be studied using samples, containing an analyte in the range of QL (Quantitation limit).

7.4 Recommended Data

- The quantitation limit and the method used for determining the quantitation limit should be presented.
- The limit should be subsequently validated by the analysis of a suitable number of samples known to be near or prepared at the quantitation limit.

8. Robustness

- The evaluation of robustness should be considered during the development phase and depends on the type of procedure under study.
- It should show the reliability of an analysis with respect to deliberate variations in method parameters.
- If measurements are susceptible to variations for analytical conditions, the analytical conditions should be suitably controlled or a precautionary statement should be included in the procedure.
- One consequence of the evaluation of robustness should be that a series of system suitability parameters (e.g. resolution test) is established to ensure that the validity of the analytical procedure is maintained whenever used.

Examples of typical variations are:

- Stability of analytical solutions
- Extraction time

In case of liquid chromatography examples of typical variations are:

- Influence of variations of pH for a mobile phase
- Influence of variations on mobile phase composition
- different columns (different lots and/or supplies)

- temperature
- flow rate

In the case of gas-chromatography, examples of typical variation are:

- Different columns (different lots and/or suppliers)
- Temperature
- Flow rate

9. System Suitability Testing

System suitability testing is an integral part of many analytical procedures.

The tests are based on the concept that the equipment, electronics, analytical operations and samples to be analysed constitute an integral system that can be evaluated as such. System suitability test parameters to be established for a particular procedure depend on the type of procedure being validated.

Validation of Sterile Products and Processes

- Validation studies are an essential part of GMP's and should be conducted in accordance with predefined protocols.
- Sterile products have several unique dosage form properties
    - Free from pyrogens
    - Free from particulate matter
    - Extremely complicated high standards of purity and quality.
    - The goal in the manufacture of sterile products should be free from microbial contamination.
- Validation and manufacture of sterile pharmaceutical products is a complicated process involving numerous activities that can be grouped into the following factors.

  Process – facility – Equipment

  Services – personnel – Cleaning

- Process consistently under control requires:
    (i) less process support
    (ii) less down time
    (iii) fewer batch failures and operate more efficiently with greater outputs.

Facilities, Equipment and Services Validation

The Validation of facilities, equipment and services is called qualification. It is further classified into:

(i) Installation qualification (IQ)

(ii) Operational qualification

1. **Installation Qualification**

   Installation qualification studies establish confidence that the process equipment and ancillary systems are capable of consistently operating with in the established limits.

   This phase of validation includes:

   - Examination of Equipment design
   - Determination of Calibration
   - Maintenance requirements etc.

   Information obtained from above mentioned studies should be used to establish written procedures for:

   - Calibration
   - Maintenance
   - Product manufacturing and
   - Control equipments

2. **Operational Qualifications**

   The purpose of the operational qualification is to provide a rigorous testing to demonstrate the effectiveness and reproducibility of the process.

   - The phase of the qualification includes:
     (i) Visual checking of the Equipment
     (ii) Checking the functions of switches and indicative lights etc.
   - The application of this qualifications procedure is especially important for facilities, services and items of equipments that are used, in the manufacture of sterile products.

The critical aspects are

1. **Heating, Ventillation and Air conditioning (HVAC) of the sterile Facility**

   These systems are used for filtering air under positive pressure for maintaining desired environmental control on the manufacturing areas.

   - The features of this system that require qualification include
   - HEPA filters integrity
   - Air borne particulate control
   - Air flow direction
   - Room air pressure differential system
   - Humidity control
   - The filter installation integrity testing is done by D.G.P. method.
   - Determination of unidirectional flow can be accomplished by isokinetic smoke.

   - Positive pressure are monitored by magnetic or photonelic gauges.

2. **Pure Water Supply**

   Quality of water is very important in the production of sterile products. Different qualities of water are used for different purposes and their specifications are according to official standards.

   Compressed gasses**:** Various gases are used in sterile product manufacturing (N_2, oxygen, CO_2). The limits of contaminants are according to specifications.

3. **Container and Closures Preparation Equipment**

   The container and closure system that comes into contact with the drug product are physical barrier between contaminate and the drug. Therefore cleaning of containers and closures are required.

   - The design of cleaning must be validated
   - Container and closures should be subjected to testing prior to beginning the validation phase to determine the type and extent of contaminants found.

   Filling Equipment for aseptic processes**:** There are several types of filling equipment for sterile products.

   - Validation work therefore is essentially a study of variability at various filling rates. Validation protocols should lay down the number and duration of filling runs for each size, filling rates and filling variability limits.

- The purpose of the validation work is to determine a filling configuration i.e. line speed, fill quantity and container size.
- The object of validation work is to find out optimum control of these variables to permit consistent filling accuracy at reasonable speeds.
- Accuracy of the order of 3-5% R.S.D can be achieved depending on the nature of product and fill quantity.

***Vials Capping and Ampoule Sealing Equipments*:** Several types of tests have been described to evaluate the effectiveness.

Vial Capping	**Ampoule Sealing**
Leakage test	Vacuum dry leak test
System integrity test	Autoclave dye process
Closure displacement test	Electronic test

Sterilization Equipment

Various methods of sterilization are used in the manufacture of sterile products which should be validated.

(a) ***Steam Sterilization Validation*:** In this process first IQ, OQ are done. Various features of the autoclave are checked for proper function.

- These include pressure valves, door safety interlock systems jacket steam traps, temperature control monitoring and recording equipment.
- On completion of OQ and IQ validation, studies will consist of replicate runs of temperature distribution, container mapping, heat penetration studies.

(b) **Dry Heat Sterilization :** Items which are included to IQ Protocol are:

(i) equipment

(ii) door gaskets

(iii) critical and non-critical instruments

(iv) heaters

(v) blowers

(vi) baffles

(vii) filters

- In OQ protocol, the items included are:

(i) cycle timers

(ii) heaters

(iii) blowers

(iv) coding coils

(v) belt speed controllers and recorders

There are many types of equipment in dry heat sterilization

1. Bath over Equipment and Tunnel Sterilization Validation

(a) Air balance determination

(b) Heat distribution studies

(c) Heat penetration studies

- In dry heat sterilization the following are validated.

  (a) endotoxin destruction

  (b) Particulate Contamination

2. Validation of Ethylene Dioxide Sterilization

- Despite hazardous properties of the ethylene gas, it continues to be used as sterilizing agent in pharmaceutical industry.
- The equipment and associated control and instrumentation should be properly calibrated before validation
- The approaches for ETO validation differ from firm to firm.
- The following general considerations are

  (a) Carefully evaluate the material and type of packing to be sterilized.

  (b) Validation studies should make use of biological indicators.

  (c) Temperature distribution studies

  (d) Loaded chamber studies

3. Validation of Radiation Sterilization Process

This type of sterilization requires highly specialized equipment. The sterilized equipment should be operationally qualified.

The qualifications for radiation sterilization are:

1. Specifications of irradiator equipment
2. Reliability and calibration
3. Radiation source strength
4. Speed of conveyer
5. Dose rate

The key elements in validating radiation sterilization are load pattern, dose distribution through the load, calibration of dose timer.

4. Validation of Sterilizing Filters

Sterilization by filtration is used in aseptic process. The important aspect of filtration sterilization are pore size, pore size distribution, integrity and capacity.

- Non distructive tests are done, two procedures are used as methods of choice for non destructive filter integrity and filtration efficiency verification. These tests are bubble point test and diffusion or pressure hold test. The bacterial challenge test is also done.

Process Validation

- The EDA in its most recently proposed guidelines has offered the following definition for process validation:
- "Process validation is establishing documented evidence which provides high degree of assurance that specific process will consistently produce a product meeting its predetermined speicifications and quality characteristics."

A. Compounding

After completion of development and scale up work, a process formulation should be run on the production equipment under normal production conditions to complete the qualification projects.

(a) **Prospective process Validation :** In prospective validation, validation protocol is executed before the process is put into commercial use.

- Critical steps in manufacturing process
- Sampling plan
- Consideration of every third data
- Complete analysis of raw material
- Acceptance criteria based on product specification
- Complete in-process records

(b) **Retrospective Validation :** All equipment, facilities and subsystems should be qualified and validated, which have been used for the production of batches of numerical data of In-process and end-product testing of which are retrospective validation.

Following method is used for retrospective validation.

- Collect numerical values of In-process data and end product testing results.
- Organize these data in chronological order.
- Include data for at least 20 – 30 batches for analysis.
- Subject the data to statistical analysis and evaluation.

B. Revalidation

FDA's guidelines on general principles of process validation for revalidation whenever there is change in formulation, equipment or process which could have impact on product effectiveness or product characteristics:

The conditions which require revalidation studies are :

- Changes in critical component.

  Change in facility/or plant

  Sequential batches that fail to confirm product and process specification.

Cleaning Validation

- The objective is to minimize the possibility of significant cross contamination.
- It is considered that a cleaning procedure that consistently reduce the contaminant, to a level not exceeding one thousandth of its lower daily therapeutic dose to the highest daily therapeutic dose of the product, can be regarded as product validated.

  These sampling methods are, in general, used, namely:

  1. Swabs
  2. Rinses
  3. Placebos
- Cleaning validation can be documented either as part of an O.Q or P.V. protocol or separately.

Personal Validation

The source of particulate matter and microbial contamination is due to personnel involved.

The personnel should be validated for the following :

- Crowing Validation
- Medical Examination
- Personnel concerned are trained

Importance of Validation

- The most compelling reasons to optimize and validate pharmaceutical production and suppoting processes are quality assurance and cost reduction.
- The basic principles of quality assurance have, as their goal, the production of articles that are fit for their intended use.
- Quality can be assured only through validation and proper In-process Quality Control.
- Hence validation is a key element in assuring the quality of the product.

Validation of Ayurvedic Products and Process

- Ayurveda is the science or knowledge of life.
- Ayurveda stresses on posibite health, a blending of physical, mental, social, moral and spiritual welfare of a subject.
- The main aim of Ayurveda is to preserve the health of a healthy subject and to cure the patient of his illness.
- Rasayana therapy, an essential component of modern Ayurveda, it helps in slowing down the ageing process enhances memory, improves the functioning of vital organs and nourishes all the tissues through the use of natural plant (herbal) or crude drugs.
- Many drugs like Aswagandha, Isabgol, Amalake, Tripala, Sankapusphi, Gudachi, Madhugashri, Brahmi, Amavat, Suntni, Guggalu, Arjunaksheera find wide spread use in Ayurveda.
- Ayurvedic formulations contain more than one herbal drug in a majority cases with understanding of Scientific Validity of Rasayana therapy.
- In Ayurveda, the herbal drugs are used in chemical pharmacological and clinical investigations.

- The active principles of herbal drugs depend on many factors like:
  - Climate and region of cultivation.
  - Season of collection
  - Treatment given during collection and storage etc.
- An installation qualification (IQ) documents specifies static attributes of a facility or equipment to prove that the installation of the unit has been correctly performed.
- The information of IQ include:
  - Introduction and objectives
  - Identification Information
  - Purpose of facility or equipment
  - Design and construction details
  - Details of services required and provided and
  - Acceptance level
- An operational qualification protocol includes:
  - (i) Identification, objectives and identification information
  - (ii) Visual inspection
  - (iii) Functioning of switches and indicator lights
  - (iv) Checks and calibration of sensor, probes, gauges, air flow rate pressure, temp. etc.
  - (v) Equipment integrity and efficiency tests.
  - (vi) Cleaning procedures
  - (vii) Acceptance criteria etc.

Process validation is done in two stages.

First Stage

- Critical process parameters are identified and protocol is designed.

  The critical process parameters should relate to various aspects and manufacturing specifications.

For e.g. for a liquid product the critical parameters could be:

(i) order (or) rate of addition of ingredients

(ii) pH

(iii) Mixing time

(iv) Light sensitivity during processing

(v) Time between manufacturing and filling etc.

Second Stage

The manufacturing three batches of product, controlling the critical parameters and thoroughly testing for compliance of specifications.

Raw material validation includes identification of critical properties/characters and a protocol and design laying specifications for each.

- Some of the critical properties for raw material validation include :
  (i) Impurity profile and residual solvents
  (ii) Colour
  (iii) Polymorphism and crystal habit
  (iv) Particle size destruction
  (v) Bulk density
  (vi) Satisfactory microbial profile etc

Validation of Ayurvedic products and process

Generally Ayurvedic medicines are the combination of selected herbal/crude drugs and are manufactured under different pharmaceutical processes to result in various dosage forms such as extracts, tinctures, decoctions, pills, powders, tablets and capsules and semisolid pastes, jellies etc.

Validation of Ayurvedic products and process should include the following :

I. Raw Material Validation

Identification of the crude drug or drugs

(i) Pharmacognostical identification

(ii) Botanical taxonomy

(iii) Chemical identity/chemical tests

(iv) Analytical data such as Ash values, solubility, Extractive values, LOD(%), acid values, saponification values.

(v) Identification of adulterants and substituents.

(vi) Determination of active constituents/clinical composition

(vii) Efficacy and toxicity testing

II. Finished Product Validation

(i) Organoleptic properties : Colour, Taste, Odour, Touch etc.

(ii) Physical characteristics : Viscosity, particle size, specific gravity refractive index etc.

(iii) Chemical characteristics : Efficacy and toxicity tests.

(iv) Biological characteristics : Efficacy and toxicity tests.

(v) Microbiological characteristics : Total count, tests for the absence of pathogenic organisms.

(vi) Stability testing : shelf-life

(vii) Storage conditions.

(viii) Packaging systems/unit.

III. Process Validation

Critical procedure parameters are to be identified for each product. Some of the critical parameters, in general are as follows :

A. For Liquid/Extractive Formulations

1. Solvent/solvent blend and compositions
2. Ratio of crude drug to solvent
3. Temperature
4. Length of time of Extraction
5. Method of collection of Extractives
6. Method of concentration
7. Light sensitivity during processing
8. Storage conditions, precautions during processing

B. For Solid Dosage Formulations (powders, pills, capsule, tablets)

1. Particle size and distribution of drug.
2. Blending order and time of blending
3. Granulating fluid, breeder concentration, granulating time.
4. Drying temperature and time.
5. Moisture content
6. Tablet hardness

7. Tablet characters such as disintegration, friability etc.
8. Tablet weight and thickness control.
9. Spray rate of film coating solution.
10. Core : Coat (polymers) ratio.

C. Semi-Solid Formulations

1. Solvent blend composition
2. Extraction process parameters such as amount of solvent, temperature, length of time, method of collection of extractives etc.
3. Method of concentration
4. Semi-solid blending time
5. Blend homogeneity
6. Viscosity/rheological character
7. Light sensitivity, storage and other precautions during processing.

Conclusion

Validation is a tool for total quality management and ensures always products of best quality and hence needs to be introduced into Ayurvedic science.

CHAPTER 20

X-RAY SPECTROSCOPY

Introduction

Using visible light, it will never be possible to see atoms under even the most powerful of microscopes. In order for an object to e seen, its size needs to be at least half the wavelength of the light being used to see it. But the wavelength of visible light, though small, is much bigger than an atom, making it invisible. In order to see molecules it is necessary to use a form of electromagnetic radiation with a wave length on order of bond lengths such as X-rays, have a wavelength short enough that they can be used to see atoms.

X-ray spectroscopy is simpler to interpret than other optical spectroscopy because X-ray temperature atoms are highly ionized (most of the electrons have been taken away from atoms) leaving only a few electrons for nucleus. This makes theoretical calculations much easier. Thus it is much easier to relate the strength of X-ray lines to be abundances of various elements.

A more important reason for developing X-ray spectroscopy is that there are many classes of astronomical objects that contain high temperature gases (at millions of "K"). At that, their energies are radiated as X-ray than at other wavelength ranges.

X-ray spectroscopy is based upon measurement of emission, absorption, scattering, fluorescence and diffraction of electromagnetic radiation. X-ray fluorescence and X-ray absorption methods are widely used for the qualitative and quantitative determination of all elements in the periodic table having atomic numbers greater than that of sodium. With spectral emission, elements with atomic numbers in the range of 5-10 can also be determined.

X-Ray Absorption

A beam of X-rays is allowed to pass through the sample and the attenuation or fraction of X-ray photons absorbed is considered to be a measure of the concentration of the absorbing substance. The differing absorption of the X-rays by different materials is the basis of this method. Major discontinuities in the absorption of X-rays by an element occur when the energy of the X-rays become sufficient to knock an electron out of an inner level of an atom. This method is useful in elemental analysis and thickness measurements.

X-Ray Fluorescence

When an atom is excited by the removal of an electron from an inner energy level, it may return to its normal state by transferring an electron from some outer level to the vacant inner level. The energy of this transition appears as X-rays, X-rays are generated within the sample. Their wavelengths are characteristic of the element and their intensities are proportional to the number of excited atoms.

This method is useful for both qualitative and quantitative analysis and this method is non destructive and frequency requires very little sample preparation before analysis can be carried out.

X-Ray Diffraction

This is another method of using X-rays in analytical work. Diffraction of X-rays from the planes of a crystal forms a basis of this method. This method depends on the wave character of the X-rays and the regular spacing of planes in a crystal. So this method is used to identify the crystal structures of various solic compounds.

Fundamental Principles

X-rays are short wavelength electromagnetic radiations produced by the deceleration of high-energy electrons or by electronic transmission of electrons in the inner orbitals of atoms. The wavelengths range of X-rays is from about 10^{-5} A^0 to 100 A^0.

Conventional X-ray spectroscopy is however largely contained to the region of about 0.1 A^0 to 25 A^0.

($1\ A^0 = 0.1\ nm = 10^{-10}\ m$)

For analytical purposes, the range of 0.7 A^0 to 2.0 A^0 is the most useful region.

A. Emission of X-rays

For analytical purposes X-rays are obtained in 3 ways :

1. By bombardment of a metal target with a beam of high energy electrons.
2. By exposure of a substance to a primary beam of X-rays in order to generate a secondary beam of X-ray fluorescence.
3. By use of radioactive source whose decay process results in X-ray emission.

1. (A) Continuous Spectra from Electron Beam Sources

The most common source of X-rays is the Coolidge tube, which consists of a heated cathode and a massive water cooled anode (target). In this, electrons produced at a heated cathode are accelerated towards a metal anode by a potential as great as 100 KV. Upon collison, part of the energy of the electron beam is converted to X-rays. Under some conditions only, a continuous spectrum is obtained, while under other conditions a, line spectrum is obtained which is super-imposed upon the continuous.

The continuous X-rays spectrum is characterised by a well defined, short wavelength limit (l_0), which depends upon the accelerating voltage (V), but not on the target material.

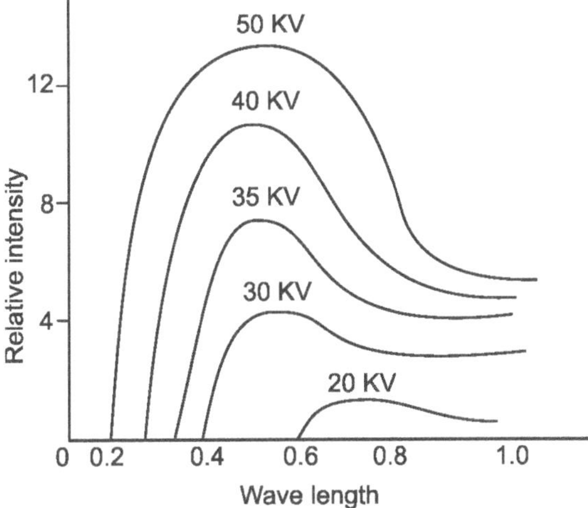

The conctinuous radiation from an electron beam source results from collisions between the electrons of the beam and the atoms of the target material. At each collision, the electron is decelerated and a photon of X-ray energy is produced. The energy of photon is equal to the difference in kinetic energies of the electron before and after the collision.

Generally the electrons in a beam are decelerated in a series of collisions, the resulting loss of kinetic energy differs from collision to collision. Thus the energies of the emitted X-ray photons vary continuously over a considerable range.

The maximum photon energy generated corresponds to the instantaneous deceleration of the electron to zero kinetic energy in a single collision.

$$hv_0 = \frac{hc}{\lambda_0} = V_e$$

V = accelerating voltage

e = charge on the electron

V_e = Kinetic energy of all electrons in beam

λ_0 = Frequency of the limiting radiation

c = Velocity of light

h = Plank's constant

V_0 = Maximum frequency of radiation at voltage V.

This equation is known as Dvane Hunt law. Upon substituting numerical values for the constants and rearranging the equation becomes

$\lambda_0 = 12{,}398/V$ [l_0 in A^0, V in volts]

(B) Discontinuous (Line) spectra from Electron Beam sources

Bombardment of a molybdenum target produces intense emission lines at about 0.63 A^0 and 0.7 A^0. An additional simple series of lines in the range of 4 A^0 to 6 A^0 is also found if spectrum of Molybdenum is examined at longer wavelengths.

The emission behaviour of Molybdenum is typical of all elements having atomic numbers larger than 23. The shorter wavelength region is called K-series and other is L-series. Elements with atomic numbers smaller than 23 produce only a K-series.

X-ray line spectrum consists of a few sharp and intense lines superimposed on a polychromatic background called "White radiation". The sharp spectral lines comprise the characteristic radiation of the target material. These lines are produced due to electron transitions which are resulted due to the complete ejection of electrons of the target atom by the incident electron beam.

X-ray line spectra result from electronic transitions that involve the innermost atomic orbitals. The short wavelength K series is produced when the high energy electrons from the cathode removes electrons from those orbitals nearest to the nucleus of the target atom.

The orbitals of principal quantum number n = 1 is called the K-shell, n = 2 in L-shell and so on. The lines in the K-series involve electronic transitions between higher energy level and the K-shell. The L-series of lines result when an electron is lost from the 2nd principal quantum level, either as consequence of ejection by an electron from the cathode or from the transition of an L-electron to the K-level that accompanies the production of a quantum of K-radiation.

The energy difference between the L and K-levels is larger than that between the M and L levels, because energy scale is logarithmic. The K-lines therefore appear at shorter wavelength. The energy differences between the transitions labelled a_1 and a_2 and those between β_1 and β_2 are so small that only a single line is observed even in highest resolution spectrometer.

The difference in energies between the levels increases regularly as the atomic number increases.

So the important characteristic of X-ray line spectrum is that the minimum acceleration voltage required for excitation of the lines of each element increases as the atomic number increases. This is due to increasing charge on the nucleus.

Because X-ray line spectra arise from electronic transition of the innermost electrons only, the wave-length of characteristic lines are independent of chemical combination in all elements, except those having the lowest atomic weights.

2. Fluorescence of X-Rays

The wavelength of fluorescent lines are always greater than the wavelength of the corresponding absorption edge. The absorption of X-rays produces electronically excited ions which return to their ground state by transitions involving electrons from higher energy levels. Thus an excited ion with a vacant k-shell is produced when the atom absorbs radiation of wavelength shorter than 0.14 A^0. The ion returns to its ground state after short interval via a series of transitions characterised by the emission of X-radiation (fluorescence) of wavelength that are identical to those that result from excitation produced by electron bombardment.

3. Radio Active Sources

Radiations in the X-ray are emitted from some radioactive elements by gamma radiation, which involves internuclear energy levels and so is not truly X-radiation. Electron capture (or) K-capture also produces x-radiation. Electron capture (or) K-capture also produces x-radiation. This process involves capture of a K-electron by the nucleus and formation of an element of the next lower atomic number. As a result of k-capute, electronic transitions to the vacated orbital occur, and the X-ray line spectrum of the newly formed element is observed. This process lowers the atomic number by one unit and leaves a vacancy in the K-shell. Hence true X-rays of the next lower element result. Without any significant continuous radiation, the half-lives of K-capture processes range from a few minutes to several thousands of years.

Absorption of X-rays

The absorption of X-rays means that the electrons of the atoms constituting the matter absorb energy from these rays and get excited. Then the excited electrons emit secondary radiation characteristic of those atoms.

When a narrow beam of X-rays is passed through a thin layer of matter, its intensity of power is generally diminished as a consequence of absorption and scattering. The effect of scattering for all but the hightest elements is ordinarily small and can be neglected in those wavelength regions where appreciable absorption occurs. The absorption spectrum of an element is very simple and consists of few broad, well defined absorption peaks.

The wavelengths of the peaks are characteristic of the element and do not depend largely on the chemical state of the element. The degree of absorption depends upon the nature and amount of absorbing material.

The appearance of sharp discontinuities known as absorption edges, at wavelengths immediately beyond absorption maxima are characteristic of X-ray absorption spectra.

Absorption of an X-ray quantum causes the ejection of one of the most innermost electrons from an atom and an excited ion is produced. In this process the entire energy of the radiation is partitioned between the K.E. of the photo electron and P.E. of the excited ion. The chances of absorption are highest, when the energy needed to remove the electron just to the periphery of the atom approaches zero (i.e., KE of ejected electron).

The absorption of X-rays follows the Beer's law

$$I = I_0 \, e^{mlp}$$

I_0 = Incident intensity of X-rays

I = Intensity after passing through the absorbing sample

L = Thickness of material (cm)

μ = Mass absorption co-efficient (cm^2/g)

ρ = The density of the absorbing material g/cm^3.

μ is also called linear absorption co-efficient, It represents the fraction of energy absorbed per cm. It is nearly independent of the physical and chemical nature of the element.

However, it decreases rapidly with decreasing wavelength of the X-rays according to this following relationship.

$$\mu = \frac{CN}{A} Z^4 A^3$$

C = Proportionality constant

N = Avogadro's number

A = atomic weight of absorbing element

λ = wavelength of X-ray radiation

If mass absorption co-efficient are plotted against wavelength of X-rays, the curves obtained are not smooth but show a series of discontinuities known as absorption edges which occur at definite wavelength for each element. At these wavelengths the energy of X-ray beam is sufficient to cause ejection of electrons from the lower atomic orbital and the mass absorption co-efficient therefore rises sharply.

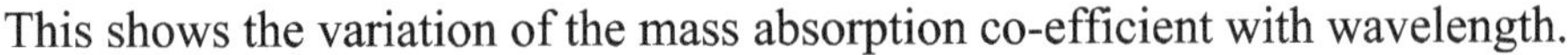

This shows the variation of the mass absorption co-efficient with wavelength.

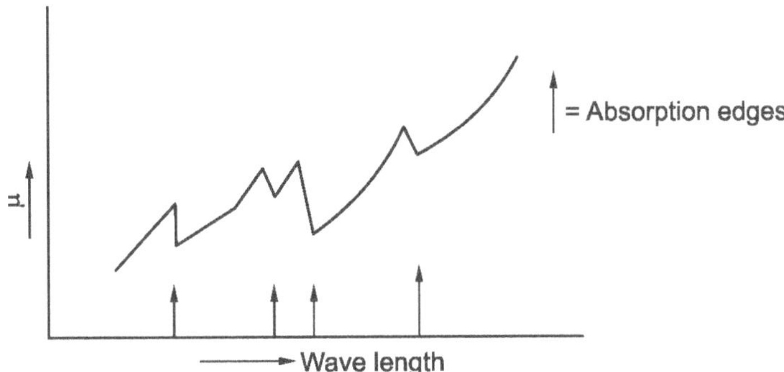

From this we know that the extent of absorption by a given element depends upon the number of atoms of that element in the path of X-rays but not on the physical (or) chemical state of that element.

There are 2 principal types of X-ray Absorption :

(a) **Photo electric X-ray absorption:** Where all the energy of the incident X-ray quantum is transferred into kinetic energy of the photoelectron, resulting in characteristic X-rays.

(b) **Scattering X-ray absorption:** whereby the incident X-ray intensity decreases because of scattering.

The linear absorption co-efficient for an element is equal to the sum of the photo electric absorption (T) and the scattering co-efficient σ. The t predominates except for low values of atomic number and high values of wavelengths.

Diffraction of X-Rays

When X-rays are scattered by the ordered environment in a crystal, interference (both constructive and destructive) takes place among the scattered ray because the distance between the scattering centres are of the same order of magnitude as the wavelength of the radiation, diffraction is the result.

Every crystalline substance scatters the X-rays in its own unique diffraction pattern producing a finger print of its atomic and molecular structure.

The conditions for diffraction are governed by Bragg's law and the diffracted beams are often referred to as reflections.

When an X-ray beam strikes a crystal surface at som angle θ, a protion is scattered by the layer of atoms at the surface. The unscattered portion of the beam penetrates the second layer of atoms where again a fraction is scattered, and the remainder passes on to the third layer.

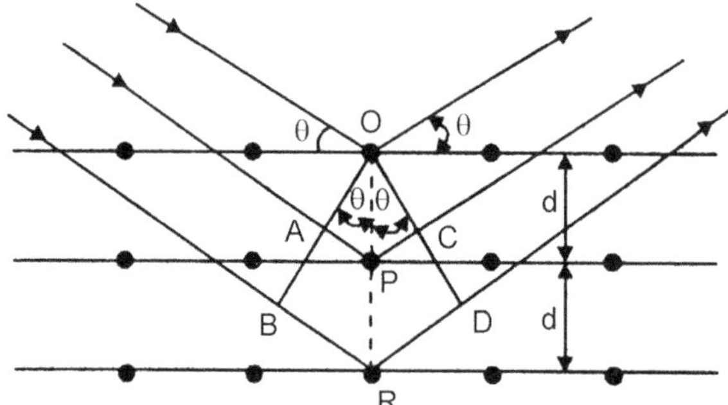

The cumulative effect of this scattering from the regularly spaced centres of the crystal is diffraction of the beam in much the same way as visible radiation is diffracted by a reflection grating.

The requirements for X-ray diffraction are :

1. The spacing between layers of atoms must be roughly the same as the wavelength of the radiation and
2. The scattering centres must be spatially distributed in a highly regular way.

W.L. Bragg treated the diffraction of X-rays by crystals. Here, a narrow beam of radiation strikes the crystal surface at angle q, scattering occurs as a consequence of interaction of the radiation with atoms located at O.P. and R. If the distance

$$AP + PC = n\lambda$$

where n = an integer

The scattered radiation will be in phase at OCP, and the crystal will appear to reflect the X-radiation.

But

$AP = PC = d \sin \theta$

d = the interplanar distance of the crystal.

Thus we may write the equation for constructive interferences of the beam at angle θ as

$$n\lambda = 2d \sin\theta$$

This equation is known as Bragg's equation.

Note : X-rays appear to be reflected from the crystal if the angle of incidence satisfies the condition that

$$\text{Sin}\theta = \frac{n\lambda}{2d}$$

At all other angles, distructive interferences occur.

Instrumentation

X-ray absorption, X-ray emission (or) fluorescence and X-ray diffraction find application in analytical chemistry. Only optical system varies in each case although component parts of the equipment are same.

The main components are :

1. Production of X-rays (source)
2. Collimator
3. Monochromator
   (a) Filter
   (b) Crystal monochromator
4. Detectors
5. Read out devices

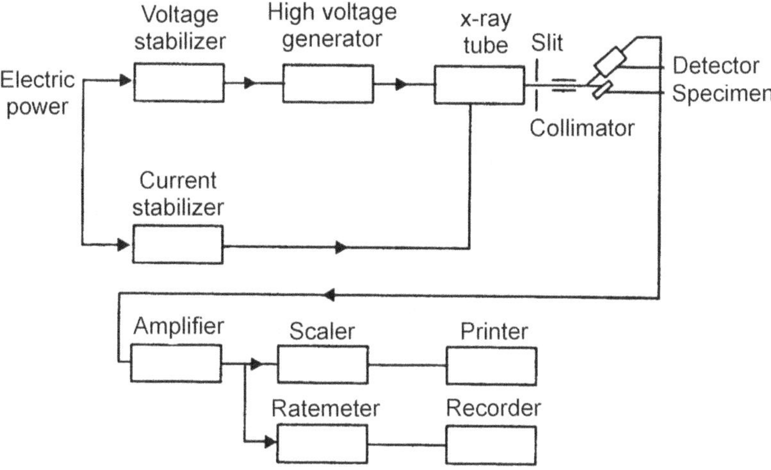

Schematic Representation of X-ray spectroscopy

1. Production of X-Rays (Sources)

X-rays are generated with high velocity electrons impinges on a metal target. Approximately, 1 percent of the total energy of the electron beam is converted into X-radiation, the remainder being dissipated as heat.

Three types of X-ray sources are encountered in X-ray instruments such as : tubes, radio-isotopes and secondary fluorescent sources.

(a) ***Coolidge tube*****:** The most common source of X-rays for analyte work is the X-ray tube (or) Coolidge tube. It is a highly evacuated tube which is available in variety of shapes and forms. This tube is mounted with a tungsten filament catode and a massive anode, which is constructed of tungsten, copper, molybdenum, chromium, silver, nickel, cobalt or iron. The anode generally consists of a heavy block of copper with a metal target plated on or embedded in the surface of the copper. Separate circuits are used to heat the filament, due to this electrons emitted by the cathode are accelerated through a high-voltage field between the target and cathode. The heater circuit provides the means for controlling the intensity of the emitted X-rays while the accelerating potential determines their energy, or wavelength.

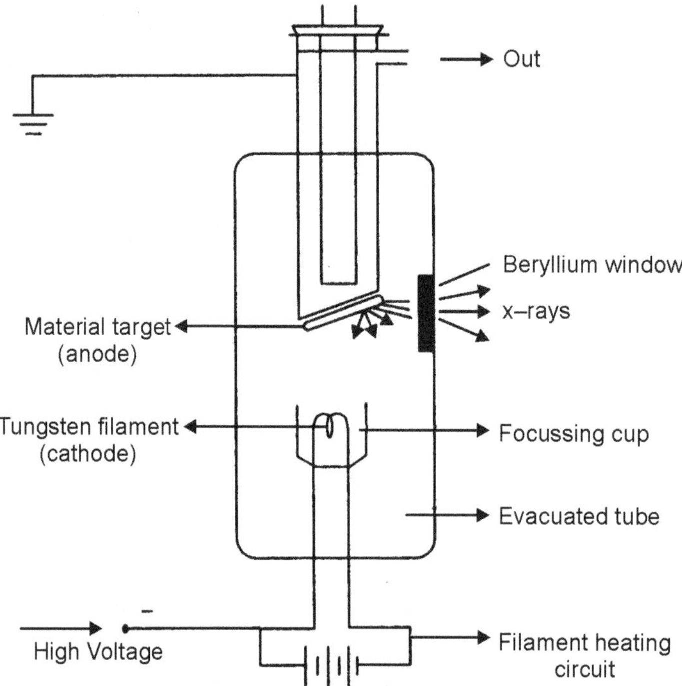

Schematic Diagram of Coolidge Tube

In Coolidge tube, which is generally self-rectifying a high voltage are source is connected directly to the cathode in order to provide accelerating potential.

The X-ray spectrum resulting from electron bombardment consists of a broad band of continuous wave lengths and a number of sharp characteristic spectralo lines. The wavelength distribution in continuum depends upon the atomic number of the target element and the applied voltage. The voltage required for the characteristic lines of each series increases as the atomic number increases.

X-ray tubes are operated at voltages upto 60 KV. This voltage is quite sufficient in exciting effectively the K-series spectra of all elements upto atomic number 50 and all L-series lines for all higher atomic number elements.

The target is viewed from a very small angle above the surface. If the focal spot is a narrow ribbon, the sources appears to be very small when viewed from the end, which leads to the sharper definition demanded in diffraction studies.

For Fluorescence work the focus is much larger, about 5 × 10 mm, and is viewed at a larger angle (20°).

On striking the target, the electrons transfer their energy to its metallic surface which then gives off X-ray radiations.

Generally, the target gets very hot in these condition which is used due to collisions of high-energy electrons. This problem can be overcome to some extent by cooling the tube with water and is sometimes rotated when a very intense X-ray beam is generated i.e. rotate the target at high speed so that the production of localized heating is reduced.

Schematic Diagram of Coolidge Tube

The choice of a target material depends upon the sample to be examined. The rule is that one should select the target material whose atomic number is greater than that of elements being examined. The choice of target material also depends on the energy of X-rays emitted by the target material which should be greater than that required to excite the elements being irradiated.

Advantage

It permits the production of X-rays of intensity much greater than that obtainable from stationary target.

Disadvantage

There is lack of focussing of the electrons so that whole surface becomes a source of X-rays.

(b) *Radio-isotopes*: A variety of radioactive substances have been used as source in X-ray fluorescence and absorption methods. Generally, the radio-isotope is encapsulated to prevent contamination of the laboratory and shielded to absorb radiation in all but certain directions.

Many of the best radioactive sources provide simple line spectra, others produce a continuum. Because of the shape of X-ray absorption curves, a given radio-isotope will be suitable for excitation of fluorescence or for absorption studies for a range of elements.

For e.g.: a source producing a line in the region between 0.3 and 0.47 A^0 is suitable for fluorescence or absorption studies involving the K absorption edge for silver, Sensitivity imoproves as the wavelength of the source line approaches the absorption edge.

(c) *Secondary Fluorescent Sources*: In some applications the fluorescence spectrum of an element that has bee excited by radiation from an X-ray tube serves as a source for absorption of fluorescence studies. This arrangement has the advantage of eliminating the continuum emitted by a primary source. For example : An X-ray tube with tungsten target could be used to excite the K_a and K_b lines of molybdenum.

2. Collimators

Radiation from an X-ray tube is collimated either by a series of closely spaced, parallel metal plates or by a bundle of tubes, 0.5 mm or smaller in diatmeter. The X-rays produced by the target material are randomly directed. They form a hemisphere with a target at the center. In order to get a narrow beam of X-rays generated by the target material are allowed to pass through a collimator which consists of two sets of closely packed metal plates separated by a small gap. The collimator absorbs all the X-rays except the narrow beam of X-rays that pass between the gap.

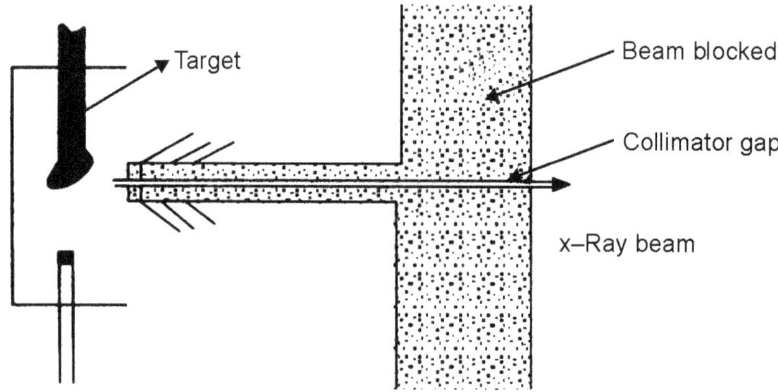

A Scheme for achieving a Narrow Beam of X-Rays

In a fluorescence spectrometer, one collimator is placed between the specimen and the analyser crystal to limit the divergence of the rays that reach the crystal. The second collimator, usually coarser is placed between the analyser crystal and the detector.

It is particularly useful at very low reflection angles for preventing radiation that has not been reflected by the crystal from reaching the detector.

Increased resolution is obtained by decreasing the separation between the metal plates of the collimator or by increasing the length of the unit, but this is achieved at the expense of diminished intensity.

3. Monochromator

For monochromatization of X-rays, two methods are available such as :-

(a) Filter

(b) Crystal monochromator

(a) *Filter*: The X-ray beam may be partly monochromatized by the insertion of the suitable filter.

A filter is a window of material that absorbs undersirable radiation but allows the radiation of request wavelength to pass

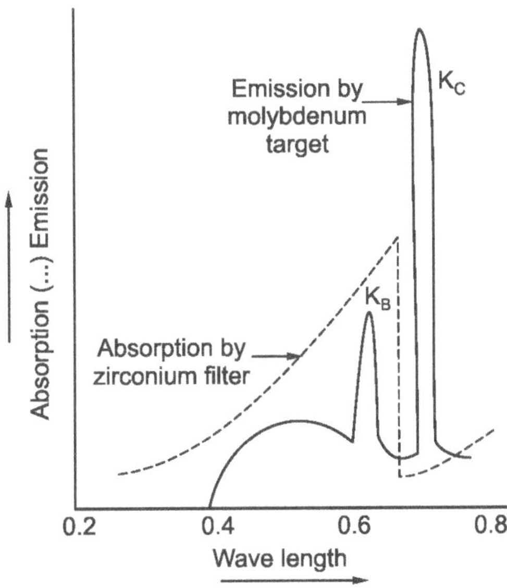

When the wavelength of two spectral lines are nearly the same and there is an element with an absorption edge at a wavelength between the lines, the element may be used as a filter to reduce the intensity of the line with the shorter wavelength.

This figure illustrates a common technique for producing a relatively monochromatic beam by use of a filter. Here the K_a line and most of the continuum emitted from a molybdenum target is removed by a zirconium filter having a thickness of above 0.01 cm. The pure Ka line is then available for analytical purposes.

Severe other target-filter combinations of this type have been developed, each of which serves to isolate one of the intense lines of a target element.

Monochromatic radiation produced in this way is widely used in X-ray diffraction studies.

Disadvantages

The choice of wavelengths available by this technique is limited by the relatively small number of target-filter combinations that are available.

Filtering the continuum from an X-ray tube is also feasible with thin strips of metal.

Glass filters are used for visible radiation, relatively broad bands are transmitted with a significant attenuation of the desired wavelengths.

(b) *Crystal Monochromator*: The monochromator consists of a pair of beam collimators, which serve the same purpose as the slits, and a dispersing element.

The dispersing element is a single crystal mounted on a goniometer or rotatable that permits variation and precise determination of the angle θ between the crystal face and the collimated incident beam.

A crystal monochromator is made up of a suitable crystalline material positioned in the X-ray beam so that the angle of the reflecting planes satisfies the Bragg's equation ($n\lambda = 2d \sin \theta$) for the required wavelength. i.e. the radiation emerges from the monochromator at an angle that is twice the angle of incidence θ. In other words, analysing crystals must have $2d$ spacing values without exceeding the maximum 2θ angle. [The beam is split up by the crystalline material into the component wavelength in the same way as a prism splits up the white light into a rainbow such a crystalline substance is known as analysing crystal.

In order to produce a spectrum it is necessary that the exit beam collimator and the detector be mounted on a second table that rotates at twice the rate of the first, i.e. the crystal rotates through an angle 2 θ. Clearly the interplanar spacing d for the crystal must be known precisely.

Crystal monochromators are of two types

(i) Flat crystal monochromator

(ii) Curved crystal monochromator

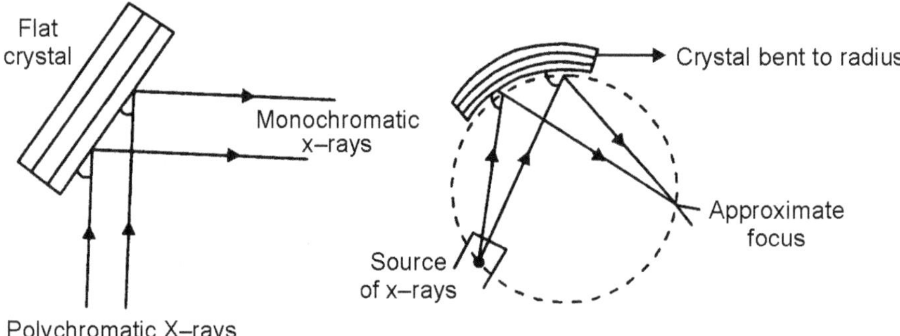

Flat Crystal Monochromator

Curved crystal Monochromator

The loss of intensity is high in flat crystal monochromator because as much as 99% of the radiation is sufficiently divergent to be absorbed in the collimators. Increased intensities by as much as a factor of ten, have been realized by using a curved crystal monochromator. The curved crystal not only acts to diffract but also to focus the divergent beam from the source on the exit collimator.

Most analytically important X-ray lines lie in the region between 0.1 and 10.A^0. No single crystal satisfactorily disperses radiation over this entire range. As a consequence an X-ray monochromator must be provided with atleast two (and preferably more) interchangeable crystals.

4. Detectors

The X-ray intensities can be measured by detectors (or) X-ray transducers.

The detection and determination of the relative intensity of X-radiation can be accomplished in three different ways:

(a) By the darkening of a photographic plate of film.

(b) By measuring the ion currents produced when the beam is absorbed by a gas and

(c) By measurement of the visible radiation produced when the beam is allowed to strike a suitable surface.

There are 3 types of detectors which have been used in X-ray absorption and emission analysis.

(a) Photographic detectors

(b) Gas ionization detectors

(c) Scintillation detectors

(d) Semiconductor detectors

(a) ***Photographic detectors*****:** X-rays affect the photographic emission almost in the similar way as an ordinary light dose. In order to record the position and intensity of X-ray beam, a plane or cylindrical film is used. X-rays were first detected by their latent image production in photographic materials. The film after exposing to X-rays is developed. The blackening of the developed film is expressed in terms of density units D given by

$$D = \log \frac{I_0}{I}$$

I_0 = incident intensity of X-rays

I = transmitted intensity of X-rays

D is related to the total X-ray energy that causes the blackening of the photographic film. The value of D is measured by the densitometer.

Photographic method is no longer used for quantitative purposes. This method is mainly used in diffraction studies since it reveals the entire diffraction pattern on a single film.

Limitations

- This method is time consuming and uses exposures of several hours.
- Rarely used for quantitative estimation because it involves the use of a densitometer, the operation of which can be both time consuming and subject to considerable error.

(b) ***Gas Ionization detectors*****:** When X-radiation passes through an inert gas such as argon. Xenon or krypton, interactions occur that produce a large number of positive gaseous ions and electrons for each X-ray quantum.

Gas ionization detectors are widely used for the detection and measurement of both X-radiation as well as the radiation produced by the decay of radioactive isotopes.

Gas filled (or) Gas ionization detectors are of 3 types :

- Ionization chambers
- Proportional counters
- Geiger-Muller tube counter

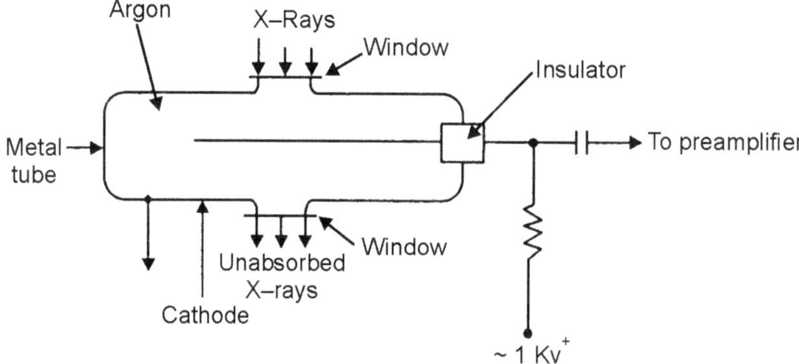

- In the Ionization chamber region between V_1 and V_2 the number of electrons reaching the anode is reasonably constant and represents the total number formed by a single photon.
- In the proportional counter region between V_3 and V_4 the number of electrons increases rapidly with applied potential.

  In the proportional counter region between V_3 and V_4 the number of electrons increases rapidly with applied potential.

  This increase is the result of secondary ion-pair production caused by collisions between the accelerated electrons and gas molecules : amplification of the ion current results.

- In the Geiger range V_5 to V_6, amplification of the electrical pulse is enormous but is limited by the positive space charge created as the faster moving electrons migrate away from the slower positive ions. Because of this effect, the number of electrons reaching the anode is independent of the type and energy of incoming radiation and is governed instead by the geometry and gas pressure of the tube.

Amplification of gas for various types of Gas ionization detectors.

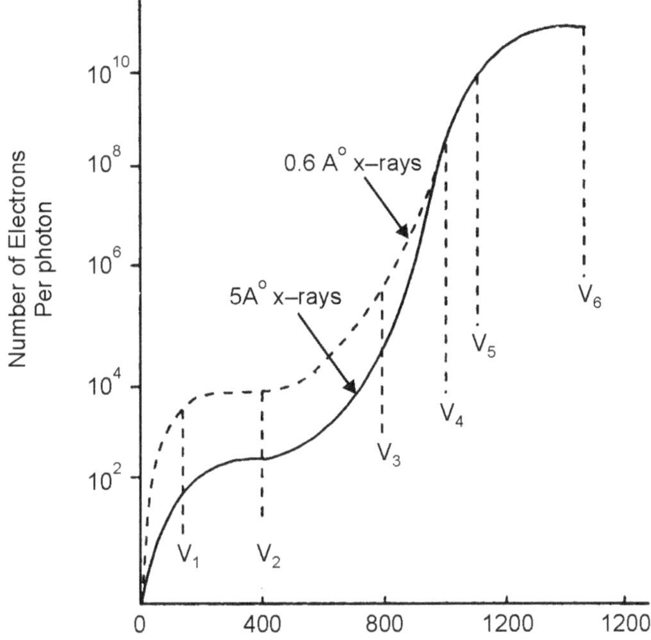

(i) *Ionization Chambers*: Since X-rays are capable of ionising a gas through which they pass, their presence can be detected by the conductivity of the gas. This can be done with an ionization chamber, a metallic container filled with dry gas. Ionization chambers are operated in the voltage range from 100-400, here the currents are small and relatively independent of applied voltage. The resulting current is measured with electrometer.

The potential across the electrodes is adjusted to minimize recombination of the ion pairs without causing amplification the the production of additional ion pairs by energetic ions that collide with neutral gas molecules.

An ionization chamber is an accurate, quick acting detector even for weak radiation. These chambers are not employed in X-ray spectrometry because of their lack of sensitivity. However, these are applied in radiochemical measurements.

(ii) *Proportional Counter*: When the electric field strength at the center electrode of an ionization chamber is increased above the saturation level, but under that of the Geiger region, the size of the output pulse from the chamber starts to increase but remains proportional to the initial ionization. A device operated in this manner is called proportional counter.

A proportion counter is filled with a heavier gas like Xenon or Krypton. Heavier gas is preferred because it is easily ionized. A proportional counter is operated in the voltage range of 800-1100 i.e. at a voltage below Geiger plate. The output pulse of a proportional counter is dependent upon the intensity of X-rays falling on proportional counter. With the proper electronic circuits, one can count X-rays of a particular energy, selectively.

The pulse produced by a photon is amplified by a factor of 500-10,000 but the number of positive ions produced is small enough so that the dead time is only about the 1 μs. In general, the pulses from a proportional counter must be amplified before being counted.

The number of electrons per pulse, which is proportional to the pulse height, produced in the proportional region, depends directly on the energy and thus the frequency of the incoming radiation.

Proportional counters are widely used in X-ray spectrometry.

Advantages

As the dead time of the proportional counter is very short (-0.2 μs), it can be used to count high rates without significant error.

A proportional counter can be made sensitive to a restricted range of X-ray frequencies with a pulse height analyser, which counts a pulse only if its amplitude falls within certain limits.

Disadvantages

The associated electronic circuit is complex and expensive. Thus the advantages of the proportional counters outweigh the extra cost.

(iii) *Geiger-Muller tube Counter (or) Geiger counter (or) GM tube*: The Geiger tube is a gas-filled transducer operated in the voltage range 800-2500 V. This potential is applied to a central wire anode surrounded by a cylindrical cathode (a glass tube that has been silvered (or) a brass cylinder). The electrodes are enclosed in a ga-tight envelope typically filled to a pressure of 80 torr of argon gas plus 20 torr of methane or ethanol or 0.08 torr of chlorine. A thin end window of mica about 2.5 cm in diameter and 2-3 mg/cm^2 thick, or a glass wall in dipping counters is the point of entry of the radiation.

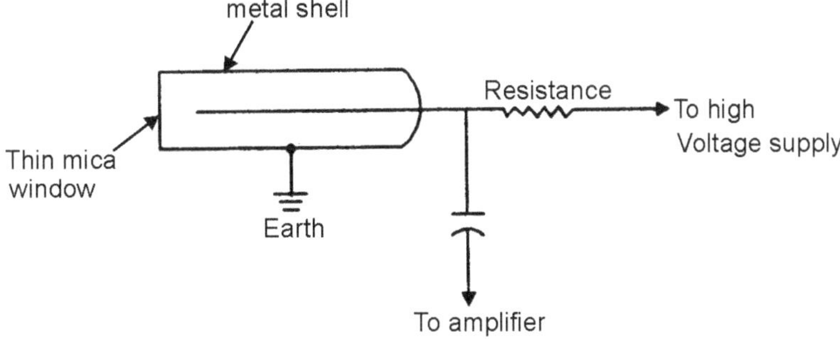

Schematic Diagram of Geiger Tube

When an X-ray enters the Geiger tube, it undergoes collision with the filling gas, resulting in the production of an ion pair : the electron produced moves towards the central anode while the positive ion moves towards the outer electrode. The mobility of the electron is quite high and under the influence of the potential gradient it soon acquires sufficient velocity to produce a new pair of ions upon collison with another atom of argon. So that the electron is accelerated by the potential gradient and causes the ionization of large number of argon atoms, resulting the production of an avalanche of electrons that are travelling towards the central anode photons, emitted when the electrons strike the anode, spread the ionization throughout the tube. These processes produce a continuous discharge, which fills the whole active volume of the counter in less than a microsecond. Each discharge builds up to a constant pulse of maximum amplitude (10 V) and 50-100 μ sec duration. These pulses are counted precisely with the aid of scalling circuits or a ratemeter with no intermediate amplification.

(c) *Scintillation Detector*: Scintillators are chemicals used to convert radiation energy into light. The most widely used scintillation detector consists of a transparent crystal of sodium iodide that has been activated by the introduction of 0.2% thallium iodide.

When an ionizing particle is absorbed in any one of several transparent scintillators, some of the energy acquired by the scintillator is emitted as a pulse of visible light or neat U.V. radiation. The light is observed by a photomultiplier tube, either directly or through an internally reflecting optic fibre. The combination of scintillator and photomultiplier tube is called a scintillation counter.

Often, the crystal is shaped as a cylinder that is 3-4 inch in each dimension. One of the plane surfaces, then, faces the cathode of a photomultiplier tube. As the incoming radiation traverses the crystal, it energy is first lost to the scintillator, this energy is subsequently released in the form of photons of fluorescence radiation. Several thousand photons with a wavelength of about 400 nm are produced by each primary particle or photon over a period of about 0.25 μs, which s the dead time. The flashes of light produced in the scintillator crystal are transmitted to the photocathode of a photomultiplier tube and are in turn converted to electrical pulses that can be amplified and counted.

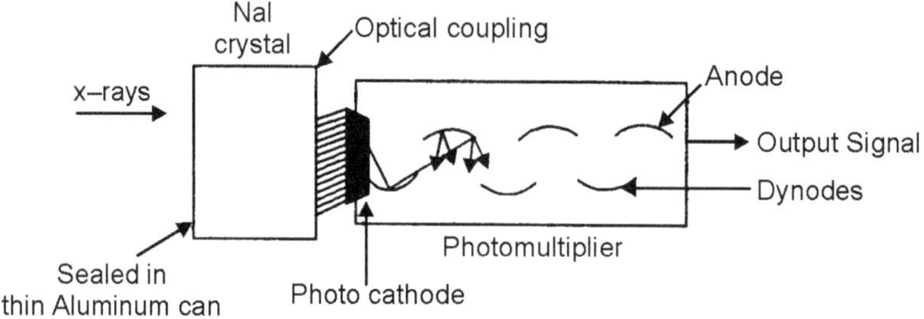

Schematic Diagram of A Scientillation Detector

An important characteristic of scintillators is that the number of photons produced in each flash is proportional to the energy of the incoming radiation. So, this counter may be used with pulse height discrimination.

The scintillation detectors is particularly useful for measuring X-rays of short wavelengths but its usefulness drops off for X-rays of longer wavelengths.

In addition to sodium iodide crystals, a number of organic scintillators like silicon, anthracene, naphthalene and P-terphenol in xylene have been used.

The conduction of electricity through a chamber operated in the Geiger region and in the proportional region is not continuous because the space charge terminates the flow of electrons to the anode. The net effect is a momentary pulse of current followed by an interval during which the tube does not conduct. Before conduction can again occur, this space charge must be dissipated by migration of cations to the walls of the chamber. During the dead time, the tube is nonconducting, response to radiation is impossible. The dead time thus represents a lower limit in the response time of the tube. The dead time of a Geiger tube is in the range from 50-200 μs.

Geiger tubes are usually filled with argon. A low concentration of an organic quenching gas, alcohol or methane, is also present to minimize the production of secondary electrons when the cations strike the chamber wall. The life time of a tube is limited to some $10^8 – 10^9$ counts by which time the quencher has been depleted.

Advantages

(a) They are simple to operate.

(b) They do not require highly stabilized electronic circuit.

(c) Physical discrimination against undesirable X-rays can be achieved by selecting the appropriate counting gas mixture.

(d) The device is applicable to all types of nuclear and X-radiation. However, it lacks the large counting range of other detectors because of its, realatively long, dead time.

Disadvantage

(a) The Geiger tube is inexpensive and is relatively trouble free detectors but the Geiger tube is used for counting low rates. This is because the dead time is 200-300 microseconds, consequently the counting loss or non linear response is significant even at moderate X-ray intensities.

(b) The efficiency of a Geiger tube falls off rapidly at wavelength below 1 A^0.

(c) As the magnitude of the output pulse does not depend upon the energy of X-ray, which causes ionization, a Geiger tube cannot be used to measure the energy of the ionizing radiation.

(d) Semi Conductor Detectors

Semi conductor detectors have assumed more importance in X-radiation. These devices are sometimes called lithium drifted silicon detectors, (or) Lithium – drifted germanium detectors.

In Semiconductor detectors, the charge carriers produced by ionizing radiation are electron-hole pairs rather than ion pairs. The ionizing radiation lifts electrons into the conduction band and these electrons travel the positive electrode with high mobilities. The positive charge travels in the opposite direction by successive exchanger of electrons between neighbouring lattice sites so that the current flow is directly proportional to the incident X-ray energy.

***Lithium Drifted Silicon Detectors*:** It is a lithium drifted detector which is fashioned from a wafer of crystalline silicon. Three layers exist in the crystal, a p-type semiconducting layer that faces the X-ray source, a central intrinsic zone and an n-type layer. i.e. A surface barrier detector consists of p-n junction formed at the surface of a slice of silicon. At the junction, there is a planer region where there are no charge carriers and no electric field. This region is called the depletion region.

The outer surface of the p-type layer is coated with a thin layer of gold for electrical contact ; often it is covered with a beryllium window that is transparent to X-rays. The signal output is taken from an aluminium layer that coats the n-type silicon. This output is fed into a pre-amplifier with an amplification factor of about 10. The preamplifier is frequently a field- effect transistor that is made an interal part of the detector.

A lithium-drifted silicon detectors are prepared by drifting of (vapour-depositing) lithium ions on the surface of a p-doped silicon crystal. Upon heating to 400° – 500°C, the lithium diffuses into the crystal because this element easily loses electrons, its presence converts the P-type region to an n-type region. While still at an elevated temperature, a dc potential is applied across the crystal to cause withdrawal of the electrons from the lithium layer and holes from the p-type layer. Current across the p-n junction requires migration or drifting of litium ions into the p-layer and formation of the intrinsic layer where the lithium ions replace the holes lost by conduction. Upon cooling, this central layer has a high resistance relative to the other layers because the lithium ions in this medium are less mobile than the holes they displaced.

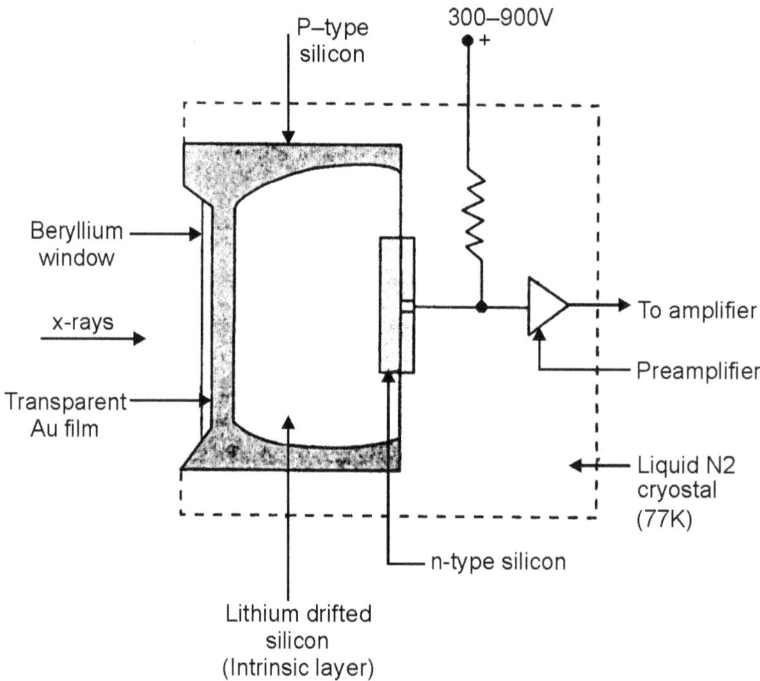

Initially, absorption of a photon results in formation of a highly energetic photoelectron, which then loses its kinetic energy by elevating several thousand electrons in the silicon to the conduction ban, a marked increase in conductivity results. When a potential is applied across the crystal, a current pulse accompanies the absorption of each photon. The size of the pulse is directly proportional to the energy of the absorbed photons.

Limitations

- The detector and preamplifier of lithium – drifted detector must be thermostated at the temperature of liquid nitrogen to decrease electronic noise to a tolerable level.
- These detectors had be to cooled at all times because at room temperature, the lithium atoms would diffuse throughout the silicon thereby degrading the performance of the detector. This problem is overcome by modern detectors which need cooling only during their use.
- Lithium drifted Germanium Detector

The lithium drifted germanium detector consists of a virtually windowless crystal, a vacuum crystal maintained by cryosorption pumping, a liquid nitrogen Dewar and a preamplifier.

The preparation is similar to lithium drifted silicon detector. In this, silicon is replaced by Germanium. The drifting process is discontinued while a layer of p-type germanium still remains. When ionizing radiation enters the intrinsic layer, electron hole pairs are created, and the charge produced is rapidly collected under the influence of bias voltage. The completed detectors must be maintained at liquid nitrogen temp (77 k) at all times to prevent precipitation of lithium.

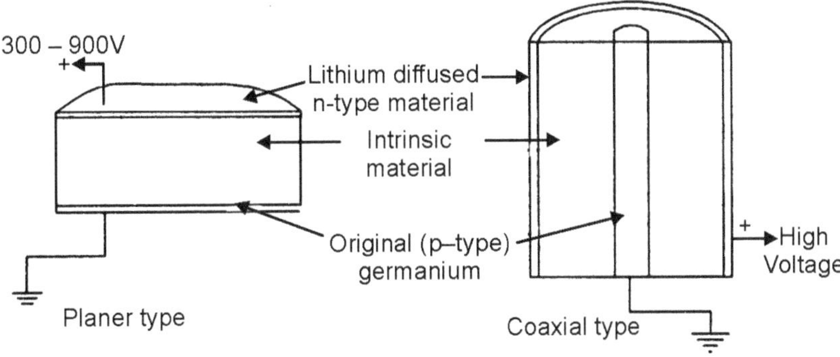

Lithium Drifted Germanium Detectors

Silicon detectors are preferred for X-rays longer than 0.3 A^0. Due to its low atomic number silicon cannot absorb the X-rays effectively in the depth of crystals available where as Germanium detectors are preferred for shorter wave lengths.

The lithium drifted silicon detectors and intrinsic germanium detectors have increased the popularity of energy-dispersive analysis. In energy-dispersive analysis of X-ray, the sample is irradiated with X-rays, gamma radiation from a radionuclide source or ions to produce secondary X-radiation characteristic of the elements present in the sample. These characteristic X-rays pass through a hollow shield onto a semiconductor detector. The purpose of the shield is onto to prevent any X-rays from hitting the edges of the detector where they may not be completely absorbed. The output of the detector is amplified by a preamplifier.

5. Signal Processors (or) Read out Devices

The signal from the preamplifier of an X-ray spectrometer is fed into a linear fast-response amplifier whose gain can be varied by a factor upto 10,000. The result is voltage pulses as large as 10V.

Pulse Height Selectors: All modern X-ray spectrometers are equipped with discriminators that reject pulses of about 0.5V or less. In this way, detector and amplifier noise is reduced significantly. Pulse height selectors are electronic circuits that reject not only pulses with heights below some predetermined minimum level but also those above a present maximum level. i.e. they remove all pulses except those that within a limited channel or window of pulse heights.

Whenever the amplitude of the pulse is proportional to the energy dissipation in the detector, the measurement of pulse height is a useful tool for energy discrimination. Current pulses are first fed into a linear amplifier of sufficient gain to produce voltage output pulses in the amplitude range of 0-100V. These amplified pulses are then sorted into groups according to their pulse heights. Pulsdes then sorted into groups according to their pulse heights. Pulses then sorted into groups according to their pulse heights. Pulses associated with particular energy must be amplified sufficiently so that their amplitudes exceed the discriminator setting. In practice this is accomplished by adjusting a combination of the gain of the amplifier and the dc voltage applied to the detector.

Pulse Height Analysers: Pulse height analysers consist of one or more pulse height selectors that are configured in such a way as to provide energy spectra. A single-channel analyzer typically has a voltage range of perhaps 10V or more with a window of 0.1 – 0.5 V. This second discriminator called the window width, the channel width, or the acceptance slit. The window can be manually or automatically adjusted to scan the entire voltage, range, thus providing data for an energy dispersion spectrum. Now all pulses above the sum of the baseline and window setting are also rejected. Only pulses with an amplitude within the confines of these settings, pass onto the counting stages.

Multi-channel analyser typically contain upto a few thousand separate channels, each of which acts as a single channel that corresponds to a different voltage window. The signal from each channel if then accumulated in a memory location of the analyser corresponding to the energy of the channel thus permitting simultaneous counting and recording of an entire spectrum.

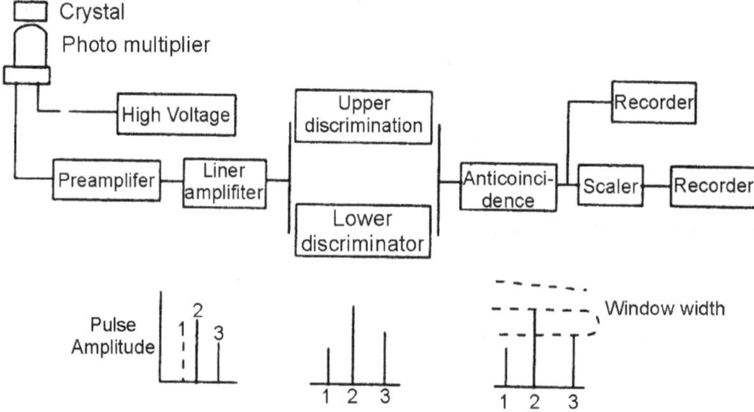

Block Diagram of Single Channel Pulse Height Analyser

With circuits for pulse height discrimination, it is possible to discriminate electronically against unwanted wavelength of different elements. Discrimination between elements eight to ten atomic numbers apart is possible with a scintillation detector. A proportional detector can discriminate between elements four to six atomic numbers apart because of its narrower pulse amplitude distribution. With semiconductor detectors, even better resolution is possible one or two atomic numbers apart.

For precise quantitative measurements, simple energy dispersion measurement, even with semiconductor detectors are not sufficient. So we must use wavelength dispersion from reflecting crystals, an energy dispersion detector, and pulse height discrimination. The pulse height analyser is used to pass either line of super imposed spectral lines, serving in-effect as, secondary monochromator. It is particularly useful for rejecting higher order scattered radiation from elements of higher atomic number when determining the elements of lower atomic number. Modern pulse height analysers make finer non-dispersive analyser with ever improving resolution.

***Scalers and Counters*:** To obtain convenient counting rates, the output from an X-ray transducer is sometimes scaled – i.e. the number of pulses is reduced by dividing by some multiple of ten.

The X-ray spectrometer-absorptionomer consists of a high intensity X-ray tube, a sample chamber, a goniometer with collimator and analyser crystal and a detector (which is also associated with power supply, scaler-ratemeter, linear amplifier, single channel pulse amplitude discriminator and stip chart recorder).

For emission analysis, the absorption cell is replaced by a parallel plate collimator.

In monochromatic absorptiometry, the secondary emitter is an element that has a strong characteristic spectral line of the desired wavelength.

In absorption edge technique, a secondary emitter is selected that has strong spectral lines on both sides of the absorption edge.

In polychromatic absorptiometry, secondary emitter is removed and output of the X-ray tube is directly passed through a sample to the detector.

***Fundamental Methods and their Applications of X-Ray Spectroscopy*:** The methods (X-ray absorption, X-ray emission and X-ray diffraction) and their applications are simpler to interpret because X-ray temperature atoms are highly ionised (most of the electrons have been taken away from atoms) leaving only a few electrons for nucleus. This makes theoretical calculations much easier, the principle easier to relate the strength of X-ray line to the abundances of various elements.

A more important reason for developing X-ray spectrometery is that there are many classes of astronomical objects that contain high temperature gases. At these temperatures, more of their energies are radiated as X-rays than at other wavelength ranges so it makes sense to observe them in X-rays.

1. X-Ray Absorption Methods

As an analytical tool, X-ray absorption is of great importance where the element to be determined is the sole heavy component in a material of low atomic weight. The application of X-ray absorption to analysis is more limited than that of X-ray emission or optical absorption, due to the overlapping of absorption spectra of various elements. While absorption measurements can be made relatively free of matrix effects, the required techniques are somewhat cumbersome and time consuming when compared with fluorescence. Thus most applications are confined to sample in which the effect of the matrix is minimal.

Direct absorption methods can be divided into 3 classes:

(a) ***Polychromatic Absorptiometry*:** This technique is mainly used for qualitative determination. This techinique is limited for which matrix changes but slightly from sample to sample. This is due to the fact that absorption of polychromatic radiation is not specific for any element. The utility of polychromatic X-rays depends upon their ability of distinguishing differences in ultimate composition and in thickness. The advantage of polychromatic analysis for control analysis lies in the extremely high beam intensity which is capable of allowing instantaneous observation and feed back for control purposes.

(b) ***Monochromatic Absorptiometry*:** Monochromatic X-rays provide greater flexibility as well as ease in interpretation of data.

This is mainly used for quantitative determination.

(c) ***Absorption Edge Method*:** This method is based on the large change in the mass absorption co-efficient across the absorption edge. In this method, the change in the mass absorption co-efficient of a sample at an absorption edge is used as a measure of the concentration of the element responsible for the edge. Hence this method of applying X-ray absorption makes use of critical absorption edges as means of identification and quantitative analyses.

Applications involved are:

(a) ***Quantitative analysis*:** This is based upon the simple fact that there is a large difference in the mass absorption co-efficient of an element on either side of an absorption edge. This method is known as absorption edge method. Since the absorption of an element in a sample is markedly greater at a wavelength just below one of its absorption edges than just above it, and since the location of such edges on the wavelength of the edge will serve to determine both the presence and the amount of the element.

For a sample having an element A, we can write as follows:

$$\ln\frac{I_x}{I_y}\alpha W_A M$$

I_x and I_y denote the extrapolated transmitted intensities at the absorbance edge.

M denotes the mass per unit area of the sample

W_A denotes the weight fraction of A.

The values of I_x and I_y are obtained from a plot of intensity transmitted vs wavelength.

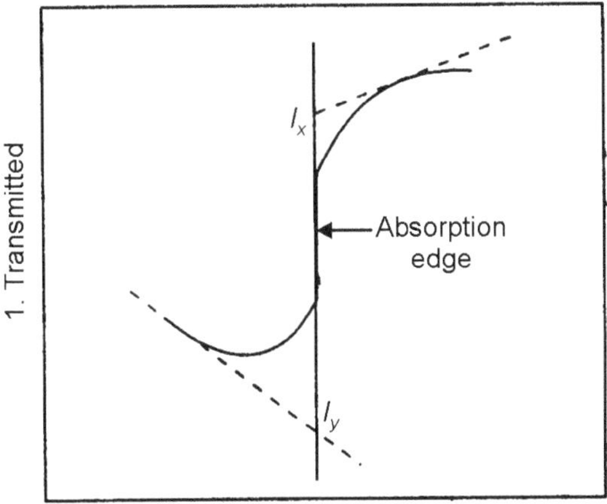

If a plot of $\ln\frac{I_x}{I_y}$ is drawn against W_AM a straight line passing through the origin will be obtained.

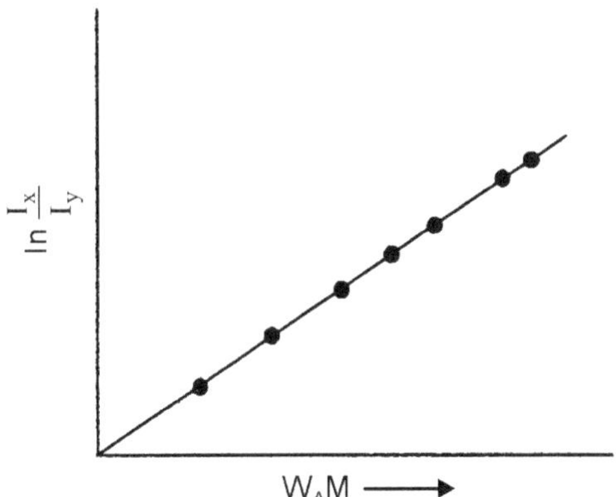

If the concentration of an unknown sample of A is to be determined, its $\ln\frac{I_x}{I_y}$ is determined by X-ray absorption method and its corresponding value of W_A can be noted.

Now consider a system having two components. At wavelengths not equal to an absorption edge, the total mass absorption co-efficient of a two component system is :

$$U \text{ total} = u_A W_A + (1 - WA)\mu B$$

$$\ln\frac{I_0}{I} = [W_A\mu_A + (1 - WA)\ \mu B]\ \rho \text{ total } l$$

This equation is relationship between

I_0 = incident intensity

I_r = transmitted intensity and

where l = thickness of the sample

ρ total is its density.

It the intensities at two wavelengths 11 and 12 are on either side of an absorption edge the formula we write is :-

$$\frac{\ln(I_0/I_1)_1}{\ln(I0/I1)_2} = \frac{W_A(\mu\mu_1 - \mu B_1) + \mu B_1}{W_A(\mu\mu_2 - \mu B_2) + \mu B_2}$$

If all samples receive the same incident intensity, it is observed that (ln $I_1/l\ I_2$] is a function of W_A so that the calibration curve can be prepared from samples of known concentration.

The error as low as 17 can be obtained and at concentrations down to 0.1 for many elements.

By this method, lead as the tetraethyl lead (TEL) in gasoline can be determined by M_0 Kα X-ray absorption. Lead absorbs more strongly than does carbon at this wavelength by a factor of about 250.

This method is subject to interference from sulphur present in gasoline. Generally, the sulphur must be determined separately.

This method has precision of ± 1 percent on samples containing as little as 2 ppm of lead.

X-ray absorption method is non destructive and is independent of chemical state of the element concerned. But its sensitivity is low. So it is useful for major constituents than for trace elements.

(b) *Qualitative Analysis*: Different elements absorb the X-rays to different degrees. This property has been widely used to detect broken bones, impurities, segregations, etc.

If a substance has more than one element and X-rays are allowed to pass through it, the photographic plate on developing shows the patches of various intensities of grey colour on it. The heavy elements absorb strongly and their presence will be revealed by the light patches on the photographic plate. On the other hand, light elements do not absorb strongly and their presence will be revealed by the dark patches on the photographic elements.

This property is widely used in industry and medicine.

1. This has been widely used to detect broken bones in surgery.
2. It is used to locate trace elements, such as barium and iodide in the body. These elements are taken by the patient. Then, their movement in the body is followed by X-ray absorption. This method helps the doctor to detect the activity of the body tissue towards barium and iodine.
3. It is used to detect blow holes or the segregation of impurities such as oxides in welds and other joints. These blow holes reveal that the weld is weak and may be breaking in use.
4. This has been widely used to measure the volume of liquids in closed vessels or pipes without opening or breaking the vessels or pipes.

2. Non-dispersive X-ray Absorption Method

In non dispersive X-ray absorptiometer a tungstem X-ray tube is employed which operates at 15-45 kV. A synchronous motor-driven chopper is kept between cell and attenuator which alternatively interrupts one half of the X-ray beam. Between the chopper and reference sample compartment, there is a variable thickness aluminium attenuator.

There are duplicate reference and sample cells upto 65 cm in length.

If liquids or gases are to be analysed, there are special arrangements for continuous flow of process streams. Both halves of X-ray beam are allowed to fall on a common phosphorus-coated photomultiplier tube which is protected from visible light by a thin metallic filter.

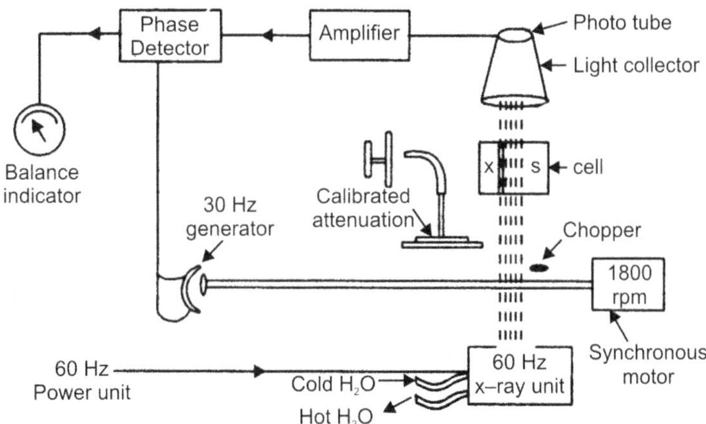

A Non-dispersive X-ray Absorptiometer

Working: A reference sample is kept in the reference cell whereas the sample to be analysed is kept in the sample cell.

Then, the adjustment is made in the alternator until the absorption in the two X-ray beams if brought into balance.

The change in thickness of aluminium required for different samples is a function of the difference in composition.

In most of the samples to be analysed, a calibration curve is prepared. Then, the unknown concentration of the sample to be analysed is obtained from the calibration curve.

Applications: This method has been widely used to determine any sample that contains one element markedly heavier than the others.

1. It has been used to determine chlorine in hydrogen plastics, and hydrocarbons.
2. It has been used to determine barium fluoride in carbon brushes and barium or lead in special glass.

X-ray absorption spectroscopy is useful for concentration from about 10 ppm to major elements. As such it is useful to speculate trace elements such as contaminants absorbed to pure minerals, soils and sediments and is also valuable tool for studying the mineralogical composition of the soil or sediment.

X-ray absorption spectroscopy results from the abosorption of a high energy X-ray by an atom in a sample. This absorption occurs at a defined energy corresponding to the binding energy of the electron in the material. The ejected electrons interact with the surrounding atoms to produce the spectrum that is observed. Occasionally, the electron can be excited into vacant band electronic states near the valence bond. As a result, distinct absorptions will result at these energies. Often these features are diagnostic of coordination and are of use for geochemistry, e.g. : This feature is diagnostic for more toxic form of chromium.

2. X-Ray Fluorescence Methods

In this method excitation is more commonly brought about by irradiation of the sample with a beam of X-rays from an X-ray tube or a radioactive source. Under these circumstances the elements in the sample are excited by absorption of the primary beam and emit their own characteristic fluorescence X-rays. This procedure is thus properly called an X-ray fluorescence or emission method.

The fluorescent emission of X-rays provides one of the most potential tools available to the analyst for the identification and measurement of heavy elements in the presence of each other and in any matrix.

The combinations of basic instrument components leads to several recognizable types of X-ray fluorescence instruments – mainly – wavelength dispersive, energy dispersive and non dispersive.

1. Wavelength Dispersive X-ray Emission Spectrometer

Wavelength dispersive instruments employ tubes as a source because of the large energy losses suffered when X-ray beam is collimated and dispersed into its component wavelength. Radioactive sources produce X-ray photons at a rate less that 10^{-4} that of an X-ray tube. The added attenuation by a monochromator would then result in a beam that was difficult or impossible to detect and measure accurately.

Wavelength dispersive instruments are of two types:

- Single channel (or) sequential
- Multichannel (or) simultaneous

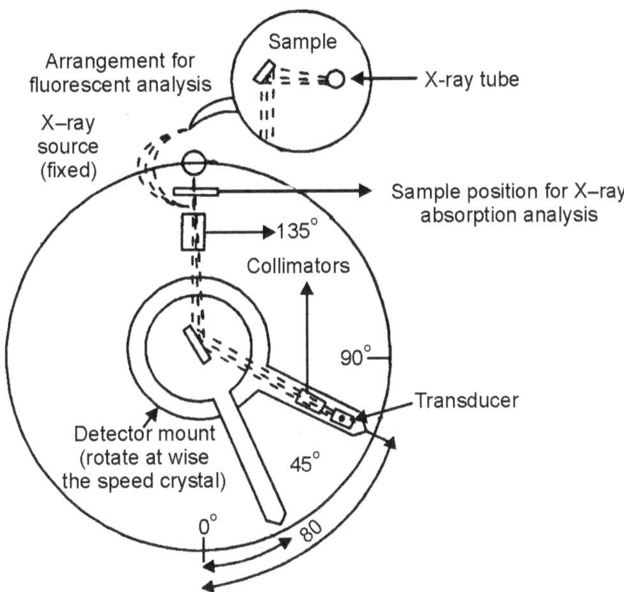

Sequential Wave length Dispersive X-Ray Emission Spectrometer

- Sequential instrument can be readily employed for X-ray fluorescence analysis. The sequential instruments are of two types:

(a) Manual and

(b) Automatic

(a) Manual instruments are entirely satisfactory for the quantitative determination of few elements. In this the quantitative determination of few elements. In this the crystal and detector (transducer) are set at the proper angles (q and 2q) and counting is continued until sufficient counts have accumulated for precise results.

(b) Automatic instruments are much more convenient for qualitative analysis, where an entire spectrum must be scanned. Here, the electric drive for the crystal and detector is sychronized, and the detector output is connected to the data acquisition system.

Most modern sequential (or) single channel spectrometers are provided with two X-ray sources, typically, one has a chromium target for longer wavelength and the other a tungsten target for shorter wavelengths. For wavelengths longer than $2A^0$, it is necessary to remove air between the source and detector by pumping or by displacement with a continuous flow of helium. Some means must also be provided for convenient interchange of dispersing crystals.

Multi channel dispersion instruments are large, expensive installations, which permit the simultaneous detection and determination of as many as 24 elements. Here, individual channels, consisting of an appropriate crystal and a detector are arranged radially around an X-ray source and sample holder. Ordinaritly, the crystals for all or most of the channels are fixed at an appropriate angle for a given analyte line : in some instruments one or more of the crystals can be moved to permit a spectral scan. Each transducer in a multichannel instrument is provided with its own amplifier, pulse height selector and counter or integrator. These instruments are ordinarily equipped with a computer for instrument control, data are ordinarily equipped with a computer for instrument control, data processing and display of analytical results. A determination of 20 or more elements can be completed in a few seconds or a few minutes.

Multi channel instruments are widely used for the determination of several components in materials of industry such as steel, other alloys, cement, ores and petroleum products.

Both multi channel and single channel instruments are euipped to handle samples in the form metals, powdered solids, evaporated films, pure liquids, or solutions.

2. Energy Dispersive Instrument

The energy dispersive spectrometer consists of a polychromatic source, which may be either an X-ray tube or a radioactive material, a sample holdr, a semiconductor detector, and the various electronic components required for energy discrimination.

An obvious advantage of this system is the simplicity, and lack of moving parts in the excitation and detection of components of the spectrometer. Furthermore, the absence of collimators and a crystal diffractor, as well as the closeness of the detector to the sample, results in a 100-fold or more increase in energy reaching the detector. The features permit the use of weaker sources such as radioactive materials or low-power X-ray tubes, which are cheaper and less likely to cause radiation damage to the sample. Their cost is $1/4^{th}$ of wavelength dispersive systems.

In a multichannel energy dispersive instrument, all of the emitted X-rays are measured. Simultaneously, increased sensitivity and improved signal-to-noise is advantageous.

The principal disadvantage of energy dispersive systems when compared with crystal spectrometers, is their lower resolution at wavelengths longer than about $1A^0$. On the other hand, at shorter wavelengths, they exhibit superior resolution.

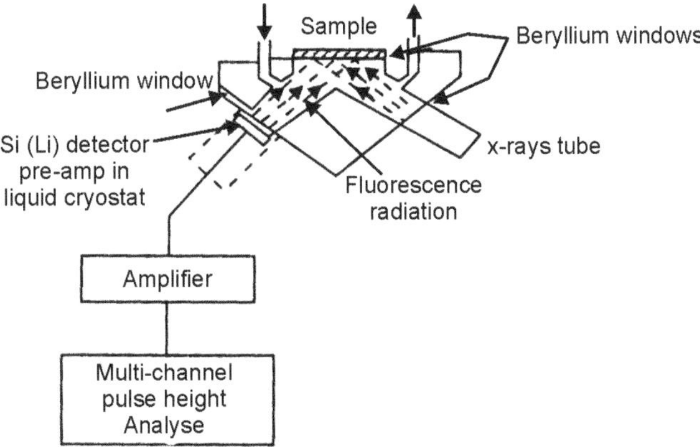

Energy dispersive X-ray fluorescence spectrometer where X-ray tubes are used for excitation of X-rays

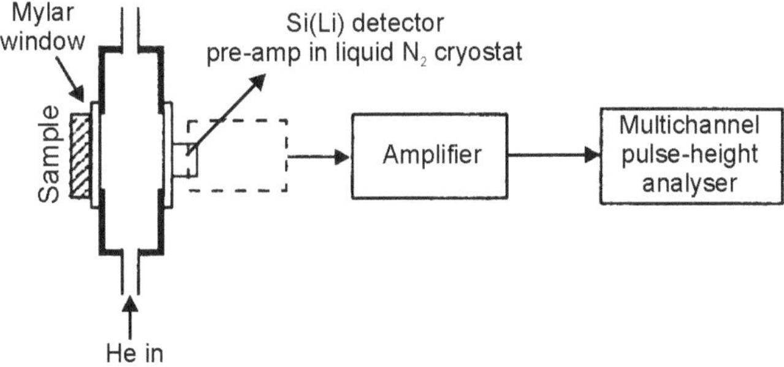

Energy dispersive X-ray fluorescence spectrometer where Radioactive substance is used for Excitation of X-rays

Non-Dispersive Instruments

Non-dispersive instruments have been employed for the routine determination of sulphur and lead in gasoline. For sulphur determination, the sample is irradiated by

X-rays produced by an iron-55 radioactive source. This radiation in turn generates a sulphur fluorescence line at 5.4 A^0. The analyte radiation then passes through a pair adjacent filters and into twin proportional counters. The absorption edge of one of the filters lies below 54 A^0 while that the other is just above it. The difference between the two signals is proportional to the sulphur content of the sample. The required time for sulphur determination by this technique is about 1 min. Relative standard deviations of about 1% are obtained for replicate measurements.

Various methods used in Applications of X-ray Fluorescence

X-ray fluorescence is one of the most widely used of all analytical methods for the qualitative identification of elements having atomic number greater than oxygen. In addition, it is often employed for semiquantitative or quantitative elemental analysis as well. In contrast to most other elemental techniques, X-ray fluorescence is non-destructive of the sample.

(a) ***Qualitative and Semiqualitative Analysis*:** Qualitative analysis by X-ray fluorescence can be illustrated with the following figure :-

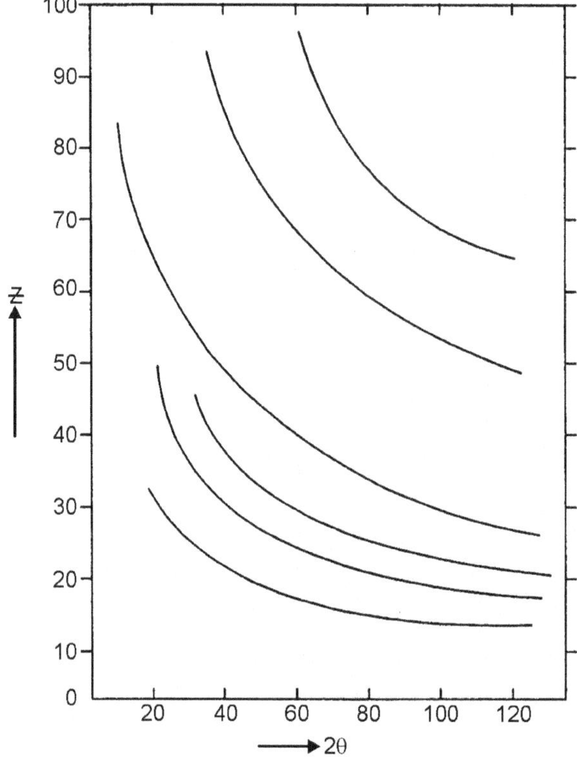

X-ray dispersion curves for a number of crystals

Here the untreated sample, which was excited by radiation from an X-ray tube, was subsequently recovered without any change. The abscissa has been plotted in terms of angle 2θ, which can be readily converted to wavelength using the equation,

$$n\lambda = 2d \sin \theta.$$

Identification of peaks can then be made by reference to tables of emittion lines of the elements. This can be done with wavelength dispersive instrument.

With an energy dispersive instrument, the spectrum is obtained when the abscissa is generally calibrated in channel number or energy in keV. Each dot represents the number of counts accumulated in one of the several hundred channels.

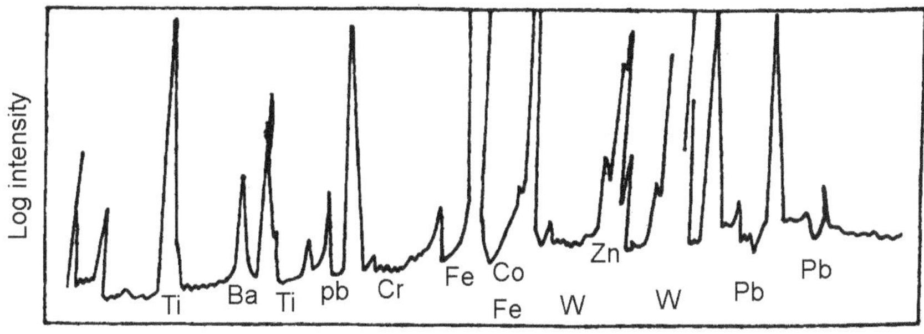

X-Ray Fluorescence for a genuine bank.
Note : recorded with a wavelength dispersive spectrometer

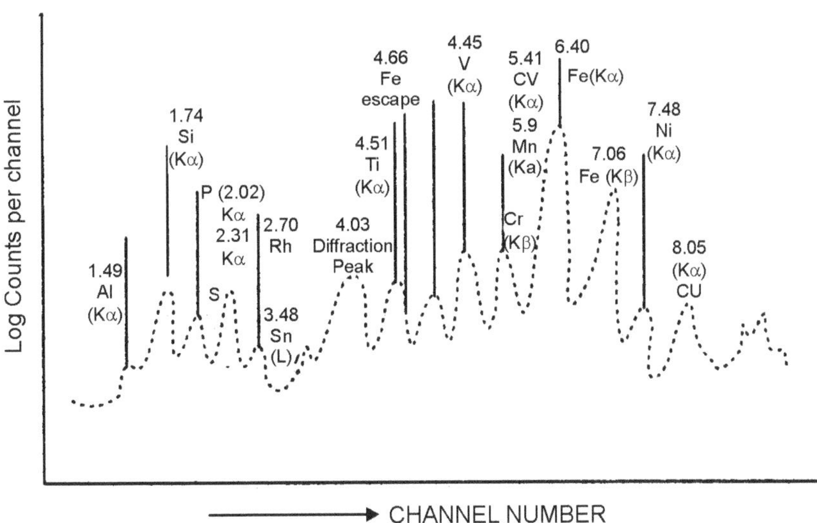

X-Ray Flourescence of an Iron Sample obtained with and Energy Dispersive instrument

Qualitative information such as gained from the above figures can be converted to semiquantitative data by careful measurement of peak heights. This measurement consists in setting the goniometer to the appropriate angle 2θ and then counting for a suitable length of time.

The concentration can be roughly estimated by using the relation :

$$P_x = P_s W_x$$

where

P_x = is relative line intensity measured in terms of number of counts for a fixed period.

W_x = is the weight fraction of the desired element in the sample.

P_x = is the relative intensity of the line that would be observed under identical counting conditions when W_x is unity.

The value of P_s be calculated by using a sample of pure element or a standard sample of known composition with reference to the element being determined.

Here it has been assumed that the emission from the species of interest is not affected by the other elements in the sample.

Quantitative Analysis

Modern X-ray fluorescence instruments are capable of producing quantitative analysis of complex materials. The accuracy of such an analysis, however, requires either the availability of calibration standards that closely approach the samples in overall chemical and physical composition or suitable methods for dealing with matrix effects.

Matrix Effects

It should be noted that the X-rays produced in the fluorescent process are generated both from atoms at the surface of the sample and atoms well below the surface of the sample. Consequently, a part of both the incident beam and the resulting fluorescent beam traverses a significant thickness of sample, within which absorption and scattering of either beam is attenuated depending upon the mass absorption coefficient of the medium can can be determined by the mass absorption co-efficient of the element and also by the co-efficients of all the other elements in the sample. Hence net intensity of a line reaching the detector in an X-ray emission analysis depends upon the concentration of the element producing the line and concentration and mass absorption co-efficients of the matrix elements.

If the matrix contains a significant amount of an element that absorbs either the incident or the emitted beam more strongly than the elements being determined, then W_x in the equation ($P_x = P_s W_x$) will be low, because P_s was calculated with a standard in which absorption was smaller, On other hand, if the matrix elements of the sample absorb less than those in the standard, high values of W_x are obtained.

When the sample contains an element whoch characteristic emission spectrum is excited by the incident beam and this spectrum in turn causes a secondary excitation of the analytical line, a second matrix effect, known as enhancement effect, gives results which are greater then expected.

These absorption and enhancement effect cause the intensity of the analytical line to depend upon the concentration of the element being determined and also upon the concentrations of the various elements comprising the sample matrix.

Several techniques has been developed in order to conpensate for absorption and enhancement effects in X-ray fluorescence analyses.

There are 5 general methods that have been used to eliminate or correct these effects.

(a) Comparison standards
(b) Internal standards
(c) Addition standardisation
(d) Dilution techniques
(e) Preparation of thin films.

(a) *Comparison Standards*: The most widely used method in emission analysis is the comparison of intensities from unknowns with those from standards of similar compositions. In this technique, the relationship between analytical line intensity and the concentration is determined empirically with a set of standards that closely approximate the samples in overall composition.

Here, it is assumed that absorption and enhancement effects are identical for both samples and standards. Empirical data are then used to convert emission data to concentration. The degree of compensation archieved in this manner, depends upon the closeness of the match between the samples and the standards.

When the unknowns and standards are very close in composition, a simple ratio of

$$\frac{I_v}{I_s} = \frac{C_u}{C_3} \text{ is adequate}$$

u for unknowns

s for standards

Calibration curves are prepared by measuring the spectral line intensity from samples of known composition. The use of comparison standards is the basis for control analysis in the chemical, metallurgical and petroleum industries. Intensity can be related to concentration by the following three methods:

(a) Linear rating (b) Graphical and (c) Mathematical

Graphical and mathematical correction techniques are used in those applications in which the unknowns vary over a wide range of composition. Graphical methods are used extensively for binary and ternary systems i.e. the ternary mixture Nb_2O_5, Ta_2O_5 and TiO_2.

(b) *Internal Standards*: In this procedure, an element which is not present in the sample, is introduced in known and fixed concentration into both calibration standards and the samples. The ratio of the line intensity of the element being determined to the intensity of a line of the internal standard acts as the analytical parameter. It is also assumed here that absorption and enhancement effects are the same for the two lines and that the use of intensity ratios compensates for these effects.

The effects of the matrix on two lines and the relative intensities of the reference and analytical lines can be grouped into the following:

(i) The mtrix has a higher absorption for the lower wavelength line.

(ii) The element has the absorption edge between the lines.

(iii) Emission lines from the matrix preferentially excite the lower atomic number of the two elements.

(c) *Addition Standardization*: This method assumes a linear relationship between the intensity and concentration over a limited concentration range. Addition techniques are suitable for the determination of trace and minor constituents, because linear relationship is valid in this concentration range. Various techniques such as grinding the mixture together with an abrasive as silicon carbide, forming pastes or slurries and fusing by means of borax, carbonate or pyrosulphate flux, have been used to achieve intimate mixing with the sample, because intimate mixing of sample and reference material is an essential requirement.

The analysis is accomplished by measuring the intensity of a characteristic spectral line of the element before and after addition of a known amount of the element to the sample. Using the ratio of intensities, the percentage of the element in the sample can be calculated.

(d) *Dilution Techniques*: In these techniques, both sample and standards are diluted with a substace that absorbs X-rays only weakly (i.e. a substance comprised of elements with low atomic number). Dilution may thus be achieved by dissolution with an inorganic or organic solvent or by fusion with a flux of borax, carbonate or pyrosulphate.

Examples of diluents include water, organic solvents containing C, H, N and O only, starch, lithium carbonate, alumina boric acid and borate glass.

By using an excess of diluent, the matrix effect becomes constant for both samples and standards and a good compensation is achieved. Another approach is to add a heavy absorber flux. This minimizes the absorption contribution of the original sample. Dilution with or without a heavy absorber, has been successfully used on a wide variety of materials particularly for mineral analysis. Where the samples and standards are dissolved in molten borax. The fused mass is then excited after cooling.

(e) *Thin films*: Matrix effects are low or almost negligible in thin film type samples because neither the primary nor the secondary X-rays are strongly absorbed by the sample. Thus the intensity of the secondary X-rays is directly proportional to the amount of element present. The elements being determined are collected by ion exchange. Solvent extraction or precipitation, in a physical form that is suitable for X-ray analysis.

For example : metal ions may be collected on a cation exchange resin loaded paper which also acts as the supporting medium for presentation in the X-ray spectrograph.

Applications of X-ray Fluorescence

1. With proper correction for matrix effects, X-ray fluorescence spectroscopy is perhaps the most powerful tool available to the chemist for the rapid quantitative determination of all but the lightest elements in complex samples. e.g. : Barict and Henke have demonstrated that nine elements can be determined in samples of granitic rocks in an elapsed time, including sample preparation of about 12 min. The precision of this method is better than wet chemical analyses.
2. Fluorescence methods also find widespread application for quality control in the manufacture of metals and alloys. Here, the spread of the analysis permits correction of the composition of the alloy during its manufacture.
3. X-Ray fluorescence methods are readily adapted to liquid samples. This method has been devised for the direct quantitative determination of lead and bromine in aviation gasoline samples. Similary, calcium, barium and zinc have been determined in the liquid hydrocarbon samples. This method is also convenient for the direct determination of the pigments in paint samples.
4. X-Ray fluorescence methods are being widely applied to the analysis of atmosphere pollutants.

   Example: one procedure for detecting and determining the contaminants involves drawing an air sample through a stock consisting of a micropore filter for particulates and three filter paper disks impregnatedwith orthotolidine, silver nitrate and sodium hydroxide, respectively. The reagents retain chlorine, sulphides and sulphur dioxide in that order. The filter then serves as samples for X-ray fluorescence analysis.
5. X-ray fluorescence is used for quantitative determination of elements heavier than sodium in rocks and soil encountered near the landing sight.
6. Birks and Brooks have also applied X-ray emission in the determination of hafnium in zirconium and tantalum in nioblum. Emission methods have also been successfully applied in trace analysis.

7. X-ray emission methods have proved to be of immense applications in such analytical problems as iron in blood, calcium in cement, titanium in paper products, chromium in glass and selenium in plant materials.
8. The most recent development in emission application has been the on-stream process control of metallurgical systems. e.g.: addition of floatation reagents to a sphalerite concentrate is controlled by on stream analysis of heads, concentrates and tailings.

3. X-Ray Diffraction Methods

X-ray diffraction has provided a wealth of important information to science and industry. The arrangement and spacing of atoms in crystalline materials has been determined directly from diffraction studies. The distance between the atoms in crystals have been found to be roughly equal to 10^{-8} cm. So optical and electron microscopes can not be used this field. It was suggested by Von Lave that it might be possible to diffract X-rays by means of crystals, because

(a) The crystals act as a three dimensional natural grating for X-rays.
(b) X-rays act as part of the electromagnetic radiation.
(c) X-rays are actually the radiations of very small wavelengths, probably of the order of 10^{-8} cm.

Since the diffraction pattern depends upon the internal structure of the crystal, this discovery led the beginning of X-ray crystallography and attempts were, later on, made to study the diffraction effects produced when X-rays were allowed to fall on the crystals.

X-ray diffraction methods are generally used for investigating the internal structures.

The following X-ray diffraction methods are used for performing analysis:

1. Lave photographic method
2. Bragg X-ray spectrometer method
3. Rotating crystal method
4. Powder method

1. Lave Method

Lave had studied the phenomenon of diffraction of crystal by two methods

(a) Transmission method
(b) Back reflection method

(a) ***Transmission Method***: The experimental equipment required for this is relatively simple :

(i) A is a source of X-rays. This emits a beam of continuous wavelength, known as white radiation which is obtained from a tungsten target at about 60,000 volts.

(ii) B is a pinhole collimator. When X-rays obtained from A are allowed to pass through this pinhole collimator a fine pencil of X-rays is obtained.

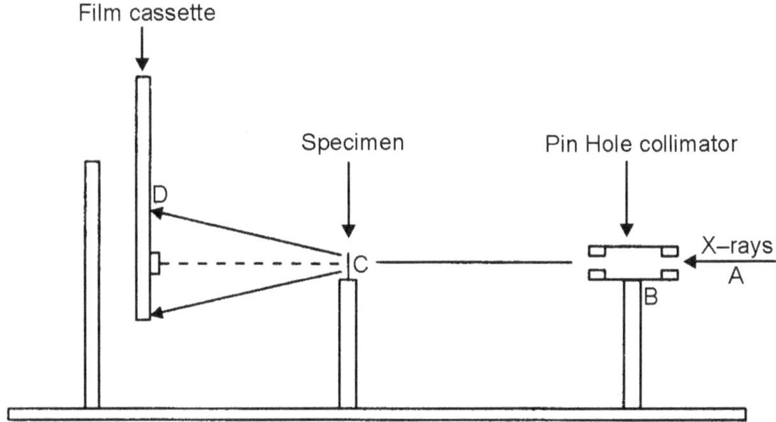

The diameter of the pinhole is importance from the stand point of detail in diffraction pattern. The smaller is the diameter, the sharper is the interference.

(iii) C is a crystal whose internal structure is to be investigated. The crystal is set on a holder to adjust its orientation

(iv) D is a film cassette arranged on a rigid base. This film is provided with beam stop to prevent direct beam from causing excessive fogging of the film.

The position of crystal is held stationary in a beam of X-rays. The X-rays after passing through the crystal are diffracted and are recorded on a photographic plate.

On examining the Lave's photograph, it is observed that the spots actually occur at the positions to be expected from the reflection law. When the X-ray beam is passed along the axis of symmetry of the crystal, the Lave's pattern would contain a series of spots whose loci are ellipses which pass through the 'cental image' made by X-ray beam. The spots on any one ellipse are produced by planes belonging to the same zone, i.e., planes which are parallel to one common direction.

Lave's pattern can be used to orient crystals for solid state experiments. Let us consider the case of a crystal with four-fold axial symmetry which is oriented with the axis parallel to the beam. Each reflecting beam then selects a wave length satisfying the Bragg equation from the incident X-ray beam. The Lave pattern obtained in this case shows the four-fold symmetry.

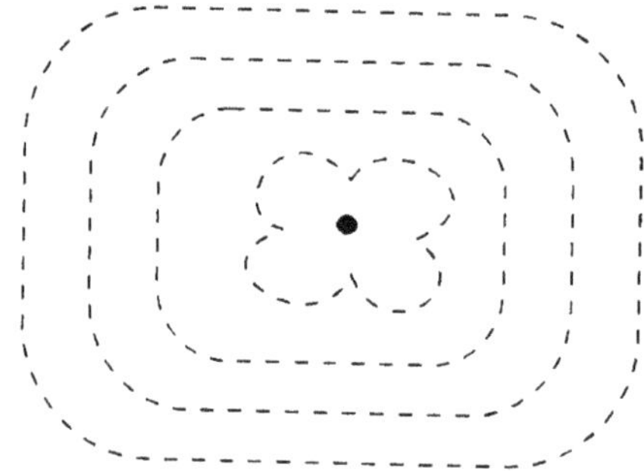

The arrangement of the spots in a Lave's photograph of a simple cublic system.

This method is most suitable for the investigation of preferred orientation sheet of fibres, particularly if the information is confined to the lower diffreaction angles. This method is also used in the determination of the symmetry of single crystals, since the Lave pattern would show the presence of rotation axes and lines of symmetry.

(b) *Back Reflection Method*: This method provides similar information as the transmission method. However the reflection method is the only method for the investigation of large and thick specimens.

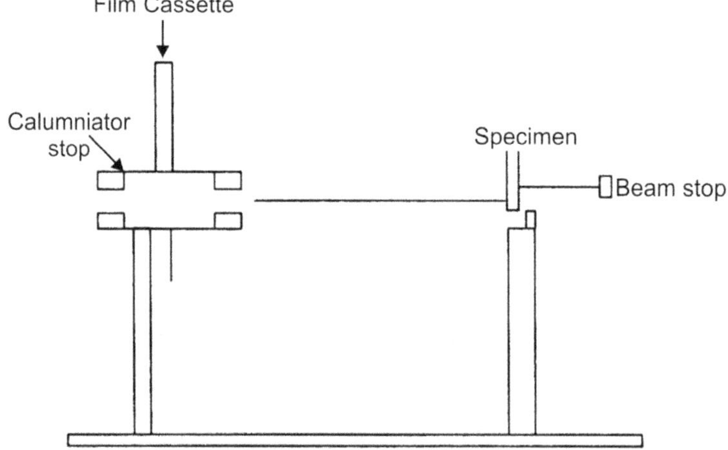

The main disadvantages of Lave's method are that a big crystal is required and furthermore there is uncertainity in the significance of reflection intensities due to un homogenous nature of X-rays.

2. Bragg's X-Ray Spectrometer Method

The interpretation of Lave's experiments and photographs proved very difficult, particularly because of the use of white X-ray having continuous range of wavelengths and lack of knowledge about the arrangement of atoms in the crystals. According to Lave, if a beam of X-rays is passed through a crystal, the emitted X-rays by the crystal are obtained on the pl. otographic plate in the form of pattern known as Lave's photograph.

W.H. Bragg and his son W.L. Bragg followed up the Von Lave's work and gave a simple explanation of the diffraction of X-rays by crystals. According to the Braggs, X-rays behave as if they are reflected. By planes of atoms in a crystal and when a beam of X-rays allowed to fall on a crystal surface at some angle θ, each atom therein acts as a source of scattered radiation of the same wavelength. Thus when an X-ray beam strikes a crystal surface at an angle θ, a portion is scattered by the layer of atoms at the surface and unscattered portion of the beam penetrates the second layer of atoms, where again fraction is scattered and the remainder passes on to the third layer. The cumulative effect of this scattering from the regularly spaced centres of the crystal is nothing but diffraction of the beam, which is almost similar to diffraction of visible radiation by a reflection grating.

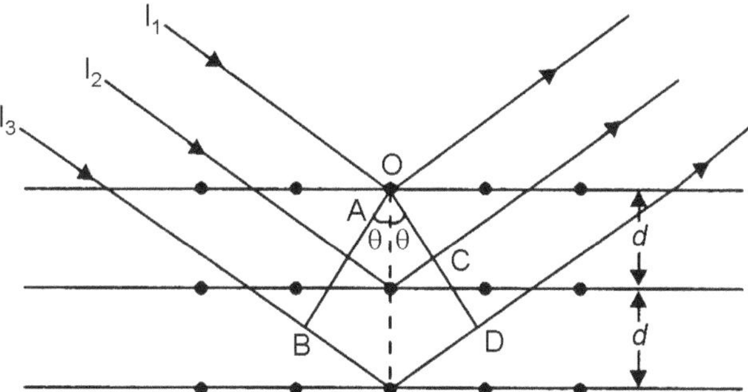

Bragg and his son developed a useful relationship between the wavelength of X-rays and the spacing between the lattice planes.

The most important requirements of diffraction are :

(a) The spacing between layers of atoms must be roughly the same as the wavelength of the radiation.

(b) The scattering centres must be specially distributed in a highly regular way.

Consider a beam of monochromatic X-rays which strikes on a set of parallel and equidistant planes called lattice planes or Bragg's planes in the crystal structure at an angle θ. Scattering occurs as a result of interaction of the radiation with atoms located at O, P and R. If the distance AP + PC = $n\lambda$.

n is known as integer 1, 2, 3 etc. known as order of reflection, the scattered radiation will be in phase OCD, and the crystal will appear to reflect the X-radiation. But AP = PC = d sin θ.

Where *d* is interplanar distance of the crystal. Thus the conditions of constructive interference on the beam at an angle q are $n\lambda = 2d \sin\theta$.

This equation is known as Bragg's equation, since sin θ cannot exceed units, the minimum spacing for which the reflection can be observed is $d = \lambda/2$.

Thus X-rays appear to be reflected from the crystal only if the angle of incidence satisfies the condition that

$$\sin\theta = \frac{n\lambda}{2d}$$

At all other angles destructive interferences occur.

For a given set of lattice planes *d* is fixed value. The study of the intensity of X-ray spectra will give the required information about the arrangement of planes of different atoms in space lattices.

Bragg obtained the positions by maximum reflection intensity by means of X-ray spectrometer.

The various components of Bragg's X-ray spectrometers are as follows :

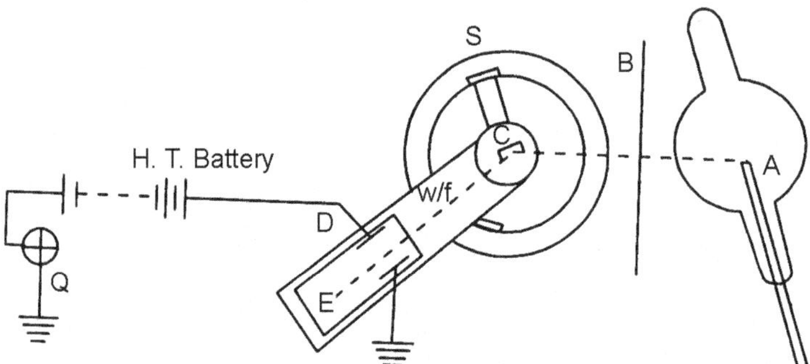

(i) X-rays from the anticathode A are allowed to pass through two adjustable slits B and B to get a thin beam of X-rays. Then, these rays are made to fall upon the crystal C.

(ii) The reflecting crystal is mounted on the table of spectrometer. The position of crystal can be adjusted by the vernier V capable of motion along the circular scale S.

(iii) The reflected X-rays from the crystal, after passing through the slit F, enter the ionization chamber E through a narrow aluminium window W.

(iv) The ionisation chamber is mounted on an W_m and its position is determined by a second vernier.

(v) One plate of ionization chamber is connected to the positive terminal of a H.T. battery while the negative terminal of the H.T. battery is connected to a quadrant electrometer Q which measures the strength of ionisation current. The other plate of ionisation chamber is emitted.

(vi) The deflection in the electrometer is a measure of ionisation and consequently gives the intensity of reflected X-rays i.e. the strength of the ionisation current is proportional to the intensity of the entering reflecting X-rays. In order to increase ionisation the chamber is sometimes filled with SO_2 (or) methyl iodide.

Working

(i) In using the Bragg's spectrometer, the crystal in mounted in such a position that $\theta = 0^\circ$ and the ionisation chamber is adjusted to receive the X-rays.

(ii) The crystal and ionisation chamber are made to move in small steps so that the angle through which the camber is moved is twice the angle through which crystal is rotated. The ionisation at first falls as θ increases but for certain values of θ it rises sharply. This corresponds to the direction of the X-ray spectrum.

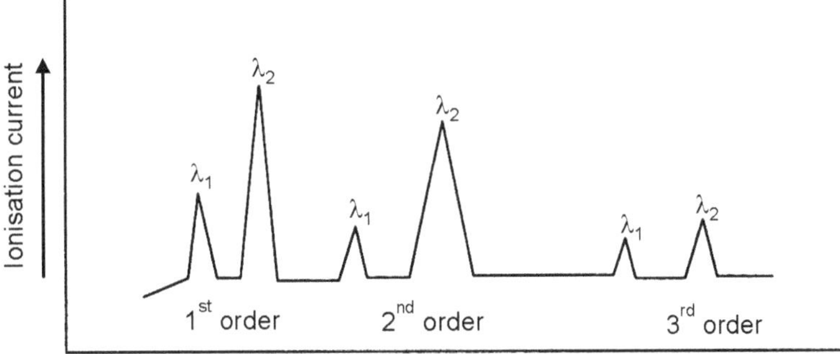

X-rays spectrum is obtained by plotting a graph between the ionisation current and the glancing angle θ. In this, the peaks correspond to Bragg's reflection, corresponding to different order glancing angles θ_1, θ_2 and θ_3.

With the known values of d and n and from the observed value of θ, λ can be measured.

***Measurement of* λ:** The wavelength of X-rays can be determined by employing the following equation:

$$2d \sin\theta = n\lambda$$

The value of θ for various order spectra produced by reflection from a crystal of (rock salt) is measured and the mean value of λ/d is determined.

Lattice constant = λ/d

Knowing d, the wavelength λ can be calculated

***Measurement of d*:** The lattice spacing *d* is connected to cell edge by the following relations:

$$d = \frac{a\sqrt{2}}{2} \text{ for simple cubic lattice}$$

$$d = \frac{a}{2} \text{ for fee crystal lattice}$$

$$d = \frac{a\sqrt{3}}{2} \text{ for bcc crystal lattice}$$

where a can be calculated by employing the following relation.

$$a = \left[\frac{\text{Molecular weight} \times \text{number of atoms in unit cell}}{\text{Avogadro's number} \times \text{Density}}\right]^{1/3}$$

Determination of crystal structure by Bragg's law

The X-rays are allowed to fall on the crystal surface. Then the crystal is rotated and X-rays are made to reflect from various lattice planes. The intense reflections are measured by Bragg's X-ray spectrometer and the glancing angle for each intense reflection is recorded. Then, on applying Bragg's equation.

$n\lambda = 2d \sin\theta$, ratio of lattice spacing for various groups of planes can be obtained. Then, the experimentally observed ratios are compared with the calculated ratios, a particular structure may be identified.

(i) $d100 : d110 : d111 = 1 : \frac{1}{\sqrt{2}} : \frac{1}{\sqrt{3}}$ for simple cubic lattice

(ii) $d100 : d110 : d111 = 1 : \frac{1}{\sqrt{2}} : \frac{2}{\sqrt{3}}$ for fcc crystal

(iii) $d_{100} : d_{110} : d_{111} = 1 : \frac{2}{\sqrt{2}} : \frac{1}{\sqrt{3}}$ for bcc crystal

***Example*:** These methods are applied to NaCl crystal.

This crystal belongs to fcc class and there are 4 atoms in unit cell.

Its density = 2.18 b/cc, M.W. = 58.5.

Avogadro's number = 6.02×10^{23}.

On substituting these values in equation

$$a = \left[\frac{\text{M.W.} \times \text{no.ofatomsinunitcell}}{\text{N} \times \text{density}}\right]^{1/3}$$

$$a = \left[\frac{58.5 \times 4}{6.02 \times 10^{23} \times 2.18}\right]^{1/3} = 5.63 \times 10^{-8} \text{ cm}$$

For fcc lattice

$$d = \frac{a}{2} = \frac{5.63 \times 10^{-8}}{2} = 2.815 \times 10^{-3} \text{ cm} = 2.815 \text{ A}^0$$

→ For maximum intensity reflections, the glancing angles are 5.9^0, 8.4° and 5.2° for 100, and 111 faces respectively for first order reflections. Thus in case of NaCl

$$d_{100} : d_{110} : d_{111} = \frac{1}{\sin 5.9} : \frac{1}{\sin 8.4} : \frac{1}{\sin 5.2}$$

$$= 1 : 0.704 : 1.115$$

$$= 1 : \frac{1}{\sqrt{2}} : \frac{2}{\sqrt{3}}$$ so NaCl is fcc crystal.

3. Rotating Crystal Method

The rotating crystal method was developed by Schiebold in 1919.

The arrangement of this method is outlined as follows :

(a) The X-rays are generated in the X-ray tube and then the beam is made monochromatic by a filter.

(b) From the filter, the beam is then allowed to pass through collimating system which permits a fine pencil of parallel X-rays.

(c) From the collimator, the X-ray beam is made to fall on a crystal mounted on a shaft which can be rotated at a uniform angular rate by a small motor.

(d) Now the shaft is moved to put the crystal into slow rotation about a fixed axis. This causes the sets planes coming successively into their reflecting positions i.e. the value of θ satisfies the Bragg's relation. Each plane will produce a spot on the photographic plate.

The photograph of a diffraction pattern up on a photographic plate perpendicular to X-ray beam or up on a film in a cylindrical camera, the axis of which coincides with the axis of rotation of the crystal.

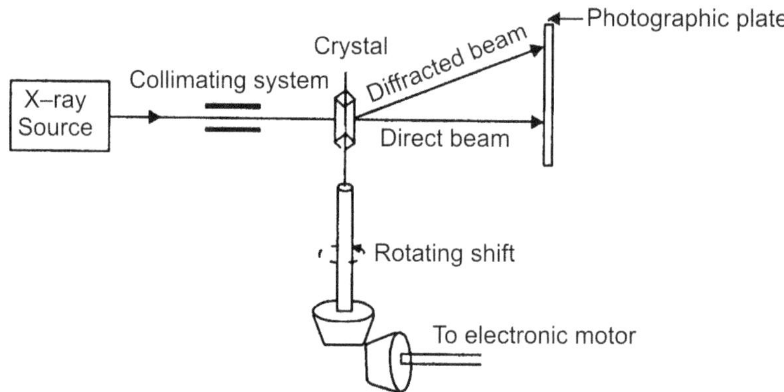

The photographs can be taken in 2 ways.

1. Complete Rotation Method

There occurs a complete series of revolutions. It is observed that each set of planes in the crystal beams are distributed into a rectangular pattern about the control point of the photograph.

2. Oscillation Method

In this, the crystal is oscillated through an angle of 15° or 20°. The photographic plate in also moved back and forth with a same period as that of the rotation of the crystal.

The position of a spot on the plate indicates the orientation of the crystal at which the spot was formed.

By the rotating crystal method, one can calculate the size of unit cell.

3. Powder Crystal Method

X-ray diffraction provides a convenient and practical means for the qualitative identification of crystals. The X-ray powder diffraction method is unique in that it is the only analytical method that is capable of providing qualitative and quantitative information about the compounds present in a solid sample.

X-ray powder methods are based upon the fact that an X-ray diffraction pattern is unique for each crystalline substance. Thus, if exact match can be found between the pattern of an unknown and an authentic sample, chemical identity can be assumed. The powder method can determine the percent of KBr and NaCl in a solid mixture of these two compounds.

For other diffraction methods, a single crystal is required, whose size is much larger than microscopic dimensions. However, in the powder method, the crystal sample need not be taken in large quantity but as little as 1 mg of the material is sufficient for the study.

The powder method was devised independently by Debye and Scherrer in Germany and by Hull in America at about the same time.

The main features of powder crystal method are :

(i) A is a source of X-rays which can be made monochromatic by a filter.

(ii) Allow the X-ray beam to fall on the powdered specimen P through the slits S_1 and S_2. The function of these slits is to get a narrow pencil of X-rays.

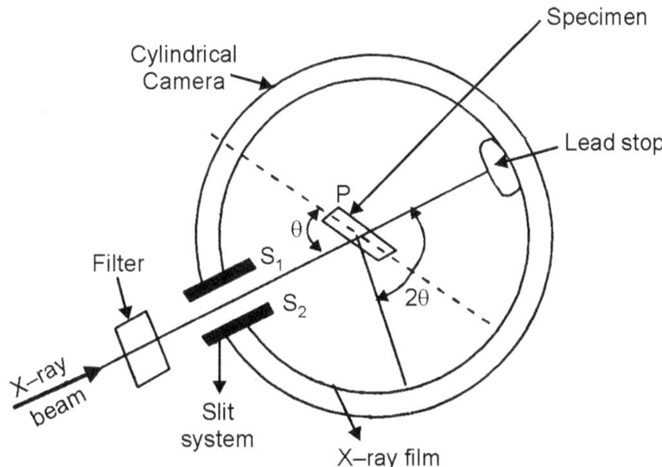

(iii) Fine powder, P, struck on a hair by means of gum is suspended vertically in the axis of a cylindrical camera. This enables sharp lines to be obtained on the photographic film which is surrounding the powder crystal in the form of a circular arc.

(iv) The X-rays after falling on the powder passes out of the camera through a cut in the film so as to minimize the fogging produced by the scattering of the direct beam.

(v) On a flat photographic plate the observed pattern consists of traces as shown in following figure:

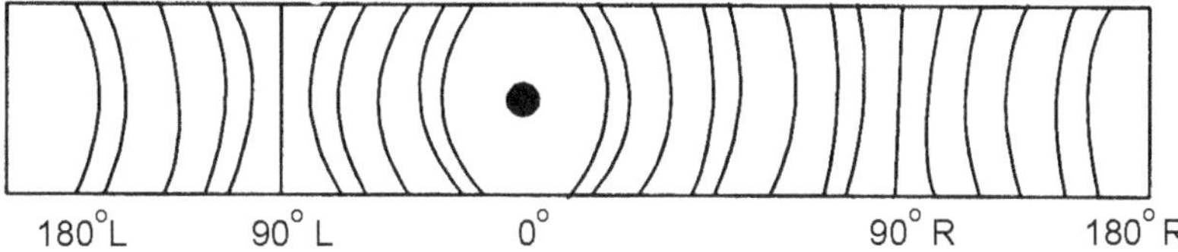

Theory: When a mono chromatic beam of X-rays is allowed to fall on the powder of a crystal, then the following possibilities may happen:

(i) There will be some particles out of the random orientation of small crystals in the fine powder, which lie within a given set of lattice planes (marking the correct angle with the incident beam) for reflection to occur.

(ii) While another fraction of the grains will have another set of planes in the correct position for the reflections to occur and so on.

(iii) Also, reflections are also possible in the different order for each set.

All the like orientations of the grains due to reflection for each set of planes and for each order will constitute a diffraction cone whose interaction with a photographic plate gives rise to a trace. The crystal structure can be obtained from the arrangement of the traces and their relative intensities.

If the angle of the incidence is θ, the angle of reflection will be 2θ.

If the film radius is r, circumference 2πr corresponds to a scattering angle of 360^0.

$$\frac{l}{2\pi r} = \frac{2\theta}{360} \Rightarrow \theta = 360 \times \frac{1}{\pi r}$$

From this the value of θ can be calculated and substituting this value in Bragg's equation ($n\lambda = 2d \sin \theta$) the value of 'd' can be calculated.

Applications of powder crystal method

(i) The method is most useful for cubic crystals.

(ii) This method is used for determining the complex structure of metals and alloys.

(iii) This method is useful to make distinction between the allotropic modifications of the same substance.

Applications of X-ray Diffraction methods

1. X-ray diffraction studies have led to a much clear understanding of the physical properties of metals, polymeric materials, and other solids.
2. X-ray diffraction is currently of prime importance in elucidating the structures of such complex natural products as steroids, vitamins and antibiotics.
3. Unit cell parameters can be measured with high accuracy. Thus constitution of compounds in which there has been partial isomorphous replacement of one or more atoms in the unit cell can be accurately determined.
4. X-ray diffraction provides a convenient practical means for the qualitative identification of crystalline compounds. Diffraction data is also employed for the quantitative measurement of a crystalline compound in a mixture example: percentage of graphite in graphite charcoal mixture which is difficult to determine by other methods.

The relative intensity of the diffraction pattern of a component in a mixture is directly proportional to the concentration and inversely proportional to the mean absorption co-efficient of the mixture. There is a linear relationship between line intensity and concentration for a mixture of compounds having same absorption co-efficients.

Quantitative analysis is carried out by comparing the intensity of a chosen diffraction line in a compound to the intensity of the same line in a standard mixture.

5. Powder diffraction method can be used to determine the degree of crystallinity of the polymer. The non-crystalline portion simply scatters the X-ray beam be give a continuous background, while the crystalline portion causes diffraction lines that are non continuous.
6. A variety of X-ray diffraction techniques are used to determine the particle size (or) crystallities.

(a) ***Spot counting method*****:** This method is used for determining size of particles larger than 5 microns. If the powder diffraction pattern of such a particle is obtained, it will consist of a series of lines or rings having a spotty appearance.

From this diffraction pattern, the size of the paticles determined by applying the following relation:

$$\nu = \frac{V.\delta.\delta\theta.co}{2n}$$

ν = the volume or size of an individual crystallite

V = the total volume of the speciment irradiated

n = the number of spots in a diffraction ring at a Bragg's angle of q.

$\delta\theta$ = the divergence of the X-ray beam and is a function of the apparatus used.

By this method determine the size of the particle with any degree of accuracy. Generally a series of samples having particles of known sizes is used to obtain diffraction rings that may be compared with those from the unknown at similar values of θ.

Disadvantages

Spots due to strained particles are difficult to count.

It the few grains present in the irradiated volume possess a preferred orientation, inaccuracies may arise.

(b) ***Broadening of diffraction lines*****:** This method is used for particles in the range 30-1000 A°. It is based upon the fact that there is broadening of the powder diffraction lines.

For a powder composed of perfect crystalline particles in this size range

$$L_{hkl} = \frac{K\lambda}{B_0 \cos\theta}$$

L_{hkl} = The mean crystalline dimension (size) perpendicular to the plance (*hkl*)

B_0 = the breadth at half maximum of a pure diffraction profile in radians.

K = a constant generally taken as unity.

The breadth of a diffraction line B_M, measured from the diffraction pattern depends upon the instrumental factors as well as on the particle size.

Thus, the measured line breadth B_M is due instrumental B_1, and small crystallite – B_0 line broadening.

The unknown sample is mixed with a standard substance having a particle size greater than 1000 A° (S_o that B_o for the standard is zero) and then the diffraction pattern is obtained which produces a diffraction line near to that from the unknown to be used in the measurement. Then, if the line profiles are considered to be Gaussian, one can wirte.

B^2M (unknown) = $B_1^2 + B_0^2$ (unknown)

BM^2 (standard) = B_1^2

hence these equations, the crystalline dimension can be estimated.

(c) ***Low Angle Scattering*****:** Low-angle scattering of X-rays is a method to reveal the distribution of particle size, which can't be revealed by spot counting and broadening of diffraction line methods.

From the Bragg's reaction $n\lambda = 2d \sin\theta$.

It follows that if one desires to have information about large structural features (large d values), attention should be focussed on small scattering angles, 2q for systems having a collection of particles identical in shape and size and separated sufficiently to eliminate inter-particle interference.

Guinier proved the following relation

$$\text{In } I_s = \text{In } I_0$$

I_s = the variation in scattered intensity with angle θ.

I_0 = the intensity scattered at '0' angle.

R = radius of gyration of the particles

If ln I_s is plotted against $(4\pi\theta/\lambda)^2$, a straight line having slope – 1/3 R^2 should be obtained. From this slope, the radius of gyration, R, can be calculated. The value of R calculated by this method is an average radius of gyration.

This method holds good for spherical and near-spherical particles.

7. Diffraction methods are also used for determination of cistrans isomerism and linkage isomerism.

X-ray diffraction study has been used to make the distinction between cis and trans isomers of a complex.

Example: The structure of bis (pyridine-2-carboxamide) nickel (II) dehydrate. $Nl(Pia)_2\ 2H_2O$.

The orange-red, diamagnetic crystals of composition $Ni(Pia)_2\ 2H_2O$ are obtained when aqueous solution of nickel (II) chloride is added to an alkaline solution of the ligand.

From X-ray studies it reveals that the complex molecule possesses a trans planar structure, and the two ligands are co-ordinated with the nickel atom through four nitrogen atoms. The water molecular do not co-ordinate directly with the nickel atom but are situated between the complex molecules. They are hydrogen bonded with each other and are linked to the amino oxygen atoms of the complex molecule.

By X-ray studies, linkage isomers of complexes are identified.

This application can be illustrated by the following example such as Biuret react with different metal ions under different conditions. Biuret may combine with a metal atoms by means of two nitrogen atoms, two oxygen atoms or one nitrogen and one oxygen atom.

(i) Viuret react with copper (π) ion in an alkaline medium to form a complex, potassium bis (biureto) cuprate (II) tetrahydrate

$$K_2\ [Cu(biv_2)_2]\ 4H_2O$$

This complex has been studied by Freeman, Smith and Taylor by X-ray diffraction method. In this complex two biuret anions are coordinated as bidentate ligands with the copper through the nitrogen atoms of the amido groups. The 4 nitrogen atoms are located at the four corners of an almost perfect square.

(ii) Biuret reacts with bivalent metals in neutral nedium forming complexes of type $M(11)\ X_2 - 2$ biv.

$$M(II)X_2 = CuCl_2,\ CuSO_4,\ Cu(NO)_2,\ NiCl_2,\ NiSO_4.\ Cd\ Cl_2$$

The crystal structure of $CuCl_2$. 2 biv has been determined. In this complex the biuret acts as a bidentate ligand but coordination occurs though two oxygen atoms.

8. Since the early part of this century to aid their studies of complex the biuret acts as a bidentrate ligand but coordination occurs though two oxygen atoms.

In 1953 when Watson and Crick looked at X-ray diffraction patterns from crystallized DNA, they were able to determine for the first time that DNA molecules exhibit a double-helical structure. But it was only in the late 50s. with the advent of computer that scientists were able to determine the precise three dimensional atomic structure of large molecules such as proteins and enzymes.

X-ray diffraction studies have great imporatance for determining the structure of biological molecules. Knowing the structure of biological molecules scientists allow to better understand how they work and can lead to better drugs out treatments for disease. For example, Rossamann and his colleagues have determined the structure of a receptor on a human cell that binds to the common cold virs. This work, and that of other laboratories, may help scientists determine how cold virus and other viruses enter and infect human cells.

9. Synctroton X-ray diffraction was developed which is similar in design to conventional X-ray diffraction. X-ray diffraction is that it is limited to crystalline materials (since amorphous materials donot diffract) Synchroton X-ray diffraction is used for analysis of these amorphous materials and thin films and this offers exceptional resolution, even on very small samples containing only a few grains of the particular mineral. This resolution and the excellent detectors for S-XRD permit the identification and quantification of trace phases not possible using other means.

QUESTION BANK

1. Explain the NMR phenomenon with the help of a neat labelled diagram, describe the various parts of a NMR instrument. Give any five applications of NMR in Pharmaceutical Analysis.

2. State and explain Beer-Lambert's law. What are its limitations?

   What is absorption maxima λ_{max} ? What is the effect of solvent polarity on λ_{max} in UV spectroscopy?

3. Write a note on sample handling in IR-spectroscopy. Indicate the region in which you expect the following functional groups to appear in IR spectrum:

   (a) CO_{str}

   (b) $C \equiv N_{str}$

   (c) $C - H_{str}$

   (d) $C - H_{def}$

   Give a neat labelled diagram of a double beam IR spectrophotometer.

4. What is fluorescence ? What are the various factors which affect the intensity of fluorescence ?

   What are the applications of fluorescence in pharmaceutical analysis ?

   What are the limitations of fluoremetric method of analysis ?

5. With the help of neat labelled diagram explain the construction and working of a flame emission spectrophotometer.

6. Explain the principle involved in Mass spectroscopy.

7. What are the various methods available for Nebulisation of sample in flame photometry?

   Give the principle and procedure involed in a Radio immuno assay.

8. Write short notes on the following :
   (a) Detectors used in UV-spectroscopy
   (b) Metastable ions and their significance in Mass spectroscopy
   (c) Bragg's equation
9. Define the terms 'σ' electrons, π-electrons, *n* electrons and antibonding orbitals.

   Describe the various electronic excitations involved in UV-spectroscopy.

   How can you distinguish between cis-trans isomers and keto-enol tautomers using UV-Spectroscopy ?
10. Give the principle involved in fluorimetry and describe the various types of fluorescence.
11. Explain why IR spectroscopy is also known as vibrational spectroscopy. Describe the various types of vibrations involved in IR Spectroscopy.
12. Mention any three nuclei other than proton which exhibit NMR phenomenon.

    Write a note on use of TMS as internal standard in NMR spectra. Explain the terms 'chemical shift, shielding and deshielding' in NMR spectroscopy with the help of one suitable example in each case.
13. What is the principle involved in Mass spectroscopy ?

    What are the different methods available to induce ionization of a sample in Mass Spectroscopy?
14. What is the principle involved in Radio-immuno Assay?

    How will you test the thyroid function in human subjects using I^{131} with the help of Radio immuno assay ?
15. Write short notes on the following :
    (a) Interference encountered in flame photometry.
    (b) 'Reciprocal Lattice' concept used in X-ray diffraction studies.
    (c) Applications of Atomic Absorption Spectrocopy.
16. What is mass spectrum ? What do you know about the formation and stability of molecular ion ? Describe in detail the instrumentation for scanning mass spectrum of an organic compound ?
17. (a) Discuss the principle involved in NMR Spectroscopy.
    (b) Explain the terms "Chemical Shift and Shielding".
    (c) Give various applications of NMR spectroscopy.

18. Give the phenomenon of Atomic Absorption Spectroscopy ? Give a schematic diagram of atomic absorption spectrophotometer? Enumerate various applications of atomic absorption spectroscopy.

19. Define the following terms :
    (a) Chromophore
    (b) Hypsochromic shift
    (c) Hyperchromic shift
    (d) Batchochromic shift
    (b) Explain various applications of ultra violet spectroscopy

20. Write notes on:
    (a) Emission Spectroscopy (b) Flame Photometry

21. (a) What is meant by X-ray diffraction ? How do you measure diffraction angle?
    (b) Explain the terms Miller indices, unit cell, Lattice energy and axis of symmetry.

22. (a) What is the difference between fluorescence and phosphorescence ?
    (b) What are various applications of Fluorimetry in pharmaceutical analysis ?
    (c) Enumerate various limitations of Fuorimetry?

23. Give the principles, construction and working of a Double beam IR spectrophotometer ?

24. (a) What are the advantages and limitations of Fluorimetry as compared to UV-spectroscopy in Pharmaceutical Analysis ?
    (b) Give any three important applications of fluorimetry in pharmaceutical Analyis.
    (c) How will you estimate 'Diphenylhydantoin, Methyl dopa and vitamin B by fluorimetry ?

25. (a) Give the principle involved in IR spectroscopy with the help of a neat, labelled diagram.
    (b) Explain the working of a double beam IR Spectrophotometer.

26. Define the terms:
    (a) Isobestic point, Hyperchromic shift, Hypsochromic shift, Bathochromic shift, with the help of one example each.
    (b) What are the applications of Colourimetry in Pharmaceutical Analysis ?

27. (a) Explain the principle involved in C^{13} NMR technique.
    (b) What are the applications of C_{13} NMR in pharmaceutical Analysis ?
28. What is radio immuno assay ? With the help of Cr^{51} tagged RBC, how will you use this technique to determine blood volume ?
29. (a) Give the principle involved in Flame photometry.
    (b) Name any four fuel-oxidant mixtures used in flame photometry. Give the temperatures, advantages and limitations of each of the above mixtures.
    (c) Give any four applications of flame photometry.
30. (a) Give the principle involved in the Atomic Absorption Spectroscopy.
    (b) With the help of a neat schematic diagram, explain the construction and working of an Atomic Absorption Spectrophotometer.
31. Write short notes on the following :
    (a) Application of Mass Spectroscopy
    (b) Wood-ward's rules in UV-Spectroscopy
    (c) Significance of Finger-print region in IR Spectroscopy.
32. (a) State and explain Beer-Lambert's law.
    (b) Describe the construction of ultra violet spectrophotometer and its various components and their functions.
    (c) Describe the estimation of a Pharmaceutical compound by spectrophotomertry.
33. (a) Explain in detail the construction and working of Infra-red spectrophotometer.
    (b) Discuss the application of Infra-red Spectrophotometric analysis.
    (c) Discuss the estimation of a pharmaceutical compound by colorimetry.
34. (a) Explain the theory of fluorimetric analysis. What are the different components and their functions in a fluorimeter?
    (b) Describe in detail, the method for the analysis of a pharmaceutical compound of your choice using a fluorimeter.
35. (a) What is flame photometry ? Give a concise account of the principle of flame photometry.
    (b) Mention the various components and their functions in a flame photometer.
    (c) Describe the applications of flame photometry.

36. Compare the principles involved, common features and differences in the techniques of nephelometry and turbilometry. Discuss their applications in Pharmacy.

37. (a) Explain the principle and methodology of TLC.
    (b) What are the common absorbents used in TLC and the method of preparing chromate plates ?
    (c) Mention the different visualizing agents for different classes of natural products.

38. (a) Explain the principle and methodology of paper chromatography.
    (b) Enumerate the applications of paper chromatography.

39. (a) Explain the basic principle and instrumentation of gas chromatrography using a diagrammatic sketch of the instrument.
    (b) Name the carrier gases and their requirements.
    (c) Give the applications of gas chromatography.

40. (a) Discuss ion-exchange resins and give their structures and characteristics.
    (b) Describe an ion-exchange resin method of analysis of compound.
    (c) Enumerate the applications of ion-exchange chromatography.

41. (a) Explain the principle and methodology of HPLC.
    (b) By means of a neat sketch, explain the instrument used in HPLC.
    (c) Enumerate the applications of HPLC.

42. (a) Explain the basic principles of radio immuno assay (RIA).
    (b) Describe the applications of this technique in Pharm. analysis.

43. Write short notes on the following :
    (a) Detectors used in gas chromatrography
    (b) Spraying reagents used in paper chromatography.

44. Write short note on the following :
    (a) Two dimensional paper chromatography.
    (b) Reference electrodes
    (c) Carrier gases in gas chromatography.

45. Attempt any three of the following :
    (a) Preparative TLC
    (b) Fluorimeter
    (c) Detector used in IR spectrophotometers
    (d) Nephelometry and turbidometry
46. Write short notes on the following:
    (a) Reverse phase chromatography
    (b) Adsorbents and solvents used in TLC
    (c) Photoelectric colorimeter
    (d) Flame photometer
47. (a) Give the different types of radiation source used in visible, UV and IR spectrometric methods.
    (b) What is vacuum UV region ? what is its significance ?
    (c) Describe the different types of bands appearing in UV spectra of organic compounds.
48. (a) Explain with a neat diagram the schematic representation of a spectrofluorimeter.
    (b) Explain the terms :
    singlet, triplet state and quenching.
49. (a) What is radio immuno assay ? Explain with one example.
    (b) What is Differential Thermal Analysis (DTA) applicable in pharmaceutical preparations ?
50. (a) What are the advantages and disadvantages of Gas chromatographic methods ?
    (b) Enumerate the different types of detectors used in GLC-analysis and briefly explain them.
51. (a) Explain the following terms :
    (b) Retention time
    (c) Column packing materials
    (d) How the principle of electrophoresis can be made applicable in chromatographic methods of separation ?

52. Discuss briefly the principles of Gas chromatography. Enumerate the materials used for stationary phase and mobile phase. Describe the construction and working of various detectors used in GC.

53. Write a brief assay on the principles and techniques for the following :

    (a) Thin layer chromatography

    (b) Ion-exchange chromatography

54. What is photoluminescence ? What is the relationship between the concentration and fluorescence ? Mention the structural features required to give fluorescence. With the help of a neat diagram, explain the construction and working of fluorimeter.

55. Derive an expression for Beer-Lambert's law as applied to solutions. Describe the general principle, construction, working and applications of a double beam UV visible spectrophotometer.

56. Define following terms used in chromatographic analysis :

    (a) Retention Time

    (b) Eluate

    (c) Eluent

    (d) Adsorbent

    (e) R_f value

    (f) Stationary Phase

    (g) Two-dimensional Chromatography

    (h) Reverse Phase Chromatography

57. (a) Discuss basic principles involved in Radio-immuno assay.

    (b) Write a note on its applications in Pharmacy.

58. Describe theory, instrumentation and analytical applications of Flame photometry.

59. (a) Explain the principles involved and applications of fluorimetric analysis.

    (b) Describe instrumentation of Fluorimeter.

60. (a) State and explain Beer-Lambert's Law

    (b) Discuss methodology and applications of UV spectrophotometric and Colorimetric methods of analysis.

61. (a) Explain the principle and methodology of TLC.

    (b) What are the common absorbents used in TLC and the method of preparing chromato plates.

    (c) Mention the different visualizing agents for different classes of products.

62. (a) Discuss with the help of an energy level diagram the phenomenon of fluorescence.

    (b) What are the structural requirements of an organic compound for exhibiting fluorescence ?

    (c) Draw a diagram of fluorimeter, label the parts and explain the function and working of each component.

63. (a) Explain in detail the construction of Infra-Red Spectrophotometer.

    (b) Discuss ion exchange chromatography and how it differs from column chromatography. Classify ion exchange resins and give their structures and characteristics.

64. (a) Discuss ion-exchange chromatography and how it differs from column chromatography ? Classify ion exchange resins and give their structures and characteristics.

    (b) Describe an ion-exchange resin method of analysis of a compound.

    (c) What is ion-exchange capacity and how is regeneration effected?

www.ingramcontent.com/pod-product-compliance
Lightning Source LLC
LaVergne TN
LVHW080849240726
843527LV00052B/286
9789352300600